Cardiac Electrosonography

Eyal Herzog · David Leibowitz ·
Yair Elitzur

Editors

Cardiac Electrosonography

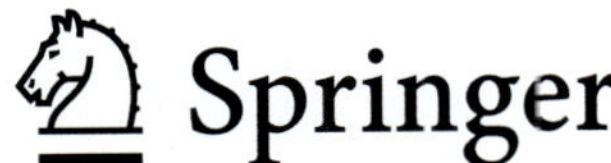
Springer

Editors
Eyal Herzog
Department of Cardiology
Heart Institute, Hadassah Medical
Center, Hebrew University of Jerusalem
Jerusalem, Israel

David Leibowitz
Department of Cardiology
Heart Institute, Hadassah Medical
Center, Hebrew University of Jerusalem
Jerusalem, Israel

Yair Elitzur
Department of Cardiology
Heart Institute, Hadassah Medical
Center, Hebrew University of Jerusalem
Jerusalem, Israel

ISBN 978-3-031-38471-4   ISBN 978-3-031-38469-1   (eBook)
https://doi.org/10.1007/978-3-031-38469-1

This Springer imprint is published by the registered company Springer Nature Switzerland AG
The registered company address is: Gewerbestrasse 11, 6330 Cham, Switzerland

Paper in this product is recyclable.

To our families, patients, colleagues, and trainees who have continuously supported us and taught us so much over the years

About This Book

We want to thank you for choosing to read our book.

As you start reviewing this book you will notice that it is written in a different format compared to other medical books.

The book has two parts.

In the first part of the book there are four tutorial chapters.

The first chapter includes novel algorithms for Cardiac Electrosonography based on cardiac symptoms, ECG, and echocardiography.

The following chapters provide tutorials for ECG performance and interpretation as well as echocardiography and chest sonography performance and interpretation. It is written in a simplified way so that all healthcare providers, at any level of their training or professional life, can study and learn.

In the second part of the book there are six chapters of clinical cases. There are total of 64 clinical cases. All cases have been written in the same format, and each case has four pages:

The first page shows an ECG and a short clinical presentation. It is published on one side of the page. The reader can use this page to test his or her ability to interpret the ECG. On the exact opposite side of that page is the second page of that case which discusses the ECG findings and includes test codes (Fig. 1) as required by the Cardiology board of the American Board of Internal Medicine in the USA. The reader will be able to compare his reading to the authors' interpretation and explanations.

The third page of each clinical case includes transthoracic echocardiography or chest sonography images with no explanations, so the reader can again test his or her ability to interpret these images. On the exact opposite side of that page the authors provide their interpretation to the images with a detailed discussion of the case and a reference.

ECG

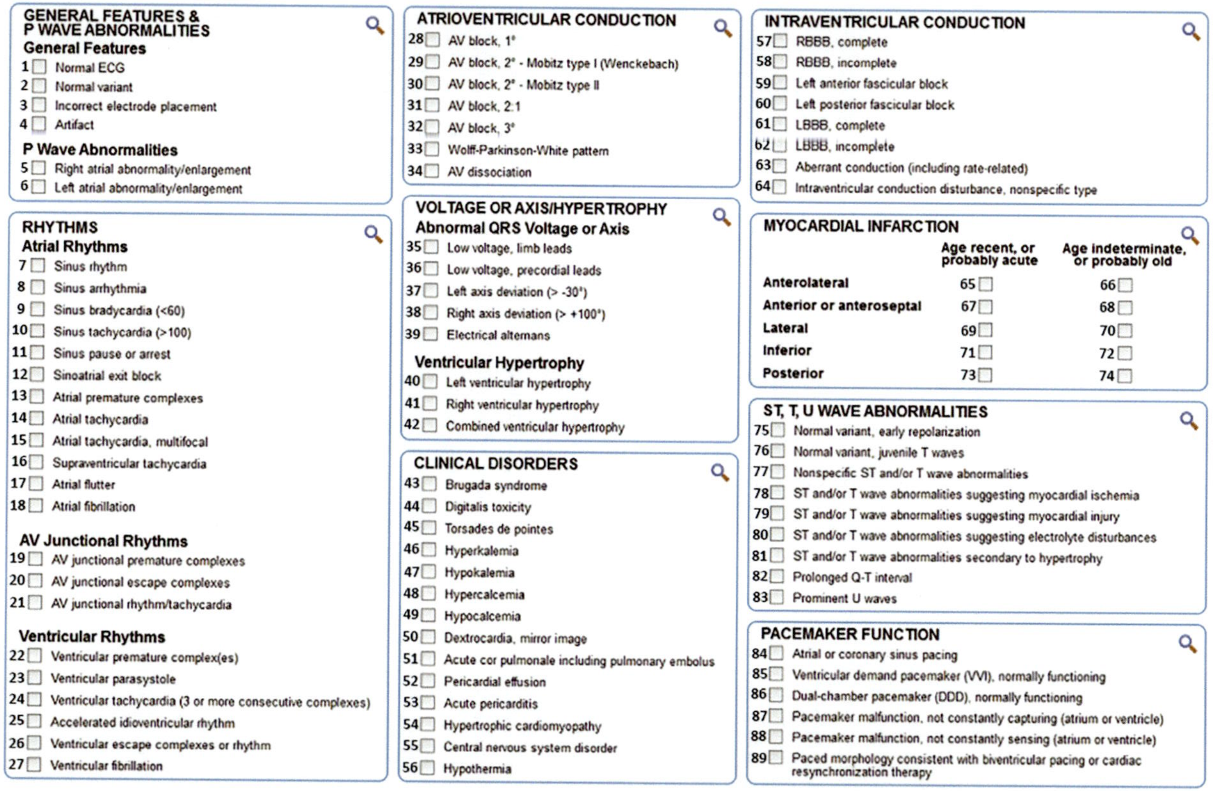

GENERAL FEATURES & P WAVE ABNORMALITIES

General Features
1. Normal ECG
2. Normal variant
3. Incorrect electrode placement
4. Artifact

P Wave Abnormalities
5. Right atrial abnormality/enlargement
6. Left atrial abnormality/enlargement

RHYTHMS

Atrial Rhythms
7. Sinus rhythm
8. Sinus arrhythmia
9. Sinus bradycardia (<60)
10. Sinus tachycardia (>100)
11. Sinus pause or arrest
12. Sinoatrial exit block
13. Atrial premature complexes
14. Atrial tachycardia
15. Atrial tachycardia, multifocal
16. Supraventricular tachycardia
17. Atrial flutter
18. Atrial fibrillation

AV Junctional Rhythms
19. AV junctional premature complexes
20. AV junctional escape complexes
21. AV junctional rhythm/tachycardia

Ventricular Rhythms
22. Ventricular premature complex(es)
23. Ventricular parasystole
24. Ventricular tachycardia (3 or more consecutive complexes)
25. Accelerated idioventricular rhythm
26. Ventricular escape complexes or rhythm
27. Ventricular fibrillation

ATRIOVENTRICULAR CONDUCTION
28. AV block, 1°
29. AV block, 2° - Mobitz type I (Wenckebach)
30. AV block, 2° - Mobitz type II
31. AV block, 2:1
32. AV block, 3°
33. Wolff-Parkinson-White pattern
34. AV dissociation

VOLTAGE OR AXIS/HYPERTROPHY

Abnormal QRS Voltage or Axis
35. Low voltage, limb leads
36. Low voltage, precordial leads
37. Left axis deviation (> -30°)
38. Right axis deviation (> +100°)
39. Electrical alternans

Ventricular Hypertrophy
40. Left ventricular hypertrophy
41. Right ventricular hypertrophy
42. Combined ventricular hypertrophy

CLINICAL DISORDERS
43. Brugada syndrome
44. Digitalis toxicity
45. Torsades de pointes
46. Hyperkalemia
47. Hypokalemia
48. Hypercalcemia
49. Hypocalcemia
50. Dextrocardia, mirror image
51. Acute cor pulmonale including pulmonary embolus
52. Pericardial effusion
53. Acute pericarditis
54. Hypertrophic cardiomyopathy
55. Central nervous system disorder
56. Hypothermia

INTRAVENTRICULAR CONDUCTION
57. RBBB, complete
58. RBBB, incomplete
59. Left anterior fascicular block
60. Left posterior fascicular block
61. LBBB, complete
62. LBBB, incomplete
63. Aberrant conduction (including rate-related)
64. Intraventricular conduction disturbance, nonspecific type

MYOCARDIAL INFARCTION

	Age recent, or probably acute	Age indeterminate, or probably old
Anterolateral	65	66
Anterior or anteroseptal	67	68
Lateral	69	70
Inferior	71	72
Posterior	73	74

ST, T, U WAVE ABNORMALITIES
75. Normal variant, early repolarization
76. Normal variant, juvenile T waves
77. Nonspecific ST and/or T wave abnormalities
78. ST and/or T wave abnormalities suggesting myocardial ischemia
79. ST and/or T wave abnormalities suggesting myocardial injury
80. ST and/or T wave abnormalities suggesting electrolyte disturbances
81. ST and/or T wave abnormalities secondary to hypertrophy
82. Prolonged Q-T interval
83. Prominent U waves

PACEMAKER FUNCTION
84. Atrial or coronary sinus pacing
85. Ventricular demand pacemaker (VVI), normally functioning
86. Dual-chamber pacemaker (DDD), normally functioning
87. Pacemaker malfunction, not constantly capturing (atrium or ventricle)
88. Pacemaker malfunction, not constantly sensing (atrium or ventricle)
89. Paced morphology consistent with biventricular pacing or cardiac resynchronization therapy

Fig. 1 Test codes as required by the Cardiology board of the American Board of Internal Medicine in the USA

Contents

Editors and Contributors

About the Editors

Dr. Eyal Herzog is a professor of Medicine at Icahn School of Medicine at Mount Sinai in New York where he was the director of the Critical Care Cardiology and Echocardiogrphy for over two decades at Mount Sinai— St. Luke's Hospital. He is currently the Director of the Department of Cardiology at Hadassah Medical Center, The Hebrew University of Jerusalem, in Jerusalem, Israel.

Over the past three decades, Dr. Herzog has developed highly respected methods for improving cardiovascular health care through the application of novel algorithmic pathways that simplify the diagnosis, treatment, and management of cardiovascular disease.

Dr. Herzog is internationally recognized for his leadership in Critical Care Cardiology and Echocardiography. He had authored many textbooks, including the "The Cardiac Care Survival Guide" and "Herzog's CCU book," that became bestsellers in the USA and around the globe.

Dr. Herzog is an outstanding teacher. He has been awarded as the "Teacher of the year" and "Physician of the year" numerous times by the Department of Medicine and the Division of Cardiology at Mount Sinai.

At Hadassah Medical Center in Jerusalem, Israel, Dr. Herzog has developed a new and novel pathway for the diagnosis and management of pulmonary embolism, which serves as a theme for his book "Pulmonary Embolism."

The cardiology department that he currently leads for the past 3 years in Jerusalem, Israel, as one of the "World's Best Specialized Hospitals" by Newsweek for these years.

Dr. David Leibowitz is an associate professor of Medicine at the Hebrew University of Jerusalem, Israel, and is the Director of Echocardiography at Mount Scopus, Hadassah Medical Center, in Jerusalem, Israel.

He graduated cum laude from Columbia College in New York City and received his MD degree from New York University. He was trained in internal medicine at Mount Sinai in New York and in cardiology and advanced echocardiography at Columbia Presbyterian Medical Center in New York where he is currently a visiting professor.

Over the past two decades, Dr. Leibowitz has developed the highly respected and prestigious clinical cardiology and echocardiography services at the Mount Scopus Hospital of Hadassah Medical Center in Jerusalem which is an integral part of the Hadassah Cardiology program which was named as one of the "World's Best Specialized Hospitals" by Newsweek for the past 3 years.

Dr. Leibowitz is internationally recognized for his leadership in clinical cardiology and echocardiography. He had authored hundreds of peer-review papers, abstracts, and book chapters in these fields.

Dr. Leibowitz is an outstanding teacher, and he has been awarded numerous teaching awards from the Hebrew University of Jerusalem.

Dr. Yair Elitzur is the associate director of the division of Cardiac Electrophysiology at Hadassah Medical Center, the Hebrew University of Jerusalem in Jerusalem, Israel, and is director of the electrophysiology services at the Hadassah Mount Scopus Hospital in Jerusalem, Israel.

Over the past decade Dr. Elitzur has developed the clinical cardiology and electrophysiology services at the Mount Scopus Hospital of Hadassah Medical Center in Jerusalem which is an integral part of the Hadassah Cardiology program, named as one of the "World's Best Specialized Hospitals" by Newsweek for the past 3 years.

He is a graduate of the Ben Gurion medical school in Beer Sheva, Israel, and was trained in internal medicine and cardiovascular medicine at Hadassah Medical Center in Jerusalem, Israel. He completed an advanced cardiac electrophysiology fellowship in both Israel and in Toronto, Canada.

His main academic interests and publications are in the fields of coronary artery disease, cardiac electrophysiology, cardiac pacemakers, and advanced cardiac devices therapy.

He was awarded numerous teaching awards for his outstanding teaching by the Hebrew University of Jerusalem and by the Hadassah Medical Center.

Contributors

Momen Abassi Department of Nephrology Hadassah Medical Center, Hebrew University of Jerusalem, Jerusalem, Israel

Ronny Alcalai Department of Cardiology, The Heart Institute, Hadassah Medical Center, Hebrew University of Jerusalem, Jerusalem, Israel

Alexander Davidovich Mount Sinai Morningside, Institute for Critical Care Medicine, Icahn School of Medicine at Mount Sinai, New York, NY, USA

Sophia Dongas Leon H. Charney Division of Cardiology, New York University School of Medicine, New York, NY, USA

Yair Elitzur Department of Cardiology, The Heart Institute, Hadassah Medical Center, Hebrew University of Jerusalem, Jerusalem, Israel

Dan G. Halpern Adult Congenital Heart Disease, NYU Grossman School of Medicine, NYU Langone Health, New York, USA

Eyal Herzog Department of Cardiology, The Heart Institute, Hadassah Medical Center, Hebrew University of Jerusalem, Jerusalem, Israel

Habib Hilo The Heart Institute, Department of Cardiology, Hadassah Medical Center, Hebrew University of Jerusalem, Jerusalem, Israel

Megan Job Leon H. Charney Division of Cardiology, New York University School of Medicine, New York, NY, USA

Tali Koren Department of Cardiology, The Heart Institute, Hadassah Medical Center, Hebrew University of Jerusalem, Jerusalem, Israel

Jonathan Koslowsky Department of Cardiology, The Heart Institute, Hadassah Medical Center, Hebrew University of Jerusalem, Jerusalem, Israel

David Leibowitz Department of Cardiology, The Heart Institute, Hadassah Medical Center, Hebrew University of Jerusalem, Jerusalem, Israel

Mohammad Mowaswes The Heart Institute, Department of Cardiology, Hadassah Medical Center, Hebrew University of Jerusalem, Jerusalem, Israel

Batel Nisan The Heart Institute, Department of Cardiology, Hadassah Medical Center, Hebrew University of Jerusalem, Jerusalem, Israel

Eldad Rachamim The Heart Institute, Department of Cardiology, Hadassah Medical Center, Hebrew University of Jerusalem, Jerusalem, Israel

Adam Rothman Mount Sinai West, Institute for Critical Care Medicine, Icahn School of Medicine at Mount Sinai, New York, NY, USA

Muhamed Saric Leon H. Charney Division of Cardiology, New York University School of Medicine, New York, NY, USA

Janet Shapiro Mount Sinai Morningside, Institute for Critical Care Medicine, Icahn School of Medicine at Mount Sinai, New York, NY, USA

Adam J. Small Adult Congenital Heart Disease, NYU Grossman School of Medicine, NYU Langone Health, New York, USA

Donna Zwas Department of Cardiology, The Heart Institute, Hadassah Medical Center, Hebrew University of Jerusalem, Jerusalem, Israel

Tutorials for Cardiac Electrosonography

Patient-Centered Care Cardiac Electrosonography

Eyal Herzog, Yair Elitzur, Tali Koren, and David Leibowitz

Abstract

In this book the authors propose a new clinical algorithmic approach for patients with acute cardiovascular syndromes based on the combination of ECG and echocardiography performance and interpretation that is termed: electrosonography. In patient-centered care, an individual's specific health needs and desired health outcomes are the driving force behind all health care decisions and quality measurements. The authors propose a novel "patient-centered care cardiac electrosonography" concept where in a patient with cardiovascular disease the patient's cardiac symptoms are in the center of the care followed by an ECG and transthoracic cardiac or chest sonography. The combination of these three elements: a detailed history and physical exam based on the patient symptoms, the ECG and the echocardiogram improves patient diagnosis and management. This chapter provides a simplified and a novel algorithmic method for ECG interpretation and three novel pathways to diagnose and manage patients with cardiovascular symptoms of chest pain, shortness of breath (dyspnea) and syncope.

E. Herzog (✉) · Y. Elitzur · T. Koren · D. Leibowitz
Department of Cardiology, The Heart Institute, Hadassah Medical Center, Hebrew University of Jerusalem, P.O. Box 12000, Jerusalem, Israel
e-mail: eyalherzog10@gmail.com

Keywords

ECG · Echocardiography · Electrosonography · Pathway · Chest pain · Shortness of breath · Syncope

1 Introduction

The electrocardiogram (ECG) is one of the oldest diagnostic tools in evaluating patients with cardiovascular symptoms. Multiple and complex criteria for its interpretation have been developed over the past decades. We propose a simplified and a novel algorithmic method for ECG interpretation as seen in Fig. 1.

In Chap. "Tutorial for ECG Performance and Interpretation" of this book, we provide a tutorial for ECG performance and interpretation.

In recent years the use of transthoracic echocardiography (TTE) and especially point of care ultrasound based on handheld echocardiography has emerged as an important clinical tool, particularly in the emergency department (ED) and intensive care unit settings. These tests are mainly performed by non-cardiologists such as intensivists and ED physicians in addition to physical exam and standard diagnostic tests such as the chest x ray and laboratory tests to evaluate patients quickly and efficiently.

In Chap. "Tutorial for Transthoracic Echocardiography Performance and Interpretation" and Chap. "Tutorial for Chest Sonography

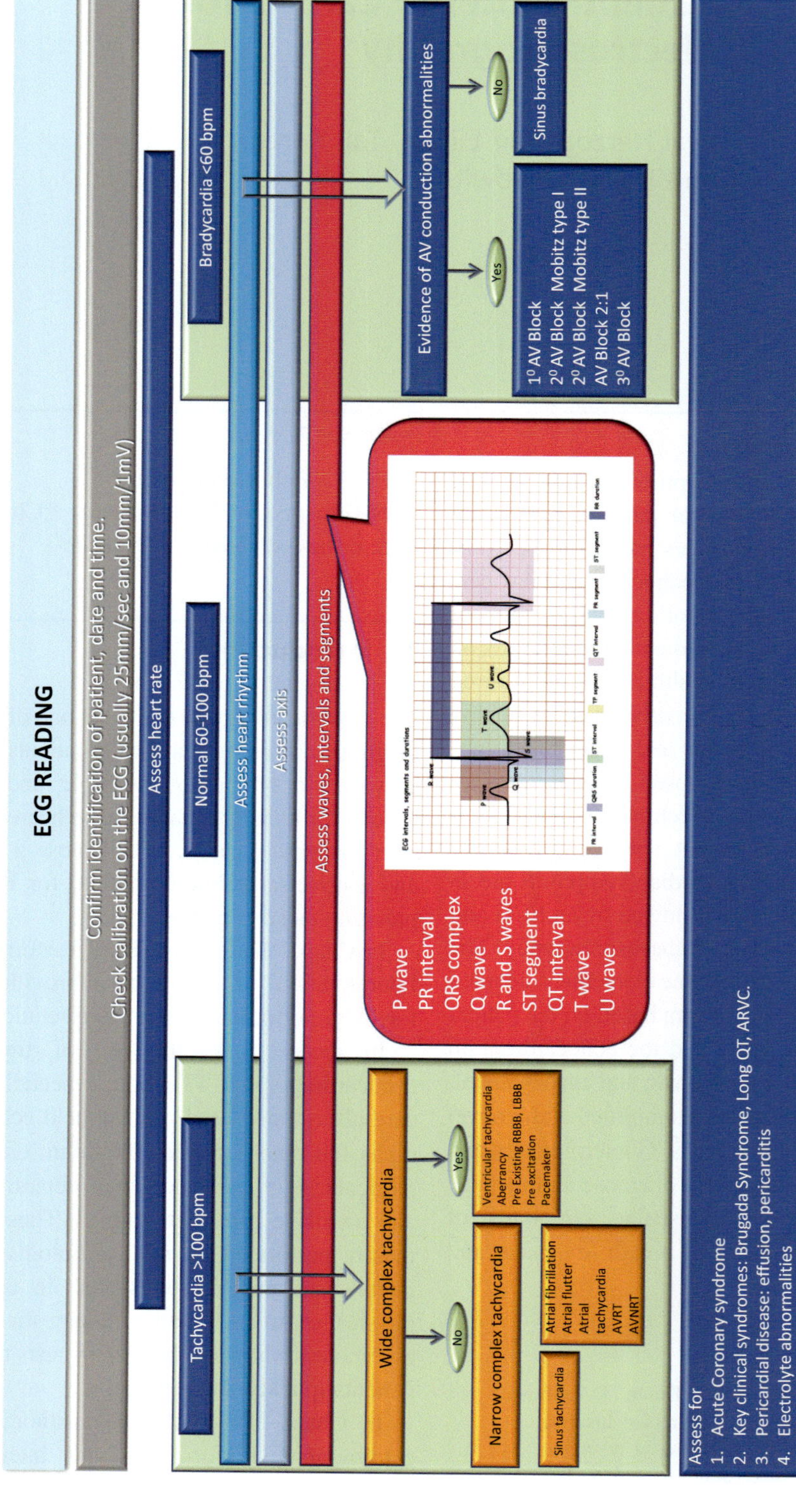

Fig. 1 A simplified and a novel algorithmic method for ECG interpretation

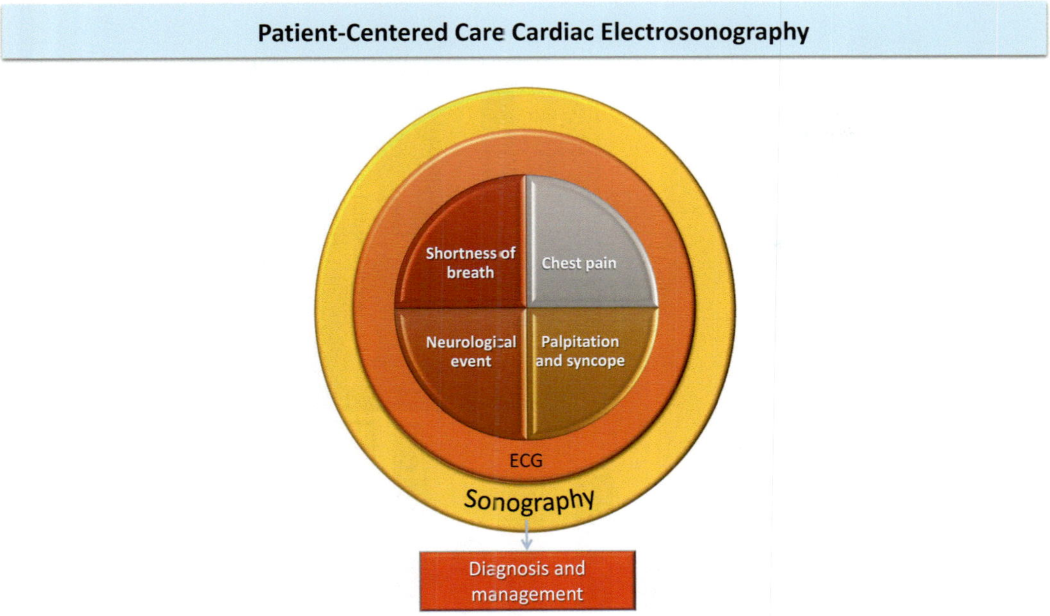

Fig. 2 Patient-centered care cardiac electrosonography

Performance and Interpretation" of this book we provide a focused tutorial for performance and interpretation of transthoracic echocardiography (Chap. "Tutorial for Transthoracic Echocardiography Performance and Interpretation") and transthoracic chest sonography (Chap. "Tutorial for Chest Sonography Performance and Interpretation").

We propose a new clinical algorithmic approach for patients with acute cardiovascular syndromes based on the combination of ECG and echocardiography performance and interpretation that we term: electrosonography. The combination of these two skills should greatly facilitate patient management by healthcare providers in the emergency setting.

In patient-centered care, an individual's specific health needs and desired health outcomes are the driving force behind all health care decisions and quality measurements.

Figure 2 shows our proposed novel "patient-centered care cardiac electrosonography" concept where in a patient with cardiovascular disease the patient's cardiac symptoms are in the center followed by an ECG and transthoracic cardiac or chest sonography. The combination of these three elements: a detailed history and physical exam based on the patient symptoms, the ECG and the echocardiogram improves patient diagnosis and management.

We outline in this chapter three main pathways to diagnose and manage patients with cardiovascular symptoms of chest pain, shortness of breath (dyspnea) and syncope.

1.1 Pathway for the Use of Electrosonography in Patients with Acute Chest Pain (Fig. 3)

In the United States it is estimated that about eight million people present each year to health care systems with complaints of acute chest pain (Eyal 2018). Initial evaluation of these patients should include a detailed history and physical examination including baseline vital signs. If the chest pain is clearly not of cardiac origin, the patient should be treated accordingly and transthoracic echo (TTE) is seldom needed.

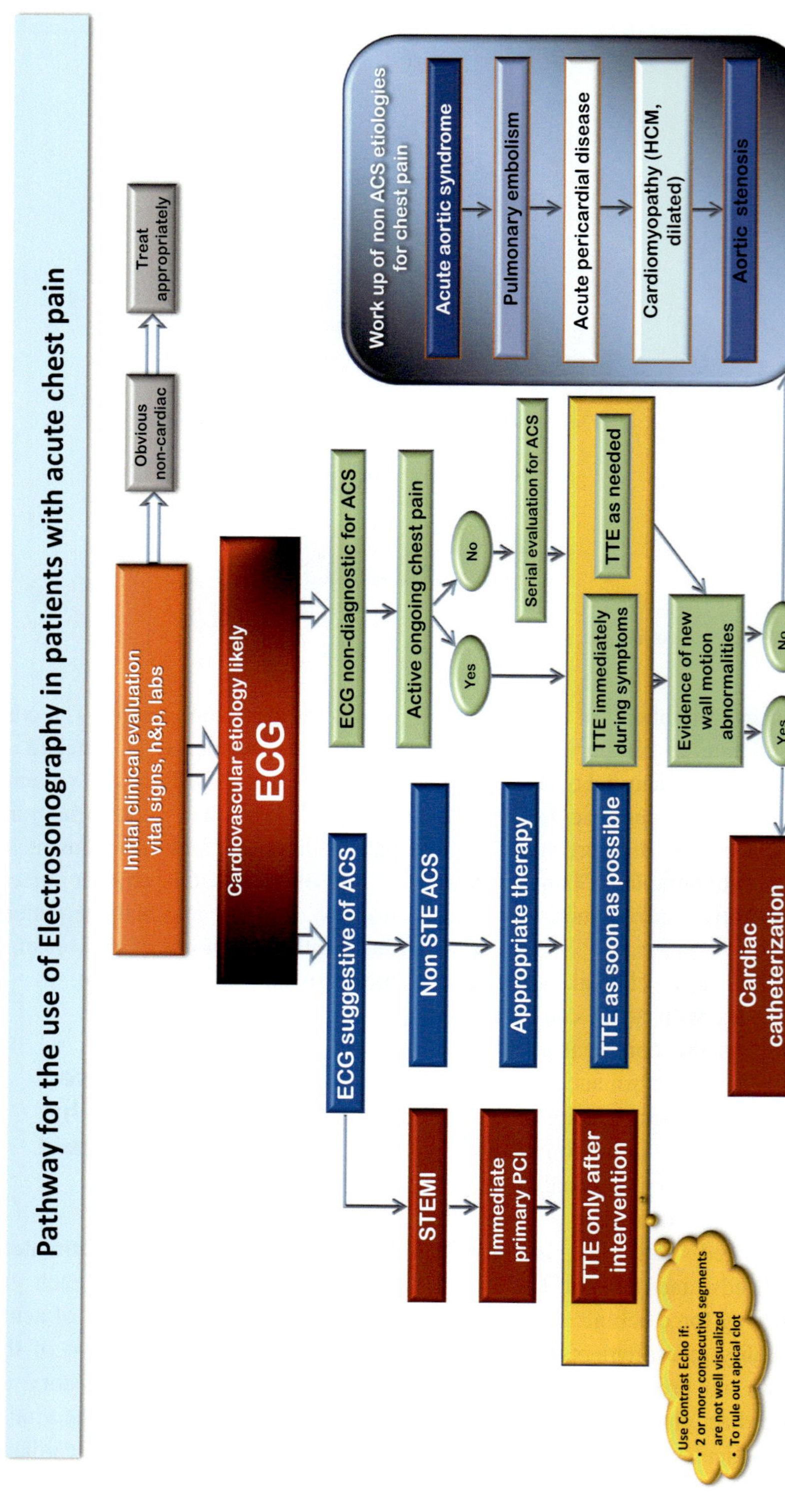

Fig. 3 Pathway for the use of electrosonography in patients with acute chest pain

If the cause of the chest pain appears to be of a cardiovascular etiology than the initial evaluation should always start with a 12-lead electrocardiogram (ECG). The ECG findings help divide patients into two groups:

1. Patients in whom the ECG is suggestive of acute coronary syndrome (ACS)
2. Patients in whom the ECG is not diagnostic for ACS.

ACS incorporates a spectrum of clinical entities ranging from unstable angina and non ST elevation ACS (non STE ACS) to ST elevation MI (STEMI). Out of all patients presenting with chest pain only the minority have ACS. Among ACS patients, most (about 75%) have non-STE ACS.

In addition to ECG, TTE is an integral part of the assessment and management of patients with ACS as seen in Fig. 3.

In patients with definitive findings of STEMI on ECG, it is well accepted that patients should preferably be referred to a site that can perform primary percutaneous coronary intervention (PCI). TTE should not be done immediately as it may delay transfer to the cardiac catheterization laboratory for PCI and should be performed only after the intervention is completed.

In contrast to STEMI cases, patients with non-STE ACS should be treated medically per current guidelines and TTE should be performed as soon as possible to evaluate for wall motion abnormalities and to exclude other structural heart disease. These patients will generally be referred for cardiac catheterization for revascularization.

Currently, the use of imaging enhancing agents (previously known as "contrast echo") is the standard of care for patients in whom two or more consecutive left ventricular endocardial segments are not visualized well, or when there is a need to rule out an apical thrombus.

For patients with persistent symptoms of chest pain suspected to be of a cardiovascular etiology other than ACS, TTE should be performed immediately.

Evidence of new wall motion abnormalities on TTE will usually mandate referral for cardiac catheterization and revascularization as needed.

If the symptoms of chest pain resolved, we recommend to continue the serial evaluation of ACS and to perform TTE as needed. If the TTE shows an evidence of new wall motion abnormalities, a diagnosis of coronary artery disease is likely and referral for cardiac catheterization is indicated. Similarly, imaging enhancing echocardiography ("contrast echo") is necessary when the endocardial definition is poor or when a clot in the apex needs to be ruled out.

For patients without regional wall motion abnormalities in whom a diagnosis of ACS has been ruled out, other cardiac etiologies should be considered. We recommend a detailed work up in the following order so as to rule out the most immediately potentially life-threatening illnesses soonest:

1. Acute aortic syndrome
2. Acute pulmonary embolism
3. Acute pericardial disease
4. Cardiomyopathy (dilated, hypertrophic)
5. Aortic stenosis.

1.2 Pathway for the Use of Electrosonography in Patients with Shortness of Breath (Fig. 4)

ECG and echocardiography are essential in evaluating patients with acute and subacute shortness of breath, occasionally termed "dyspnea". As with patients who present with acute chest pain, the initial evaluation should include a detailed history and physical examination including baseline vital signs. If the shortness of breath is clearly not of a cardiac origin, the patient should be treated accordingly and transthoracic echo (TTE) is not generally needed as part of the acute assessment.

If the cause of the shortness of breath appears to be of a cardiovascular etiology than the initial evaluation should always start with a 12-lead electrocardiogram (ECG). As in patients presenting with chest pain, the ECG findings help divide patients into two groups:

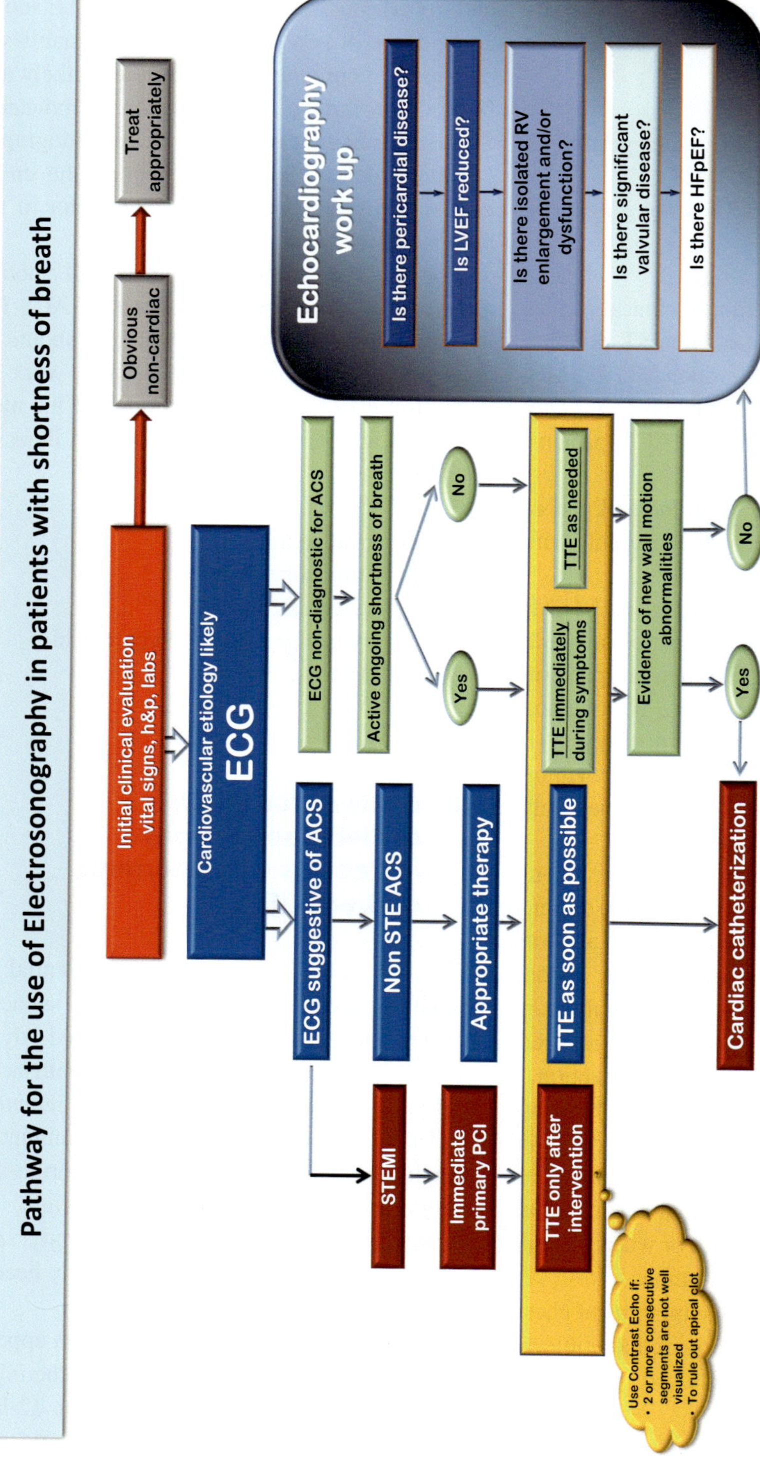

Fig. 4 Pathway for the use of Electrosonography in patients with shortness of breath

1. Patients in whom the ECG is suggestive of acute coronary syndrome (ACS)
2. Patients in whom the ECG is not diagnostic for ACS.

TTE is an integral part of the assessment and management of patients with ACS presenting with shortness of breath as seen in Fig. 4.

Our algorithm for management of patients with acute shortness of breath who have ACS is similar to the algorithm for the management of patients with acute chest pain as the shortness of breath can be a symptom of acute ischemia as well.

As outlined earlier in this chapter, in patients with STEMI, it is now well accepted that patients should preferably be referred to a site that can perform primary percutaneous coronary intervention (PCI). TTE should not be done immediately as it may delay care and the transfer to the cardiac catheterization laboratory for PCI. TTE should be performed only after the intervention is completed.

In contrast to STEMI cases, patients with non-STE ACS should be treated medically per current guidelines and TTE should be performed as soon as possible to evaluate for wall motion abnormalities and to exclude structural heart disease. Most of these patients will eventually be referred for cardiac catheterization for revascularization.

For patients for whom the shortness of breath is suspected to be of a cardiovascular etiology other than ACS, TTE should be performed immediately if the symptoms persist and the patient still has active ongoing dyspnea.

For patients in whom a diagnosis of ACS is ruled out, and they do not have evidence of new wall motion abnormalities, other cardiac etiologies for shortness of breath should be considered. We recommend a work up in the following order:

1. Is there pericardial effusion?
2. Is left ventricle ejection fraction (LVEF) reduced?
3. Is there evidence of an isolated right ventricular (RV) enlargement and/or dysfunction?
4. Is there significant valvular disease?
5. Is there heart failure with preserved ejection fraction? (HFpEF)

1.3 Pathway for the Use of Electrosonography in Patients with Syncope (Fig. 5)

Syncope is a syndrome consisting of a relatively short period of temporary and self-limited loss of consciousness caused by transient diminution of blood flow to the brain. In the United States, 1–2 million patients are evaluated for syncope annually, making up 3–5% of emergency department visits, and 1–6% of urgent hospital admissions (Emad and Eyal 2018).

Our team has developed a standardized pathway which is comprehensive, yet simple, and provides guidelines for the management of all patients presenting with syncope (Fig. 5).

The combined use of ECG and echocardiography, which we term electrosonography, is essential in managing these patients.

The initial assessment of a patient with syncope includes a meticulous and comprehensive medical history. Incorporating eyewitness accounts can help determine the cause of syncope. Orthostatic hypotension and autonomic dysfunction can be identified by measuring blood pressure and pulse rate in the upper and the lower extremities in the supine and upright positions. Basic laboratory tests, including basic metabolic panel and complete blood count should be performed in all patients with syncope. A 12-lead electrocardiogram (ECG) should be done in all patients in the initial evaluation.

Definition of True Syncope

We use the acronym **SELF-1** which reflects the four criteria that should be met for an event to be considered true syncope.

S: Short period, Self-limited, Spontaneous recovery
E: Early-rapid onset.
L: Loss of consciousness-transient.
F: Full recover, Fall.

Patients who did not lose consciousness are defined as "not true syncope".

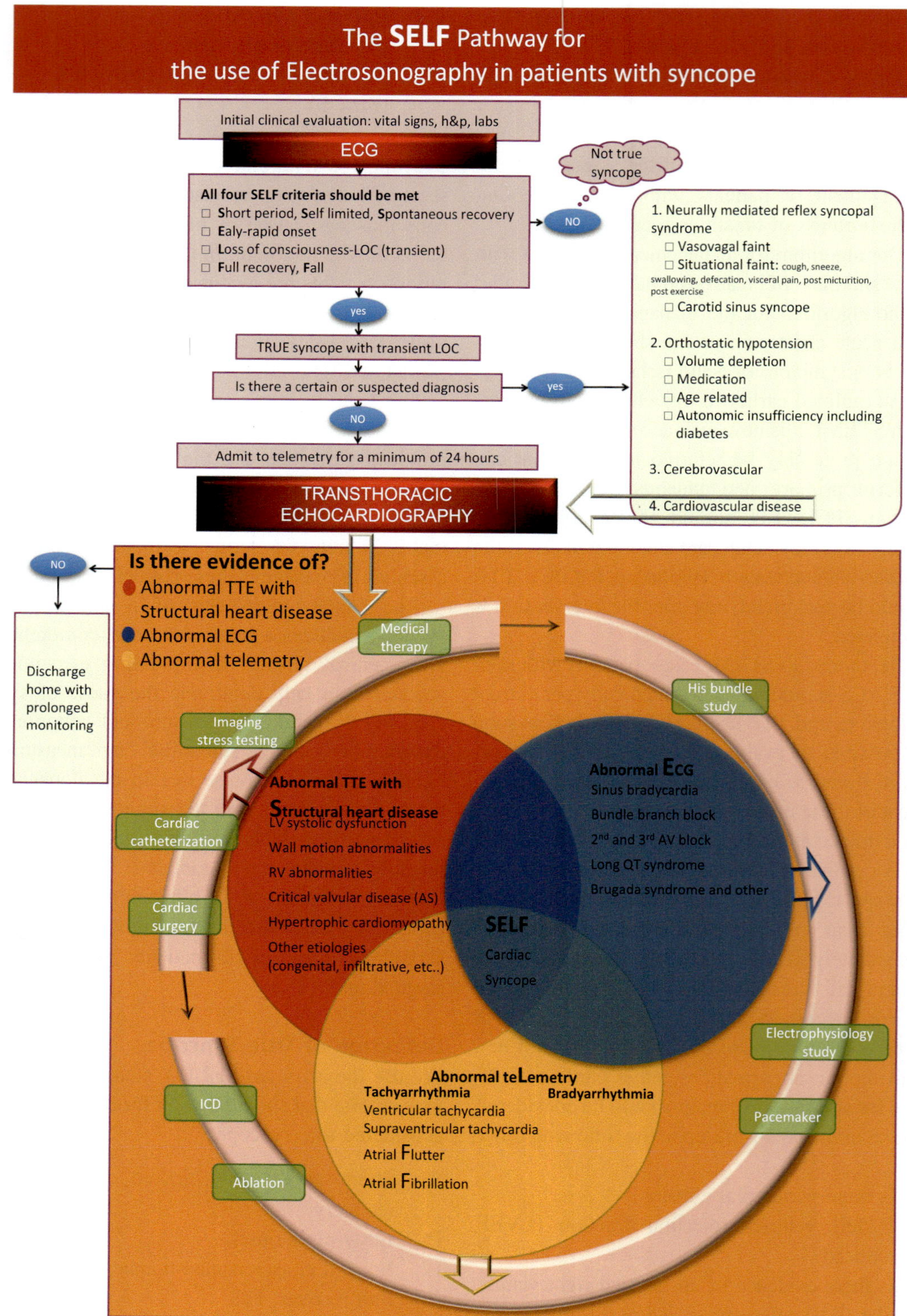

Fig. 5 Pathway for the use of Electrosonography in patients with Syncope

Classification of Syncope When There is a Certain or Suspected Diagnosis

These are certain disorders causing true syncope with transient loss of consciousness:

1. *Neurally mediated reflex syncopal syndrome* including: vasovagal faint, situational faint (such as cough, sneeze, swallowing, defecation, visceral pain, post micturition and post exercise) and carotid sinus syndrome. This reflex syncope, when triggered, gives rise to vasodilatation and bradycardia
2. *Orthostatic hypotension syncope*: syncope occurs in the assumption of an upright position. It can occur after starting of medications that can lead to hypotension, or can be due to autonomic neuropathy. Volume depletion is an important cause of orthostatic hypotension
3. *Cerebrovascular disease*
4. *Cardiovascular disease*: Structural heart disease demonstrated on electrosonography can cause syncope by multiple mechanisms generally related to impaired cardiac output due to structural disease of the myocardium or cardiac valves as well as cardiac arrhythmias.

Risk Stratification for Admission to the Hospital

One of the main dilemmas that face emergency department health care providers is whether to admit patients with syncope to the hospital or to refer them for an outpatient evaluation. Many risk assessment scores have been developed. In all these scores, there is a consensus to admit patients with abnormal ECG, hypotension, heart failure and anemia.

In our standardized SELF pathway, we use the **SELF-2** criteria to evaluate the need for admission.

These criteria include:

S: abnormal transthoracic echocardiography (TTE) with **S**tructural heart disease

E: abnormal **E**CG

L: abnormal te**L**emetry

F: atrial **F**ibrillation and **F**lutter as example of common tachyarrhythmias.

Admitted patients should be monitored for a minimum of 24 h, which could potentially reveal bradyarrhythmia or tachyarrhythmias. The management of bradyarrhythmias may include electrophysiologic testing with or without subsequent pacemaker implantation. Tachyarrhythmias include ventricular tachycardia, supraventricular tachycardia and the more common atrial fibrillation and atrial flutter. The treatment of these patients may include radiofrequency ablation or device therapy with a pacemaker or an implantable cardioverter defibrillator (ICD).

Management of Cardiac Syncope

The major goal of the evaluation of syncope in patients with heart disease is to identify a potentially life-threatening diagnosis, particularly arrhythmias. Work up and management of these patients can include medical therapy, stress testing with cardiac imaging, cardiac catheterization, and possible revascularization with percutaneous coronary intervention or cardiac surgery.

Electrosonography in Cardiac Syncope

Electrocardiogram (ECG)

Electrocardiography is essential in the workup of patients with unexplained syncope; however, it may only reveal a direct cause in 5% of patients. Abnormal ECGs may include the following findings: sinus bradycardia resulting from sinus node dysfunction or atrioventricular (AV) block resulting from AV node or His-Purkinje system dysfunction, pre-excitation patterns, a long or short QT interval and Brugada syndrome.

Echocardiography

Echocardiography should be performed in all patients with true syncope because it can identify patients with significant structural heart disease including: LV systolic dysfunction, wall motion abnormalities, RV dysfunction, critical valvular disease (like severe aortic stenosis), hypertrophic cardiomyopathy and other etiologies like congenital or infiltrative diseases.

Management of Patients with Unexplained Syncope but with no Evidence on Electrosonography for Cardiac Etiology

In the absence of underlying heart disease, syncope is not associated with excess mortality. Our recommendation for these patients is for early discharge, with consideration for prolonged monitoring.

References

Emad A, Eyal H. The approach to the patient with syncope. In: Herzog E, editor. Herzog's CCU book. USA: Wolter Kluwer; 2018. p. 285–93.

Eyal H. Echocardiographic assessment of acute chest pain in the CCU. In: Herzog E, Argulian E, editors. Echocardiography in the CCU. Switzerland: Springer; 2018. p. 3–26.

Tutorial for ECG Performance and Interpretation

Yair Elitzur, David Leibowitz, Momen Abassi, and Eyal Herzog

Abstract

Following history and physical examination, ECG reading is the initial step in the electrosonography approach. This chapter offers a concise tutorial of ECG performance and interpretation. The tutorial begins with fundamentals of the ECG as a three-dimensional, vectorial view of the electrical activity of the heart. Standard electrode placement and the resultant 12 ECG leads are discussed. We introduce an algorithmic approach to ECG reading, presented as a graphic flowchart. The chapter then presents diagnostic criteria for the different branches of the algorithm, accompanied by clear diagrams and real-world ECG examples of common cardiac disorders seen in the acute care setting.

Keywords

Electrocardiogram · ECG · Electrosonography · Ischemic heart disease · Cardiac arrhythmias · Heart block

Y. Elitzur (✉) · D. Leibowitz · E. Herzog
Department of Cardiology, The Heart Institute, Hadassah Medical Center, Hebrew University of Jerusalem, P.O. Box 12000, Jerusalem, Israel
e-mail: Elitzur1970@gmail.com

M. Abassi
Department of Nephrology Hadassah Medical Center, Hebrew University of Jerusalem, Jerusalem, Israel

1 Introduction—Generation of an ECG Tracing

The ECG is a body-surface recording of electrical signals generated by the heart. These signals are the result of a repetitive cycle of depolarization (in systole) and repolarization (in diastole) of cardiac cells. As opposed to electrical signals that may be recorded by catheters within the heart, the signals recorded on the body surface represent a summation of electrical activity of the heart as a whole. This summed activity is a vector; it has an *amplitude*, measured in millivolts, and a direction, termed the *axis*. Because the signals have a direction, they will appear different when recorded at different angles from the heart.

By convention, when an ECG is performed, the patient is connected to the device by ten different electrodes: four on the hands and feet, and six on the chest. The chest electrodes are designated V1–V6; correct placement upon the chest is crucial for precise ECG interpretation. Following is a description of correct chest electrode positioning, also shown in Fig. 1:

V1: Fourth intercostal space at the right sternal border.
V2: Fourth intercostal space at the left sternal border.
V3: Midway between V2 and V4.

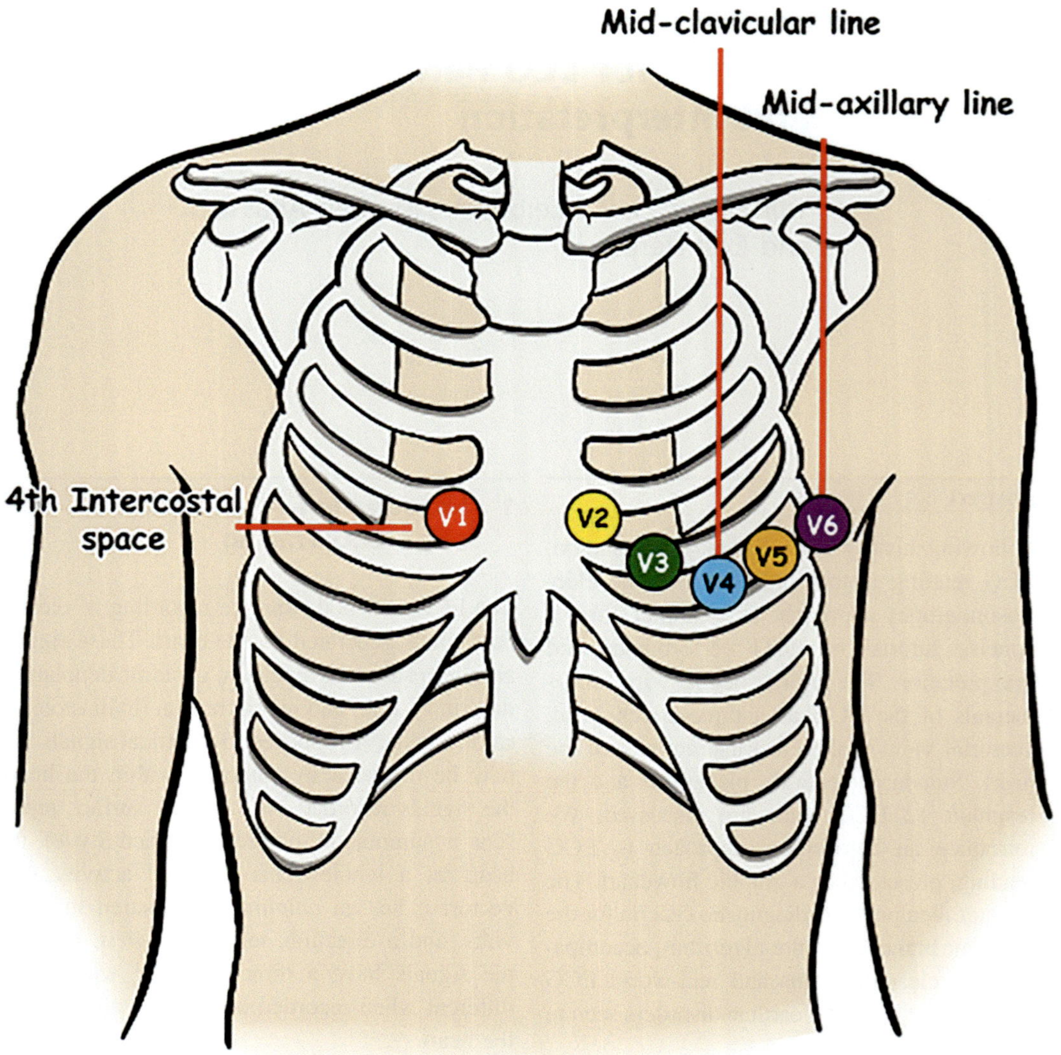

Fig. 1 Correct positioning of ECG chest electrodes

V4: Fifth intercostal space in the midclavicular line.

V5: In the horizontal plane of V4 at the anterior axillary line (or if the anterior axillary line is ambiguous, midway between V4 and V6).

V6: In the horizontal plane of V4 at the midaxillary line.

The electric current may be measured between any two poles; however, there is a standard way of measurement resulting in the standard 12-lead ECG. Each 'lead' depicts the current measured between two poles.

Thus, lead I is measured from the left (+) to the right (−) arm. Therefore, this lead 'looks' at the heart from the left side. Any component of the electric current travelling from right to left (toward the left hand) will be plotted on lead I as an upward movement. Any current component travelling from left to right will be depicted as a downward movement. Therefore, if there is a positive signal in lead I, we know that at this moment the summation of cardiac electric

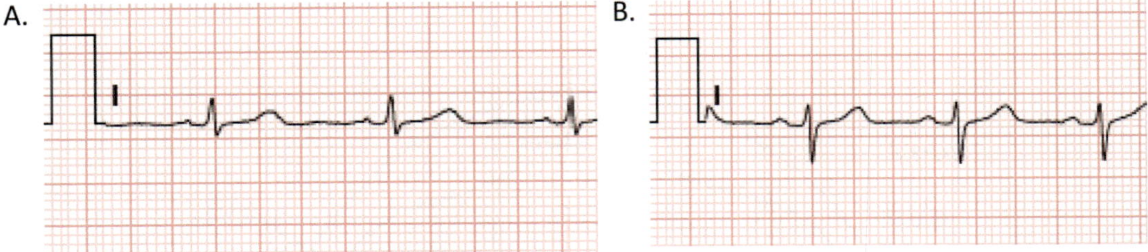

Fig. 2 In this example, the QRS complex in A is more positive than negative. This indicates that the summation of ventricular activity, or the QRS axis, is directed from right to left, which is normal. In B the QRS in lead I is more negative than positive, indicating a rightward axis, which is not normal

activity is directed to the left. This concept is illustrated in Fig. 2.

The standard 12 ECG leads comprise the following (Kligfield et al. 2007):

Lead I—right arm to left arm (0°)

Lead II—right arm to left leg (+ 60°)

Lead III—left arm to left leg (+ 120°)

aVR—right arm to average of left arm and left leg (− 120°)

aVL—left arm to average of right arm and left leg (− 30°)

aVF—left leg to average of both arms (+ 90°).

These six leads describe the direction of electrical activity in the frontal plane; showing whether the current is mainly directed up, down, right, left or any direction in between in this plane.

The chest leads provide a 'look' at the heart in the horizontal plane; showing whether the current is mainly directed toward the front, back, or any direction in between in this plane.

The chest (precordial) leads are measured from each chest electrode to 'Wilson's Central Terminal', which is the average of leads I, II and III; it is virtually the electrical center of the heart. Figure 3 describes the six frontal leads and 6 chest leads.

It is convenient to view groups of leads as showing the electrical activity from common aspects of the heart, related to the heart 'walls':

Leads I, aVL,—High lateral leads

V5, V6—Lateral leads

II, III, aVF—Inferior leads

V1, V2—Septal leads

V3, V4—Anterior leads

aVR—Right sided lead.

We thus determine the 'QRS axis' of the ECG, describing the main direction at which the heart, especially the left ventricle, is activated. Certain heart conditions may cause an abnormal axis; for example, a block in one of the left conduction fascicles (left anterior or posterior fascicular block) would typically cause a shift of the QRS axis to the left or to the right, depending on the fascicle blocked.

The normal frontal plane QRS axis is − 30 to + 90°.

1.1 ECG Waves, Segments and Intervals

Every normal heart beat is composed of several electrical events represented on the ECG:

- Depolarization of the atria
- Conduction delay in the AV node
- Depolarization of the ventricles
- Repolarization.

These events are represented by distinct inscriptions on the ECG:

P wave—atrial depolarization

PR segment—conduction delay in the AV node

PR interval—time from beginning of atrial activation to beginning of ventricular activation

QRS complex—ventricular depolarization

ST segment and T wave—ventricular repolarization

U wave—the small wave following the T wave.

By convention, a *segment* is measured between two waves and does not include the waves; an *interval* includes waves.

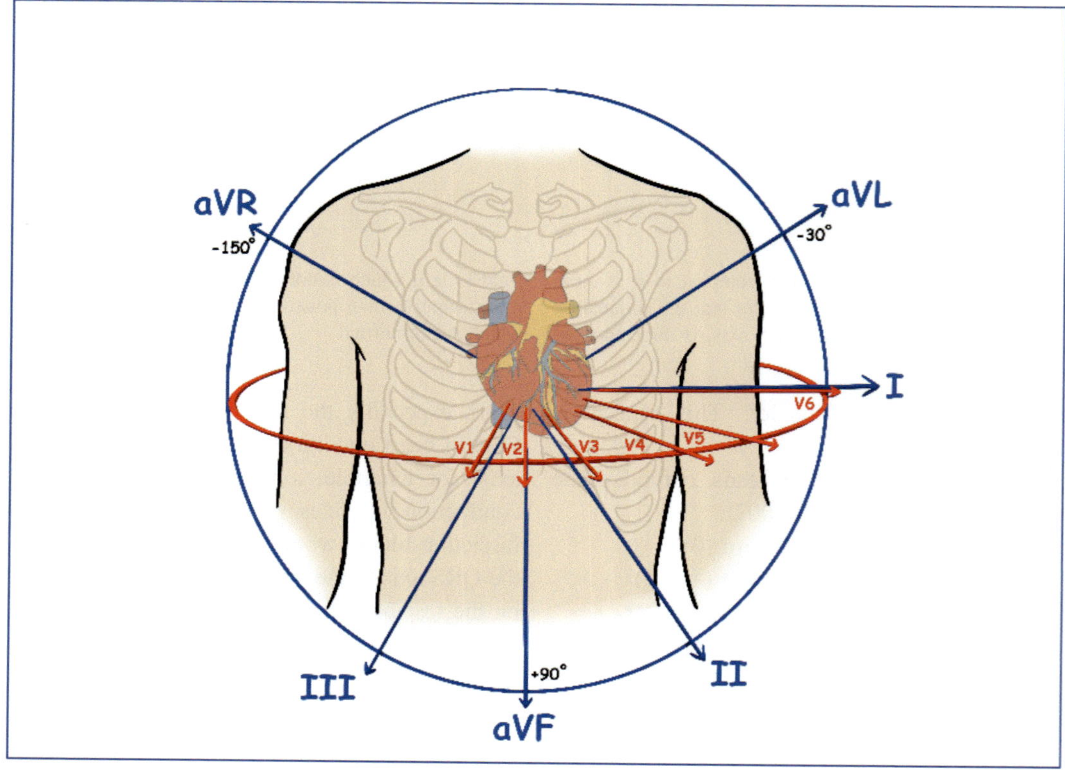

Fig. 3 The six frontal leads (blue) and 6 chest leads (red)

The ECG waves, intervals and segments are shown in Fig. 4.

Normal values are:

PR interval 120–200 ms (3–5 mm)
QRS 80–120 ms (2–3 mm)
QT 350–450 ms (the normal QT depends on heart rate).

1.2 The Normal ECG and Incorrect Lead Connection

Accidentally switching the wires of the ECG between arms and legs, as well as among the precordial leads, may lead to incorrect diagnosis.

Each possibility of wire connection misplacement will produce a distinct, typical ECG abnormality.

If any abnormality exists in the P or QRS axis, it may be useful to review the patient's prior ECG and proper wire connections.

The most obvious and common mistake is switching the left and right arm connections. This will produce a right axis deviation, positive p, QRS and T waves in aVR (an abnormal finding!), and negative P, QRS and T in leads I and aVL. Obviously, a similar pattern may suggest the uncommon condition of dextrocardia. However, in dextrocardia the progression of the QRS complex in the chest leads will be abnormal (all negative), whereas in lead reversal this will be normal. Figure 5 is an ECG example of accidental reversal of the right and left arm electrodes.

1.3 Determining the Heart Rate from the ECG

The standard paper speed when performing an ECG tracing is 25 mm/s. The ECG paper is divided into small 1 mm boxes. Every five of these comprise a larger, 5 mm box. Five of these, comprising 25 mm, contain 1 second. In each minute, therefore, there will be 5 × 60 = 300

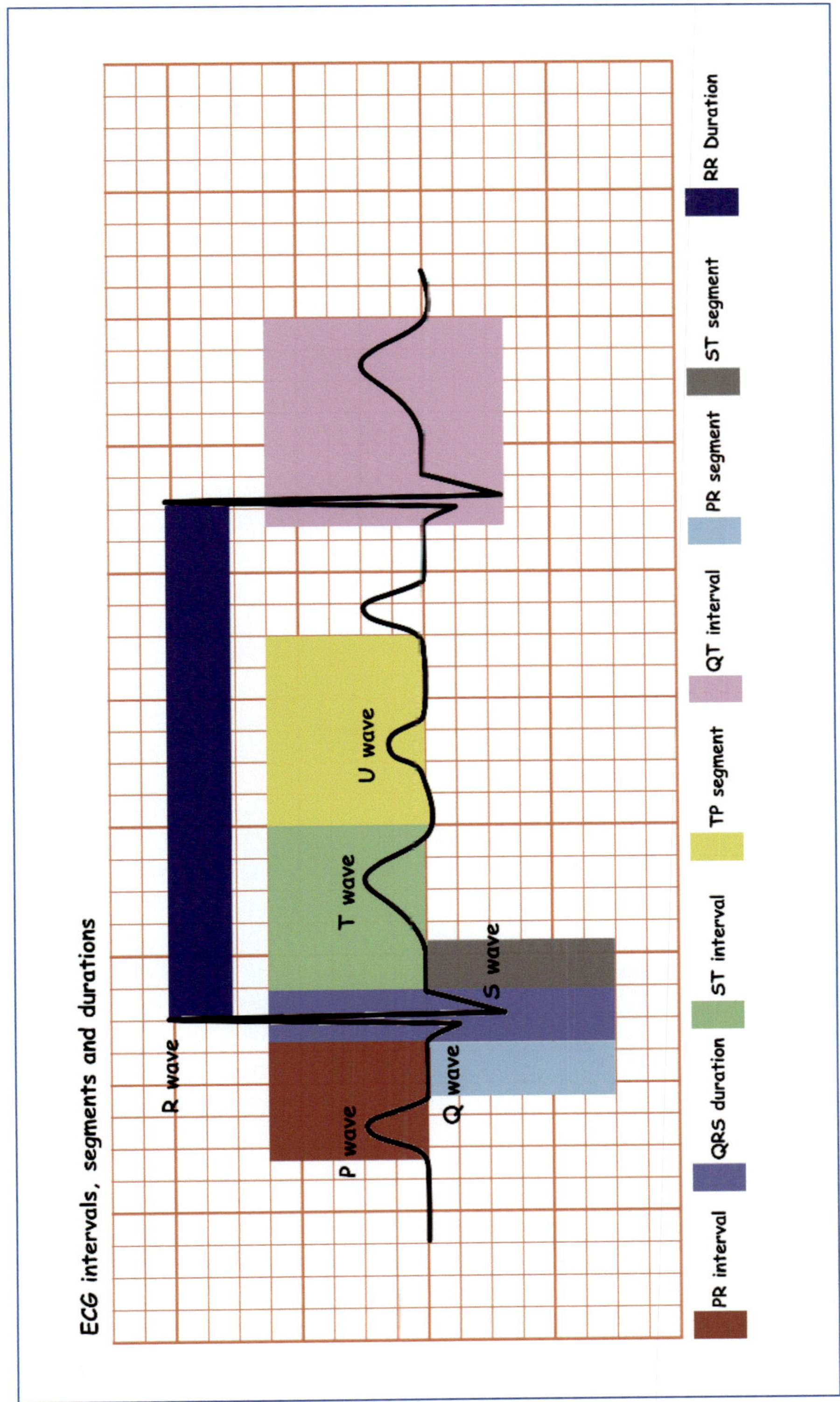

Fig. 4 ECG intervals and segments

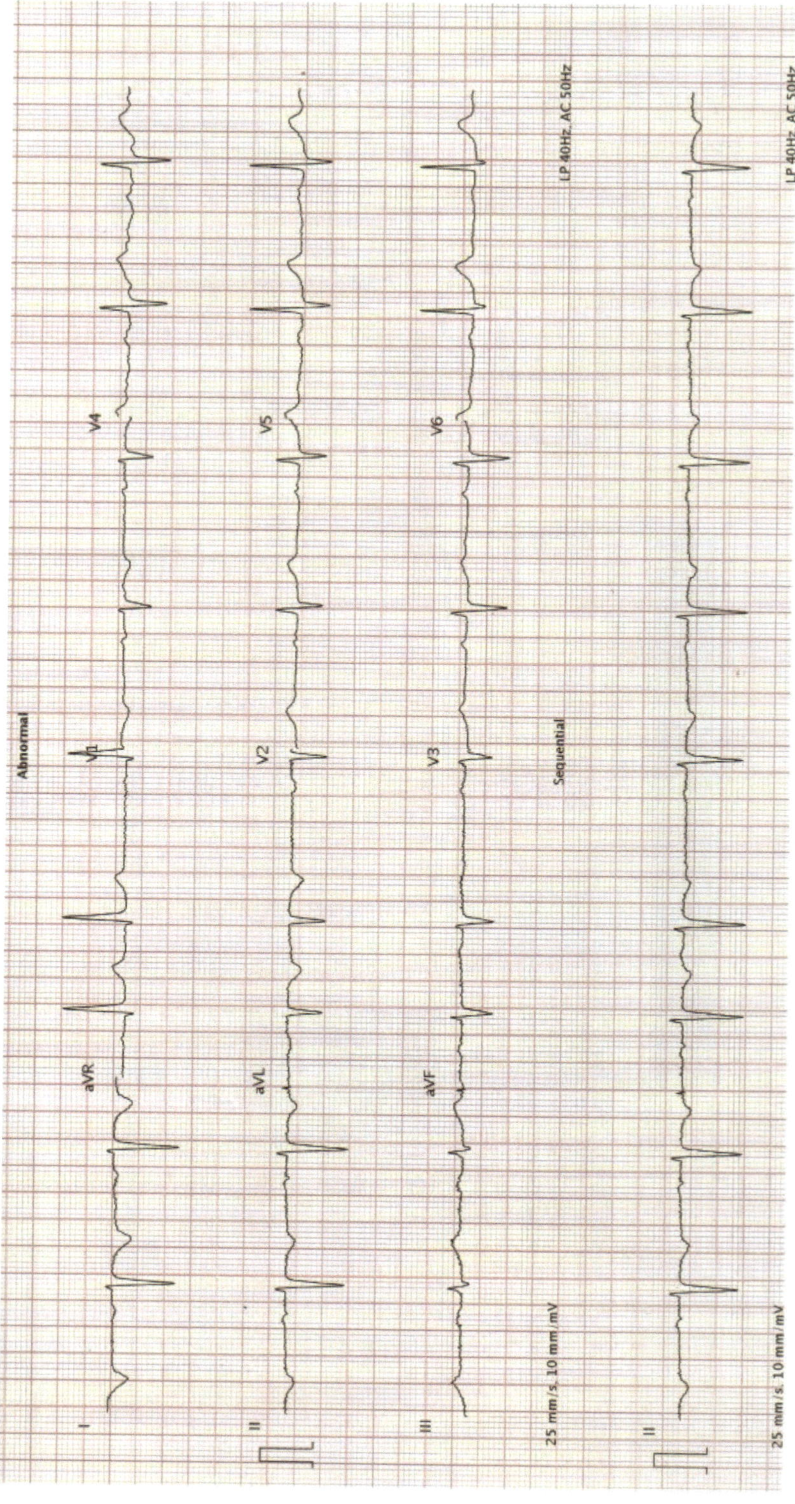

Fig. 5 ECG with right arm—left arm lead reversal. Note positive P, QRS and T waves in aVR, negative P, QRS T in leads I and aVL

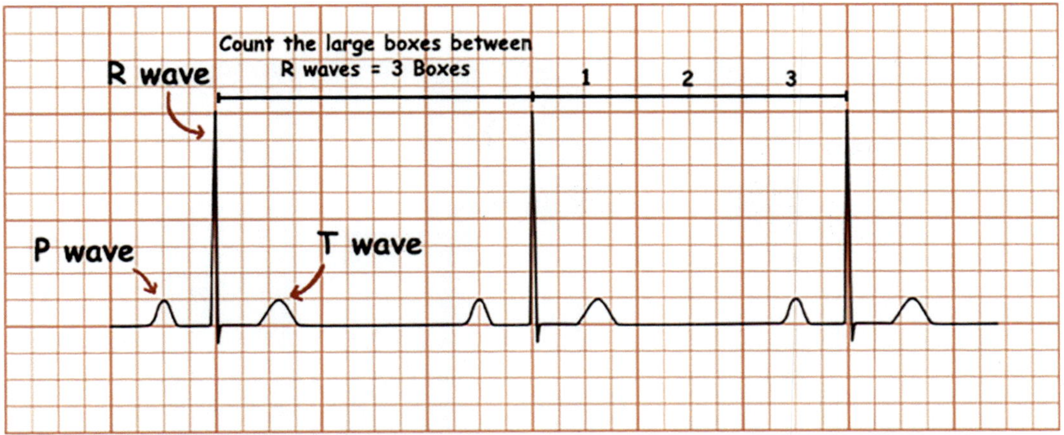

Fig. 6 Determining the heart rate from the ECG

boxes of 5 mm. Hence, to determine the number of beats per minute, one should count the number of 5 mm boxes between 2 QRS complexes (2 R waves), and divide 300 by this number (as illustrated in Fig. 6). For example, if there are three 5-mm boxes between 2 QRS complexes, then the rate is 300:3 = 100 beats per minute. Determination of the heart rate from the ECG is illustrated in Fig. 6.

2 The ECG in Heart Disease: A Systematic Approach to ECG Interpretation

When examining the ECG in different clinical scenarios, there are two possible approaches. The classical approach stresses a systematic, comprehensive and structured 'walk-through' of the whole ECG tracing, in order to never miss an abnormality. Making this a habit is very important for the caregiver in training, as is acquiring the habit of a structured history taking, physical examination, etc.

However, alongside systematic observation, there are different aspects of the ECG that require special attention in specific clinical scenarios. In order to simplify, we shall divide these into four main categories:

- Problems of heart rate and rhythm
- Ischemic heart disease
- Structural heart disease
- Extra-Cardiac disease.

Several possible approaches have been developed for ECG reading. In this book, we recommend an algorithmic thought process, depicted in the algorithm in Fig. 7. This approach aims at prioritizing emergency situations, followed by careful analysis of the ECG tracing for other common heart conditions:

I. Verification of patient identity and technical aspects of the ECG. This is an essential part of ECG interpretation. The main technical issues to look for are calibration for paper speed (25 mm/s) and voltage (10 mm/mV), and correct wire connection to the patient.

II. Analysis of the heart rate: Normal, fast (tachycardia) or slow (bradycardia).

III. Analysis of heart rhythm: Whether the mechanism controlling the heart rate is the usual one ('sinus rhythm'), or is there an abnormality in the production, or propagation, of the electrical signals that drive the heart. If the heart is driven by an abnormal mechanism, we say that the patient has an *arrhythmia*. This may be a

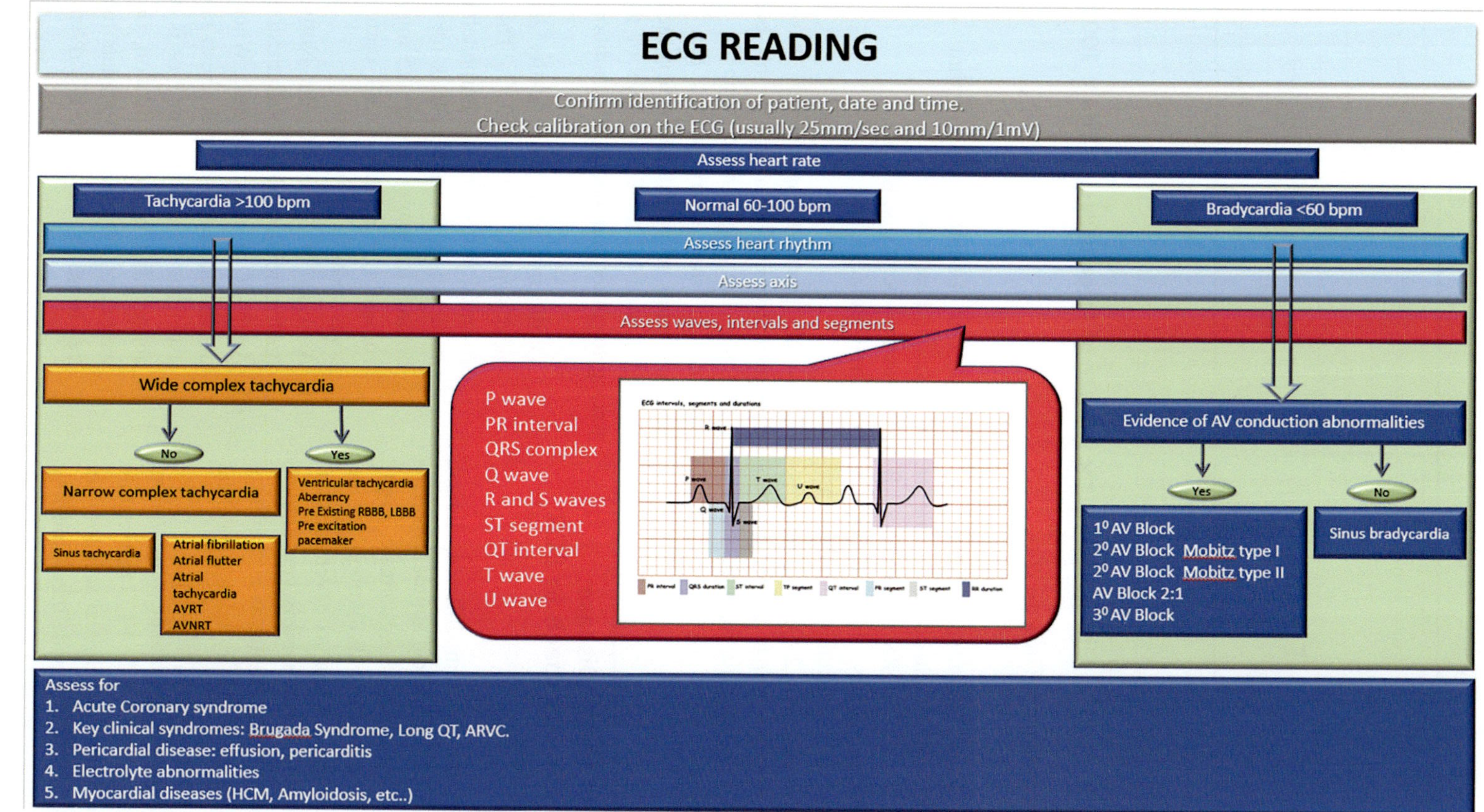

Fig. 7 ECG reading algorithm

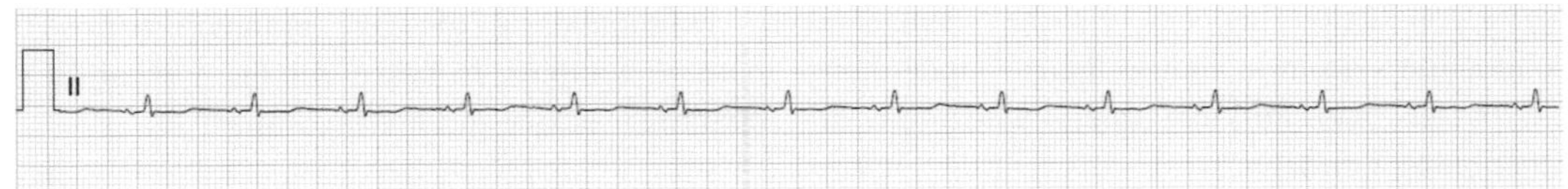

Fig. 8 Sinus rhythm

bradyarrhythmia (too slow) or a *tachyarrhythmia* (too fast). If this is the case, we then analyze the rhythm to further classify the specific arrhythmia.

IV. Following determination of rate and rhythm, we analyze the QRS axis and measure waves, intervals and segments.

V. We then search for ECG signs of other significant heart conditions, including diseases of heart muscle (e.g. hypertrophy), electrical heart disease (e.g. long QT), and extracardiac disease such as pericardial, or lung diseases.

While adoption of a standard, algorithmic routine is very important, at times one may become aware at first sight of a life-threatening condition on the ECG, such as ventricular fibrillation or acute ST elevation myocardial infarction. In this case, necessary emergency steps should be taken; however, complete analysis of the ECG should still be undertaken as soon as possible.

Figure 7 is a comprehensive algorithm describing the approach to reading an ECG.

3 Analysis of Heart Rhythm

3.1 Normal Sinus Rhythm

A fundamental step in ECG diagnosis is to determine if there is normal sinus rhythm.

Normal sinus rhythm is characterized by p waves that are upright (positive) in inferior leads (II, III and aVF). P waves will usually be visible in leads II or V1. There should be a 1:1 ratio between p wave and QRS complexes: every p wave should be followed by a QRS complex.

The rate is considered normal if it is in the range of 60–100 bpm. However, the rate should be considered in the clinical context. For example, a slower rate may be normal for an athlete, and a fast rate may be appropriate in cases of fever, stress, inflammation, etc.

Normal sinus rhythm is usually regular, however it is typically mildly fluctuating and not fixed. Figure 8 shows normal sinus rhythm.

4 Approach to the ECG with Tachycardia

The health care provider should first determine if this is sinus rhythm (in this case—sinus tachycardia) using the definition of sinus rhythm. If so, the caregiver must search for a medical condition causing the tachycardia. This is not an arrhythmia.

Uncommonly, a patient may have inappropriate sinus tachycardia or sinus node reentry which are cardiac or autonomic in origin—and not a response to a medical condition. This diagnosis can be made only after exclusion of physiologic causes for the tachycardia.

If the rhythm is not sinus, this is a tachyarrhythmia.

Regardless of the mechanism, the key question is if the arrhythmia is causing hemodynamic instability. In this case it must immediately be stopped by cardioversion or defibrillation.

Once tachyarrhythmia is determined to be of non-sinus origin and the patient is stable, a more specific diagnosis should be made.

The first step is to evaluate if the QRS complex is wide (> 120 ms) or narrow.

4.1 Narrow Complex Tachycardia

A narrow QRS complex means that during tachycardia, the spread of electrical current throughout the ventricles is rapid. This happens when conduction happens via the specialized conduction system including the AV node, bundle of His and Purkinje fibers which are all functioning normally.

Hence, the origin of this tachycardia is always supra-ventricular.

The five most common types of supraventricular tachycardia (excluding sinus tachycardia, which is not an arrhythmia) are:

- Atrial fibrillation
- Atrial flutter
- Atrial (ectopic) tachycardia
- Atrioventricular nodal reentrant tachycardia (AVNRT)
- Atrioventricular reentrant tachycardia (AVRT).

The first three tachyarrhythmias are arrhythmias which originate in the atria and are conducted to the ventricles.

The last two tachyarrhythmias result from a reentry loop: AVNRT involves two pathways within the AV node: a fast pathway and a slow pathway. This arrhythmia happens when a premature beat reaches the fast pathway while it is still refractory from the previous beat. If a person has an additional slow pathway that is not refractory at this moment, then the electrical impulse from the premature beat may go down this pathway to the ventricles. Since it is a slow pathway, by the time the signal reaches the ventricles the fast pathway may recover and not be refractory any more. The electrical impulse may then travel retrogradely from ventricle to atrium. This time, conduction is rapid since this pathway is fast; upon reaching the atrium it will again go down the slow pathway, thereby entering a vicious cycle of rapid atrial and ventricular activation. This is a brief description of AVNRT, but the same mechanism holds for any tachyarrhythmia resulting from a reentrant mechanism (such as atrial flutter, scar related VT and others).

In case of AVRT, there is only one pathway crossing the AV node; however, there is an additional pathway connecting the atria and ventricles at a different location along the mitral or tricuspid annuli. The basic mechanism of generation of the arrhythmia is similar to AVNRT.

Differentiating the five common forms of narrow complex is based on the typical ECG characteristics of these arrhythmias:

A. Atrial fibrillation is a chaotic arrhythmia. The precise mechanism by which this happens is not well defined. The result is an atrium that is not activated in a rhythmic fashion, causing impaired atrial mechanical contraction. Sampling of electric signals within a fibrillating atrium shows very rapid activity that may have different rates in different places within the atrium. As seen in Fig. 9, on the ECG there are no p waves, and there is a fibrillating isoelectric line between ventricular beats. The ventricular rhythm is 'irregularly irregular'.

B. Atrial flutter shows rapid atrial flutter waves, usually running at about 300 bpm. These may be conducted to the ventricles in a fixed ratio (commonly 2:1) or with a variable conduction ratio. If conduction is variable, the ventricular rate may be irregular; however, it would typically be 'regularly irregular', as opposed to the ventricular rate in atrial fibrillation which is 'irregularly irregular'.

- In case of 'typical' atrial flutter, these will have the classical 'sawtooth' pattern: consecutive, rapid atrial ('F') waves with no separating isoelectric line, as seen in Fig. 10. This pattern usually indicates an 'isthmus dependent flutter', meaning it is conducted over the cavo-tricuspid isthmus. Another feature of typical atrial flutter is an opposing polarity of the flutter waves in leads II and V1; more commonly, flutter waves will be negative in lead II and positive in V1. This may indicate rotation in a counter-clockwise direction. The significance of an atrial flutter being 'isthmus dependent' is related to a potentially straightforward cure using ablation at the isthmus.

C. Atrial tachycardia, AVNRT, AVRT: From a practical point of care standpoint, it usually is not very important to differentiate among these narrow complex, regular arrhythmias in

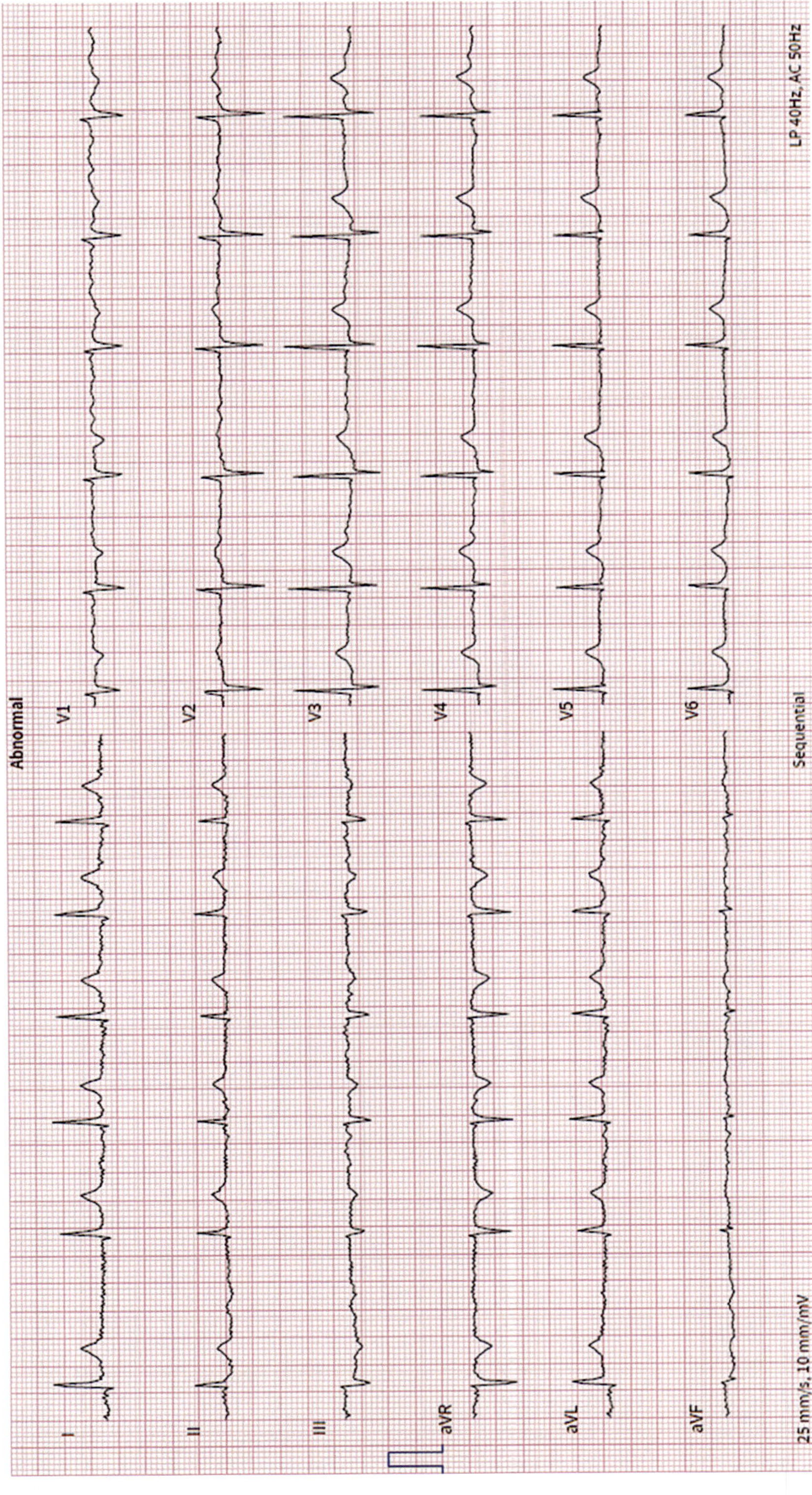

Fig. 9 Atrial fibrillation. The ventricular rate is irregular. There are no distinct p waves, and the isoelectric line has a 'fibrillatory' look—it is not a smooth line

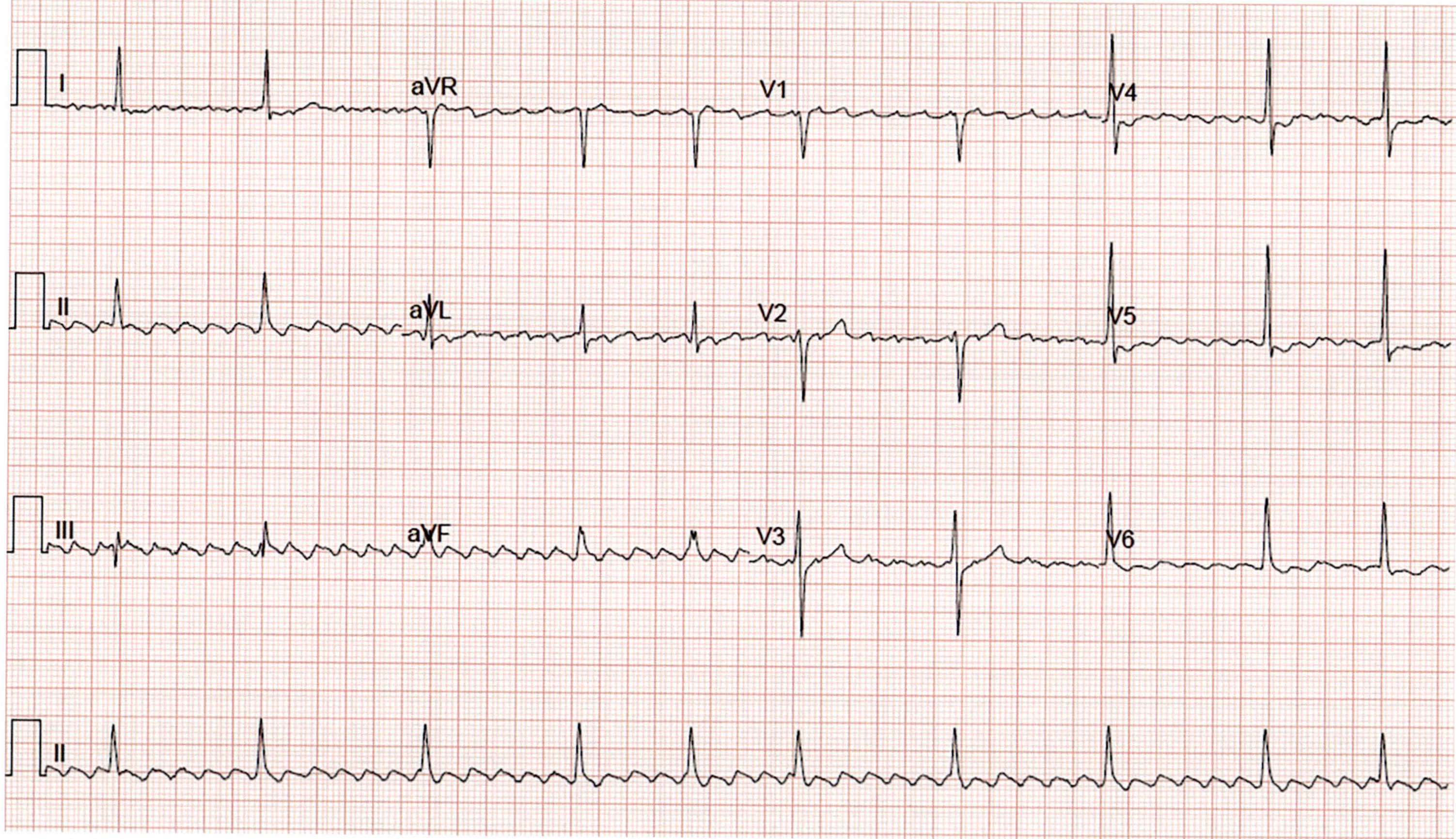

Fig. 10 Typical Atrial Flutter. Note 'Sawtooth' pattern, negative flutter waves in II and positive in V1

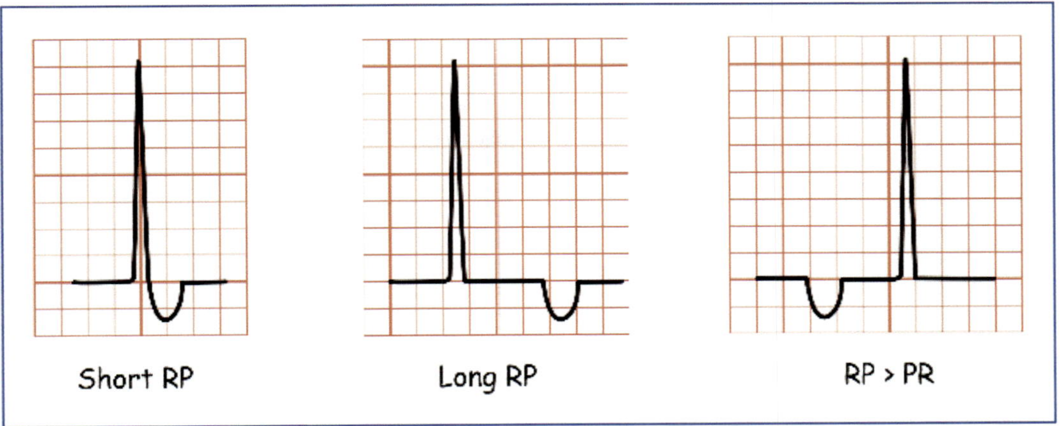

Fig. 11 Diagram showing schematically the three possibilities of RP interval in narrow complex tachycardia. Generally, short RP may favor a diagnosis of AVNRT or junctional tachycardia; long RP favors AVRT, and RP > PR favors atrial tachycardia. This sign is not specific; see text

the acute setting as initial treatment algorithms will be similar. However, for long term treatment the correct diagnosis is very important since ablation may cure many of these conditions. At times, a definite diagnosis can only be made during electrophysiological study; but often a highly probable presumption may be made based on the ECG at presentation.

A strong hint for the correct diagnosis is the RP interval. This is measured from the beginning of the QRS complex to the beginning of the following P wave. In case of AVNRT (or ectopic junctional tachycardia), the origin of tachycardia is in the AV node. Hence, activation of the atria (p wave) and ventricles (QRS) is almost simultaneous. The p wave will typically be inscribed on the QRS complex or very close after it, as seen in Figs. 11 and 12. We therefore look for a 'short RP' interval. In fact, if the RP interval is shorter than 70 ms, the diagnosis of AVNRT becomes very likely. The p wave will be negative in inferior leads since it is a retrograde p wave coming from the AV node and moving upwards. At times the RP interval may be so short, that the P wave will actually be hidden within the QRS complex and not visible. A clue for this may be a subtle difference between the QRS complex during tachycardia and the QRS complex of the same patient when in sinus rhythm: the cause of

the difference will be the hidden p wave. Figure 12 is an example of a short-RP narrow complex tachycardia, proven in the electrophysiology lab to be AVNRT.

In the case of AVRT, the electrical impulse goes down the AV node, activates the ventricle, then travels to the accessory pathway whereby it conducts retrogradely to the atrium. On the ECG, the time it takes to reach the accessory pathway causes a delay manifest as a longer 'RP' interval. However the RP will typically not be longer than the PR interval; in other words, the retrograde p wave will still be closer to the previous beat than to the next beat. An example may be seen in Fig. 13.

In atrial tachycardia, a focus is firing rapidly in the atria. Each impulse conducts to the ventricles via the regular AV node-His-Purkinje system. In terms of P-QRS relationship, this is quite similar to sinus rhythm; therefore, we may typically see a 'very long RP' interval, where RP > PR, meaning each p wave is closely followed by a QRS, as opposed to AVNRT and AVRT where each QRS is followed by a retrograde p.

This P-QRS relationship may sometimes make the healthcare provider wonder if this is not sinus tachycardia after all. The p wave in atrial tachycardia will have a different morphology than the sinus p wave, and the rate of the tachycardia is typically quite fixed when compared to the fluctuating nature of sinus tachycardia. Atrial tachycardia will have an abrupt

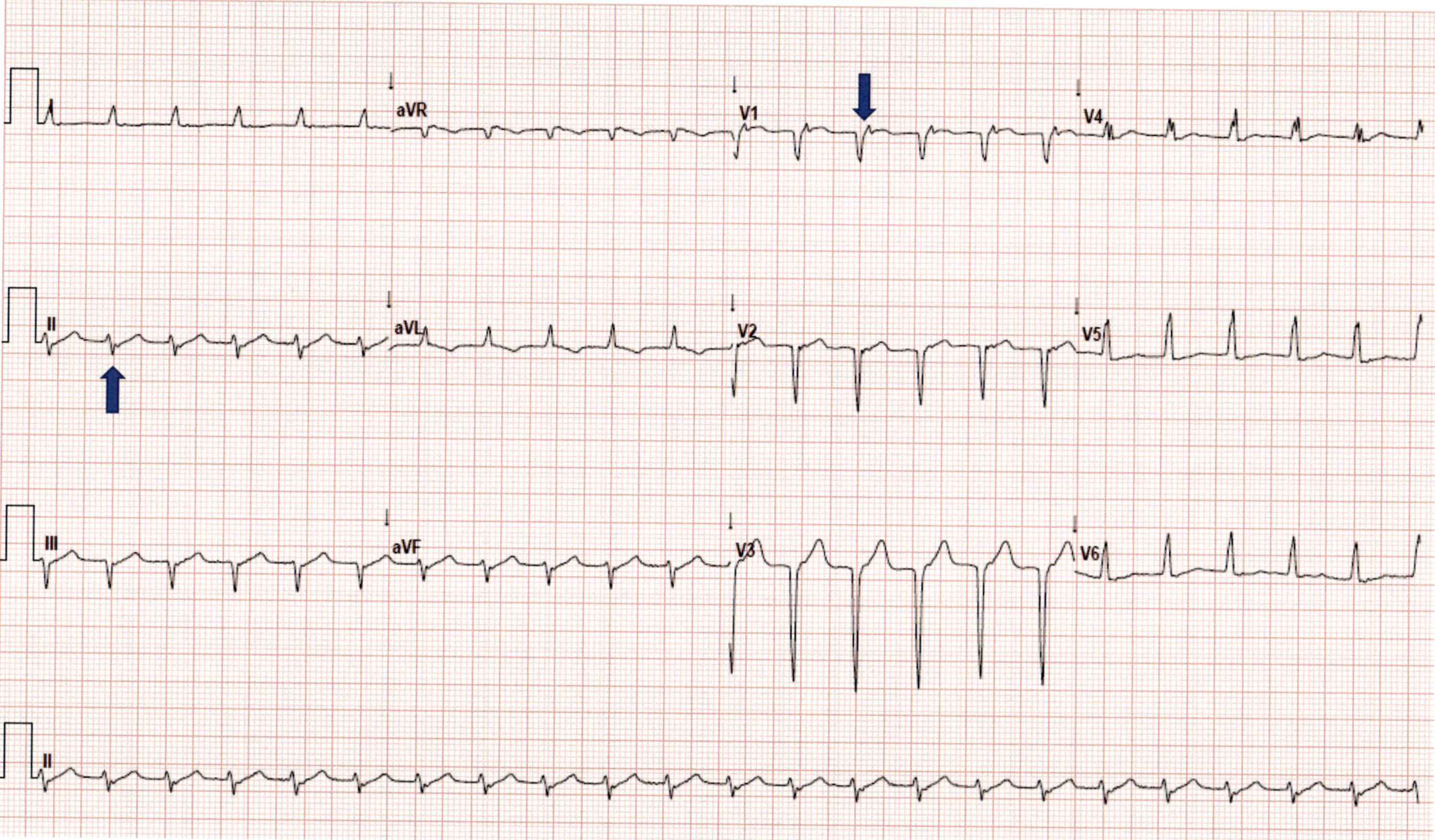

Fig. 12 Narrow complex tachycardia with a short RP interval. Arrows indicate the retrograde P wave. This turned out to be AVNRT

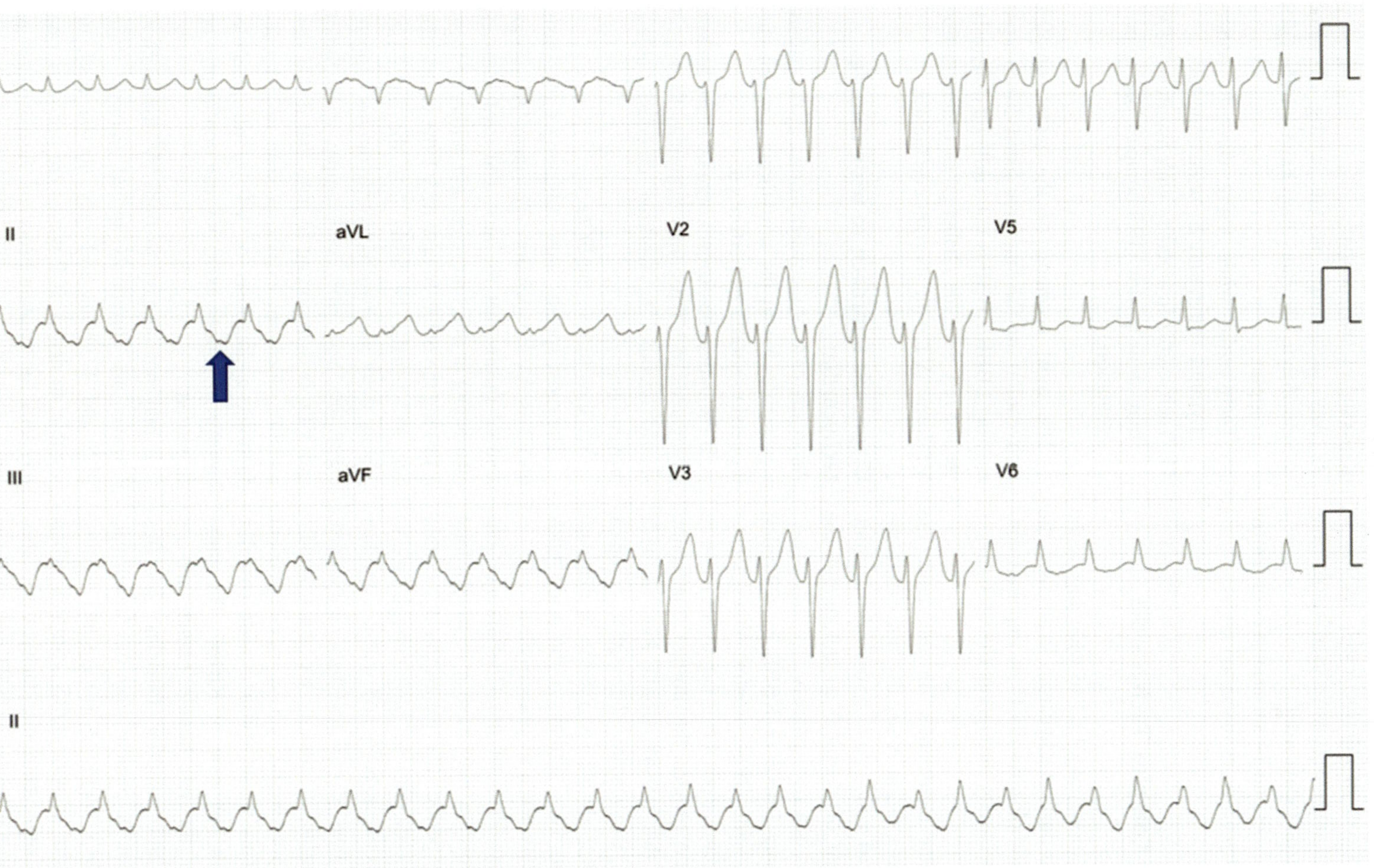

Fig. 13 Narrow complex tachycardia with a long RP interval. Arrow indicates P wave. This was AVRT utilizing a septal accessory pathway

initiation whereas sinus tachycardia increases in rate gradually. Sinus tachycardia will never have negative p waves in inferior leads, but this or other types of unusual p wave morphology may be seen in atrial tachycardia.

Figures 12, 13 and 14 are examples of narrow complex tachycardia, as discussed above.

4.2 Wide Complex Tachycardia

Several conditions may lead to widening of the QRS complex during tachycardia. In all cases, the wide QRS complex results from impaired conduction of electricity throughout the ventricles.

A. Ventricular tachycardia. In this case, the tachycardia origin is usually not within the specialized conduction system. As a result, the spread of electrical current though the ventricles is a slow process.
B. Pre-existing LBBB or RBBB by definition causes a wide QRS complex. When tachycardia occurs, even if it is supraventricular in origin and utilizes the normal conduction system, this person would have a wide complex tachycardia. The QRS complex morphology during tachycardia in this case would be very similar to the wide QRS morphology when in sinus rhythm.
C. Aberrancy: Parts of the His-Purkinje conduction system may have a relatively long refractory period. This means that at a certain rate the tissue does not have enough time to recover between beats and will not conduct the next beat. It will therefore be blocked. For example, if this is the right bundle branch, we would get a rate-dependent RBBB. This would cause a wide complex as seen in any case of RBBB. The same holds for the left bundle branch and its anterior and posterior fascicles. By this mechanism, a person who has a normal, narrow QRS complex when in sinus rhythm, will acquire a wide QRS complex when having a supraventricular tachycardia. This phenomenon is known as 'SVT with aberrant conduction'.

D. In a person with an implanted pacemaker, rapid ventricular pacing will cause a wide complex tachycardia.
E. Any tachycardia in the setting of some electrolyte disorders may have a wide QRS complex.
F. Tachycardia while using class IC antiarrhythmic drugs may be wide complex.
G. Tachycardia in a person with manifest WPW may show a wide QRS complex due to pre-excitation.

The most common of the wide complex tachycardias are the first three listed. Since a pre existing LBBB/RBBB is not a difficult diagnosis, we are left with the challenge of differentiating VT from SVT with aberrant conduction.

Diagnostic approach to wide complex tachycardia:
As in any case of tachyarrhythmia, if the patient is unstable due to the arrhythmia, prompt cardioversion should be performed.

If the patient has known organic heart disease, a diagnosis of VT becomes extremely likely and should become the working diagnosis unless proven otherwise.

We then turn to the ECG.

The most specific sign indicating a diagnosis of VT is AV dissociation. The term 'AV dissociation' means that the atria and ventricles are contracting at different rates, and neither of them is driving the other. In case of VT the ventricular rate will usually be faster than the atrial rate (unless there are two tachyarrhythmias happening at the same time; for example, atrial flutter and VT). It is important to note that if AV dissociation does not exist (not seen or 1:1 conduction), a diagnosis of VT is still possible; however if it does exist, VT can confidently be diagnosed.

It may not be easy to find AV dissociation. P waves are commonly spread amongst wide QRS and T waves and may not be easy, or possible, to detect. If P waves are not seen, one may look for 'capture beats' or 'fusion beats' as seen in Fig. 15: beats with a QRS complex that is normal, or not as wide as other tachycardia beats.

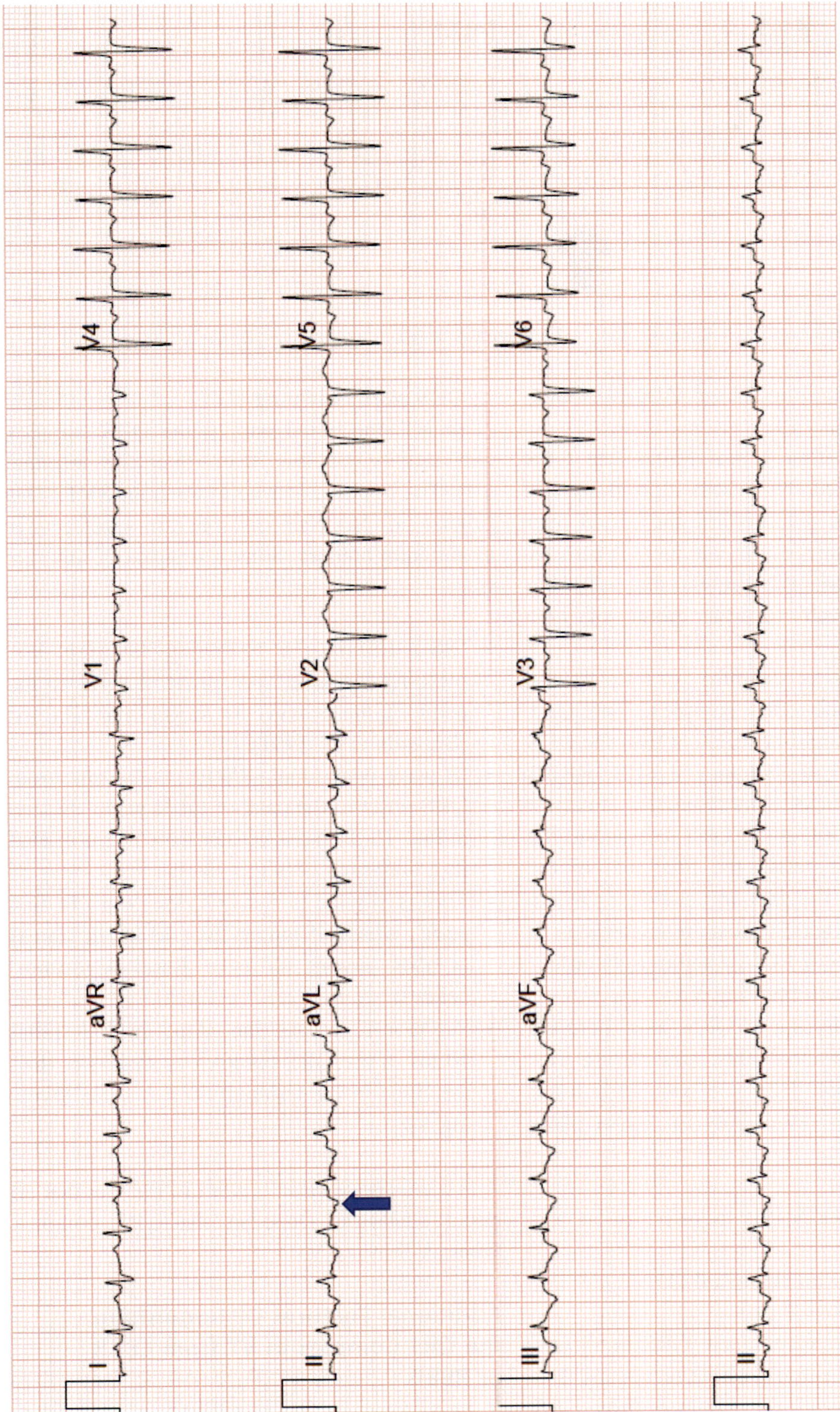

Fig. 14 Narrow complex tachycardia with a 'very long' RP, or RP > PR. Arrow indicates P wave. Note P wave is negative in lead II. This was an atrial tachycardia

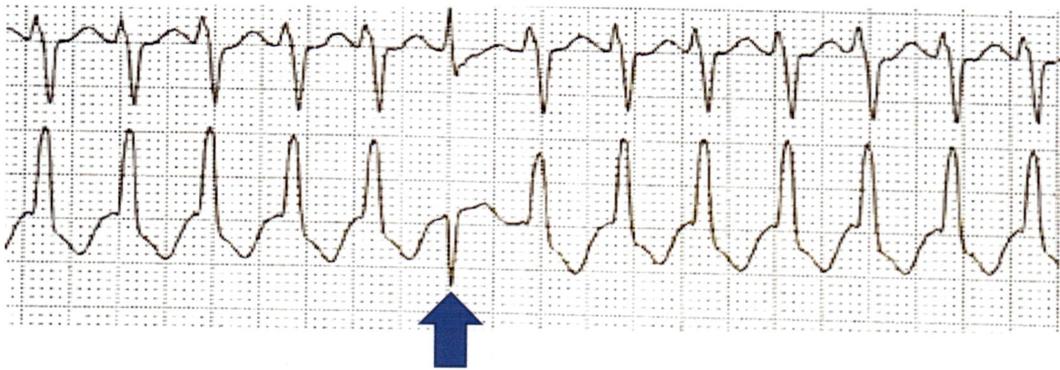

Fig. 15 **Capture beat** proving VA dissociation and a diagnosis of VT

The presence of these indicates AV dissociation, and a diagnosis of VT.

If AV dissociation is not found, the QRS should be analyzed. Numerous algorithms and criteria have been put forward and tested over the past decades, suggesting that there is actually no perfect method. We present the following simplified approach for the point of care physician.

The first step is carefully examining the morphology of the QRS complex. The QRS complex in VT should be different than the QRS complex expected in aberrancy: LBBB, RBBB or the left hemiblocks. This difference is easiest to find when looking at the QRS *axis* and at the *slopes* of the first versus the final part of the QRS. Apart from the axis and slopes, there are several distinctive features that are uncommon in a bundle branch block ECG, whether right or left.

QRS *axis* features favoring VT:

(note: when referring to QRS 'axis' here we mean three dimensional axis, considering precordial lead polarity. This is in contrast to usual terminology which refers only to frontal plane axis).

- A 'northwest' QRS axis (negative in L1 and inferior leads)
- LBBB pattern with rightward axis
- RBBB with leftward axis
- Precordial lead concordance (QRS in all precordial leads is either positive or negative)
- An initial R wave, or a mainly positive QRS in aVR.

QRS *slopes* favoring VT:

In VT, the initial part of the QRS complex will usually be less steep than the terminal part. The opposite is true in aberrant SVT. This general rule has been quantified in several ways by different authors. Some exmaples of this rule are:

- 'RS > 100 ms' is a finding favoring VT, meaning the time from onset of QRS to the nadir of the S wave is longer than 100 ms (Brugada et al. 1991).
- 'R wave peak time' (RWPT) is the time from QRS onset to the peak of the R wave, as seen in Fig. 16. If this is greater than 50 ms in lead II, a diagnosis of VT is likely.
- This is similar to the criterion 'time to first peak', which, if longer than 40 ms in lead II or aVR, favors VT (see 'Basel Algorithm' below).
- 'Vi/Vt < 1' means the slope in the initial 40 ms of the QRS complex is shallower than the slope in the terminal 40 ms, again favoring VT.

All the above criteria point to the fact that an initial shallower slope in the QRS complex favors VT over SVT.

Additional Features Distinguishing the QRS Complex in VT from LBBB or RBBB

If the tachycardia looks 'RBBB-like', it is likely VT if:

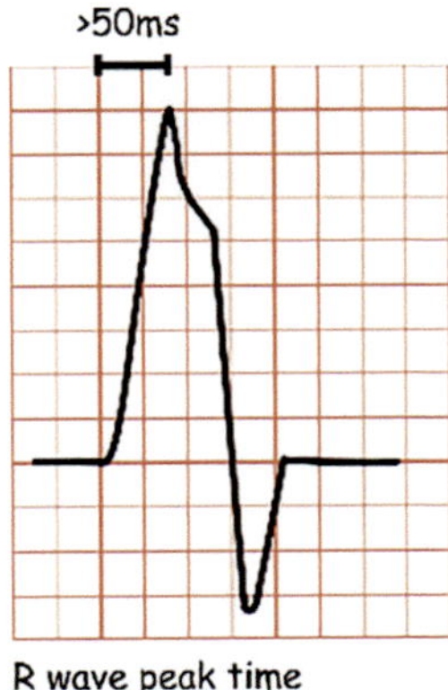

Fig. 16 Diagram showing R wave peak time. If this is greater than 50 ms in lead II, VT is more likely

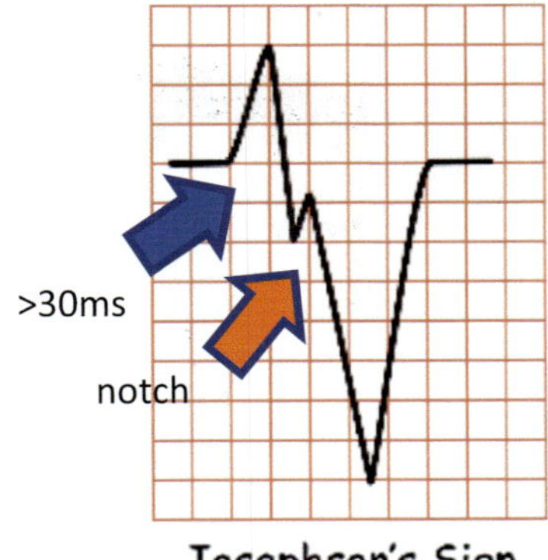

Fig. 17 'Josephson's sign'

QRS is wider than 160 ms.

The QRS complex in V1 is biphasic (e.g. qR).

If the tachycardia looks 'LBBB-like', is likely VT if:

QRS is wider than 145 ms.

In V1 there is an r wave wider than 30 ms.

There is a notch on the initial descending part of the QRS complex in V1 or V2.

(the above two criteria are sometimes referred to as 'Josephson's sign' (Kindwall et al. 1988) and are illustrated in Fig. 17.)

The Basel Algorithm

A simple algorithm has recently been published and coined the 'Basel Algorithm (Moccetti et al. 2022)'. This algorithm considers three criteria, as illustrated in Fig. 18:

- Clinical criterion: Structural heart disease, including history of myocardial infarction, reduced ejection fraction ($\leq 35\%$), or an implanted ICD or CRTD device.
- ECG criteria: in leads II and aVR, the time from beginning of QRS to the first peak should be measured. One must determine if this exceeds 40 ms (one small, 1 mm box).

The three criteria derived are:

1. Structural heart disease
2. Time to first peak in lead II > 40 ms
3. Time to first peak in lead aVR > 40 ms.

If any 2 out of the above three criteria exist, VT is likely.

4.3 Polymorphic VT and VF

Polymorphic VT is a wide complex tachycardia where consecutive QRS complexes appear different from one another. The mechanisms underlying this arrhythmia are different from those underlying the more common, monomorphic form of VT.

A specific type of polymorphic VT is Torsades de Pointes. This is polymorphic VT that is related to a prolonged QT interval, which may be a genetic or acquired condition. Torsades de Pointes has a typical form of sinusoidal 'twisting' of the QRS complexes around the isoelectric line.

Polymorphic VT should be regarded as an unstable rhythm with a chance of deteriorating to ventricular fibrillation.

Ventricular Fibrillation (VF):

Ventricular fibrillation is a chaotic and rapid rhythm in the ventricles. On the ECG there are no distinct P or QRS waves. The signals are typically of low amplitude and are irregular.

Ventricular fibrillation is not compatible with life and signifies cardiac arrest. A patient with VF should immediately receive CPR and be shocked as soon as possible.

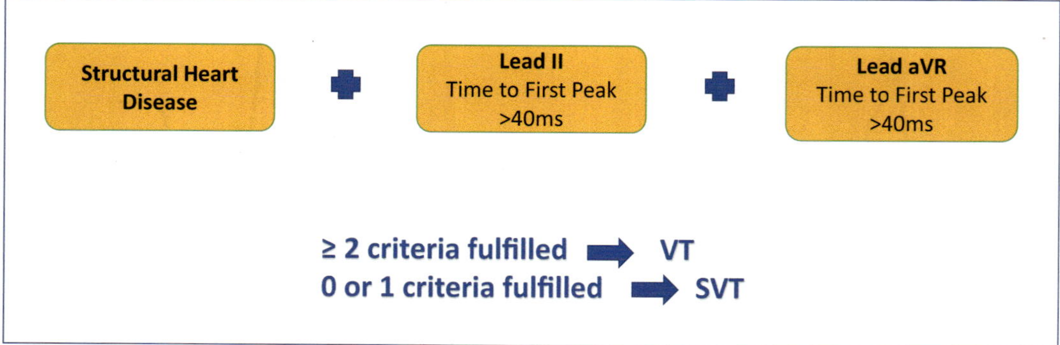

Fig. 18 The Basel algorithm

5 Approach to the ECG with Bradycardia

5.1 Sinus Node Disease

The first step when approaching an ECG with bradycardia is to determine if there is a sinus rhythm, and whether the P waves are conducted from atria to ventricles in a 1:1 ratio. As previously discussed, this means there are upright (positive) P waves in the inferior leads II, III and aVF. It also means there is a P wave preceding each QRS complex, and every P wave is followed by a QRS complex. If this is the case, the diagnosis is sinus bradycardia.

Sinus bradycardia may be normal. The most common physiologic forms of sinus bradycardia may be found in asymptomatic athletes, or during sleep.

However, sinus bradycardia is not normal if it prevents the heart from supplying an adequate cardiac output for any given condition (recall that cardiac output is the product of stroke volume and heart rate). This is a common condition, especially in old age, called 'sick sinus syndrome'. In sick sinus syndrome, the diseased sinus node is not capable of producing the required heart rate. An example of severe sinus bradycardia at rest is shown in Fig. 19. Some patients may have an adequate heart rate at rest, but are not capable of generating an adequate rate during exertion. This is termed 'chronotropic incompetence' and is another manifestation of sinus node disease. Other patients may suffer from sudden sinus pauses, causing a sudden sensation of dizziness or even loss of consciousness. A particular form of sinus node disease is the 'tachy-brady syndrome', shown in Fig. 20. In this condition there are episodes of an atrial form of tachycardia—usually atrial fibrillation or flutter. When these episodes stop, the sick sinus node requires a long time to recover, causing a typical 'conversion pause', a sinus pause at the termination of tachycardia.

Sinus node disease is commonly found in the elderly, but may also result from certain medications, or a genetic predisposition.

Escape Rhythm

When there is a prolonged sinus pause or arrest, it is important to note the 'escape' mechanism. Following the pause, the sinus node may recover, in which case the ECG will show recovery of the normal P waves. If this does not happen, electrical activity may arise from a different area within the atria; here, a P wave with different morphology will be seen preceding the QRS complexes. This is called an 'escape' rhythm. If there is no atrial escape rhythm, the AV node may produce the escape rhythm. This form is called a 'junctional', or 'nodal' escape rhythm. If the AV node produces the electrical impulse, then the ventricles and atria are activated almost at the same time, in

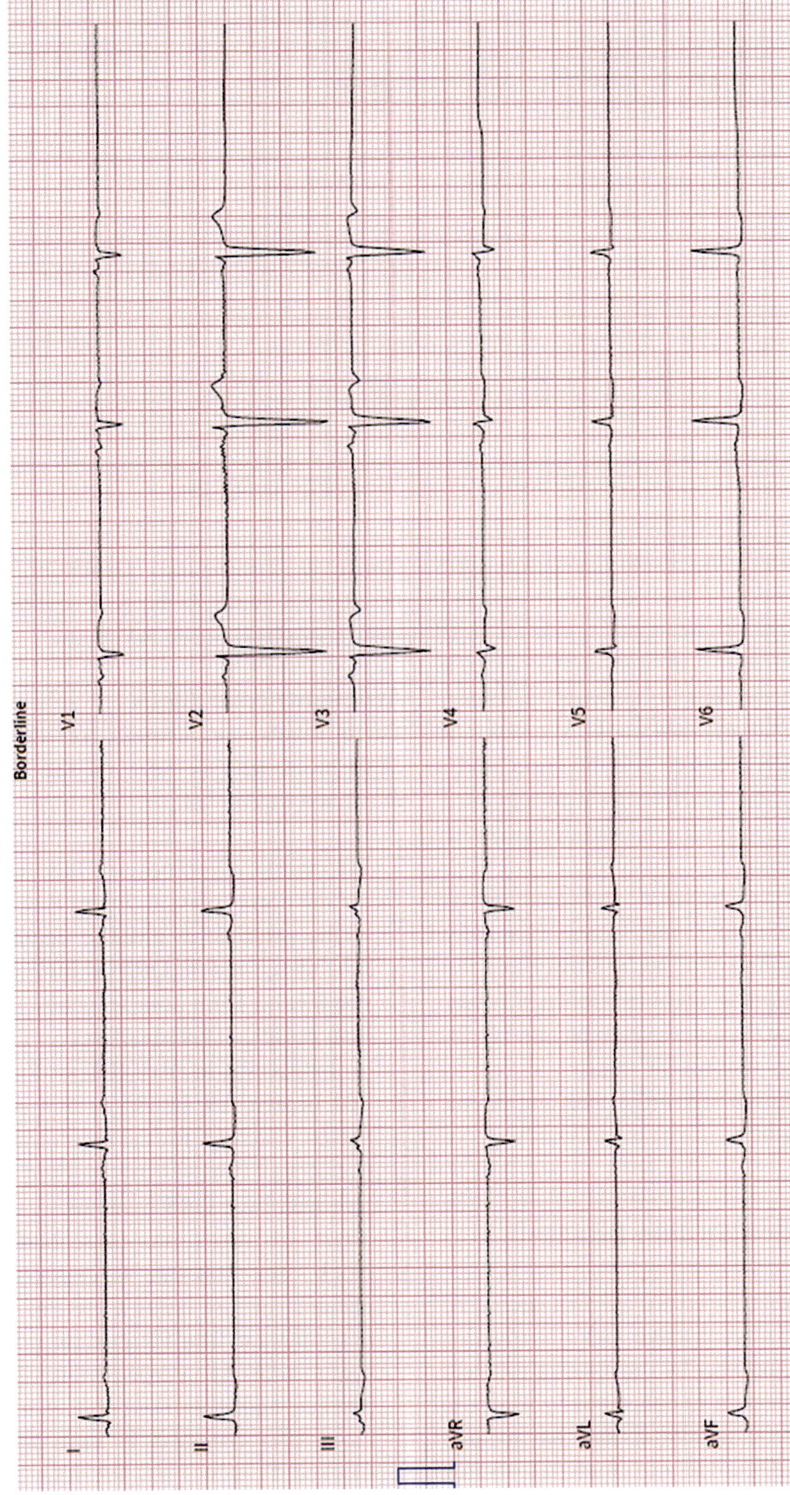

Fig. 19 ECG with severe sinus bradycardia, a result of sick sinus syndrome in an elderly patient presenting with dizziness

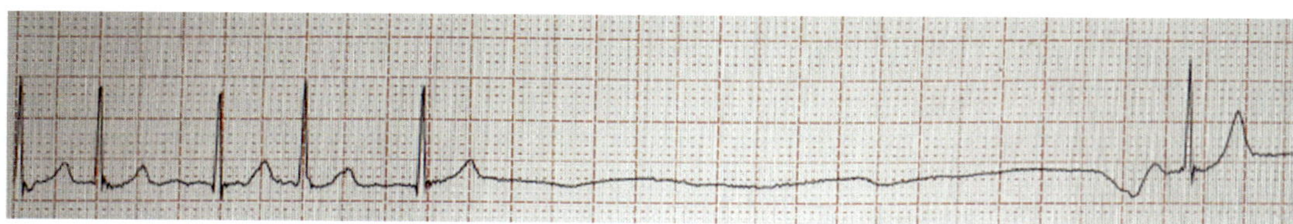

Fig. 20 Tachy-brady syndrome, a variant of sick sinus syndrome. A conversion pause is seen with eventual recovery of sinus activity. The sinus pause occurs at termination of atrial fibrillation

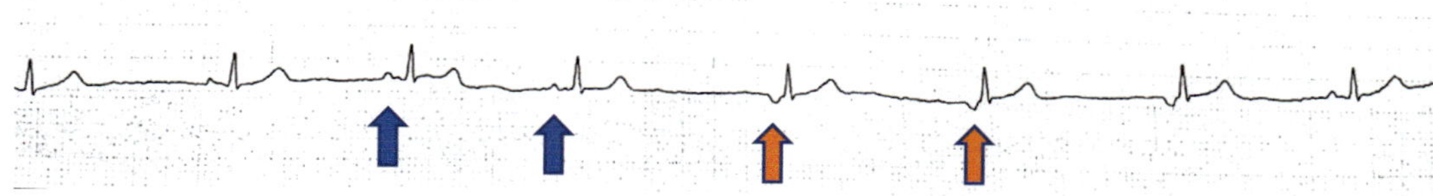

Fig. 21 Sinus bradycardia with ectopic atrial escape beats. The blue arrows indicate sinus node origin; the orange arrows point to negative p waves, resulting from an ectopic atrial escape mechanism

opposite directions. The result is a narrow QRS complex, very closely followed by a retrograde P wave. This p wave will be negative in leads II, III and aVF as opposed to a normal sinus P wave. In case the AV node fails to provide an escape rhythm, it may still arise within the ventricles. In this case the QRS complex will be wide, and it may or may not be followed by a retrograde P wave, which will be evident a short duration after the QRS complex.

The distinction between different escape mechanisms is of clinical importance. Generally, distal escape rhythms tend to be slower and less dependable than proximal ones. Hence, a patient with nodal escape rhythm tends to be more stable than one with a ventricular escape. Figure 21 demonstrates sinus bradycardia with an ectopic atrial escape rhythm.

5.2 Conduction System Disease

A different cause of bradycardia is that caused by disease of the atrio-ventricular (AV) conduction system. Conduction may be impaired at different levels of the system. It is conceptually useful to categorize AV conduction disease as nodal—occurring in the AV node, or infranodal—below the AV node at the bundle of His (practically similar to 'infrahisian'). Generally, block at the nodal level tends to be less severe than block below, or distal to the AV node.

Atrioventricular Block

Three levels, or degrees of atrioventricular (AV) block may be seen on the ECG and are illustrated in Fig. 22.

1. 1st degree AV block: in this case, 1:1 AV conduction is present. Every P wave conducts to the ventricle to produce ventricular depolarization, and a QRS complex. However, conduction from atria to ventricles is slower than normal. This manifests on the ECG as a prolonged PR interval (longer than 200 ms).
2. 2nd degree AV block: in this case, most P waves conduct to the ventricle. However, occasional P waves are blocked and are not followed by a QRS complex.
   There are two forms of second-degree AV block. The first one is characterized by a peculiar pattern known as the Wenkebach phenomenon. The PR interval prolongs from beat to beat. At a certain point, one P wave is blocked and does not conduct to the ventricles. After the next P wave following the blocked P wave, the PR interval resets to normal, and the cycle begins again. Hence,

Classification of atrioventricular block

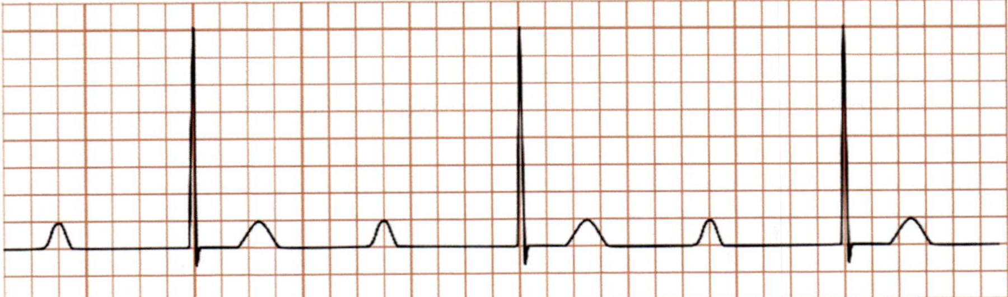

First degree AV Block

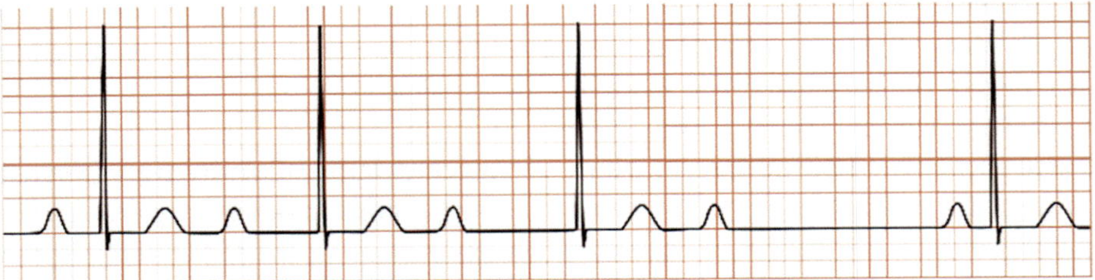

Second degree AV Block - Mobitz I (Wenckebach)

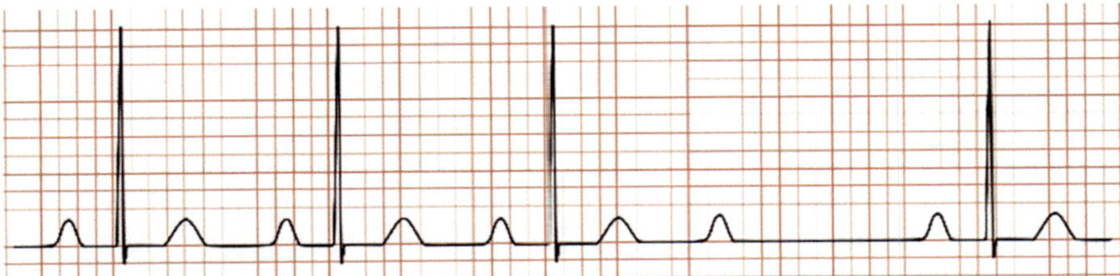

Second degree AV Block - Mobitz II

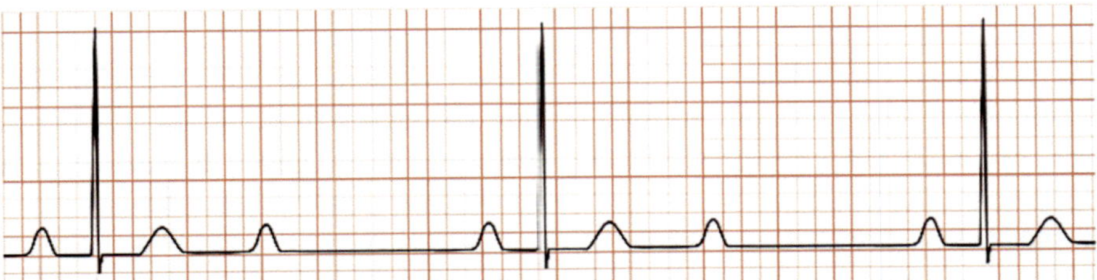

2:1 AV Block

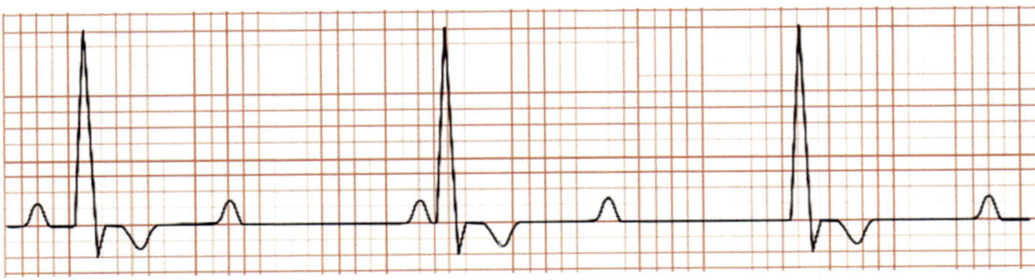

Third degree AV Block

Fig. 22 Classification of atrioventricular block

the best way to detect the Wenkebach phenomenon is to measure the last PR interval before the blocked P wave, and compare it to the PR interval in the beat immediately following the blocked P wave. With the Wenkebach phenomenon, the first PR interval following the blocked P wave will be shorter than the interval preceding the blocked P wave. When second degree AV block has Wenkebach periodicity, the condition is known as 'Mobitz type 1 2nd degree AV block'. An example of Mobitz type 1 2nd degree AV block is shown in Fig. 23.

Another pattern of 2nd degree AV block is more arbitrary, whereby some P waves are blocked in an unpredictable manner, or with a certain ratio, for example 3:1 or 4:1, without PR prolongation. This pattern is called a 'Mobitz type 2 2nd degree AV block'.

The significance of the Mobitz classification is that usually the Wenkebach phenomenon characterizes blocks at the AV nodal level. Hence, an asymptomatic patient with a Mobitz type I AV block is usually stable, and may not require any specific intervention. A Mobitz type 2 block, however, may mean that the block is infranodal; existence of this type of AV block may signify impending complete block, and should prompt consideration of pacemaker implantation.

Before describing 3rd degree, or complete AV block, two additional types of AV block will briefly be mentioned:

2:1 AV block. In this case every second P wave is blocked. Even if this block were to be at the AV node level, there is no way to see PR prolongation because the next beat would already be blocked. The distinction between Mobitz 1 and Mobitz 2 as described cannot be made and therefore, 2:1 block is regarded as a distinct entity. When more than one consecutive P waves are not conducted but there is no complete AV block, the condition is called 'high degree AV block'.

3. 3rd degree, or complete AV block. In this case, the P waves and QRS complexes have different rates and are said to be dissociated from one another. The atrial rate will usually be faster than the ventricular rate. An example of complete AV block is shown in Fig. 24. If the ventricles are dissociated from the electrical activity of the atria, there must be some escape mechanism causing them to contract in order to sustain life. As in the case of sinus arrest, the escape mechanism may arise just below the AV node, in the bundle of His or in the ventricle itself. The ECG signs of these escape beats are the same as in sinus arrest, except that an atrial escape is obviously not possible.

Intraventricular Conduction Disease

Intraventricular conduction problems may exist in any portion of the His-Purkinje system. This includes the right and left bundle branches. The left bundle branch may be completely blocked, or blocked distally at either the anterior or posterior fascicle.

Diagnosis of intraventricular conduction blocks relies on traditional, previously published criteria. The mechanisms underlying the formation of each deflection in the QRS complex have been well described and are beyond the scope of this tutorial.

Complete left or right bundle branch block causes widening of the QRS complex due to slow conduction of the electrical signal across the interventricular septum, bypassing the blocked bundle branch. Other criteria are:

Left Bundle Branch Block (Figs. 25, and 26).

1. QRS duration greater than or equal to 120 ms. (In adults).
2. Broad notched or slurred R wave in leads I, aVL, V5, and V6.
3. Absent q waves in leads I, V5, and V6. (In aVL, a narrow q wave may be present.)
4. R wave peak time greater than 60 ms in leads V5 and V6. Small r waves may be seen in leads V1, V2 and V3.
5. ST and T waves are usually opposite in direction to QRS.

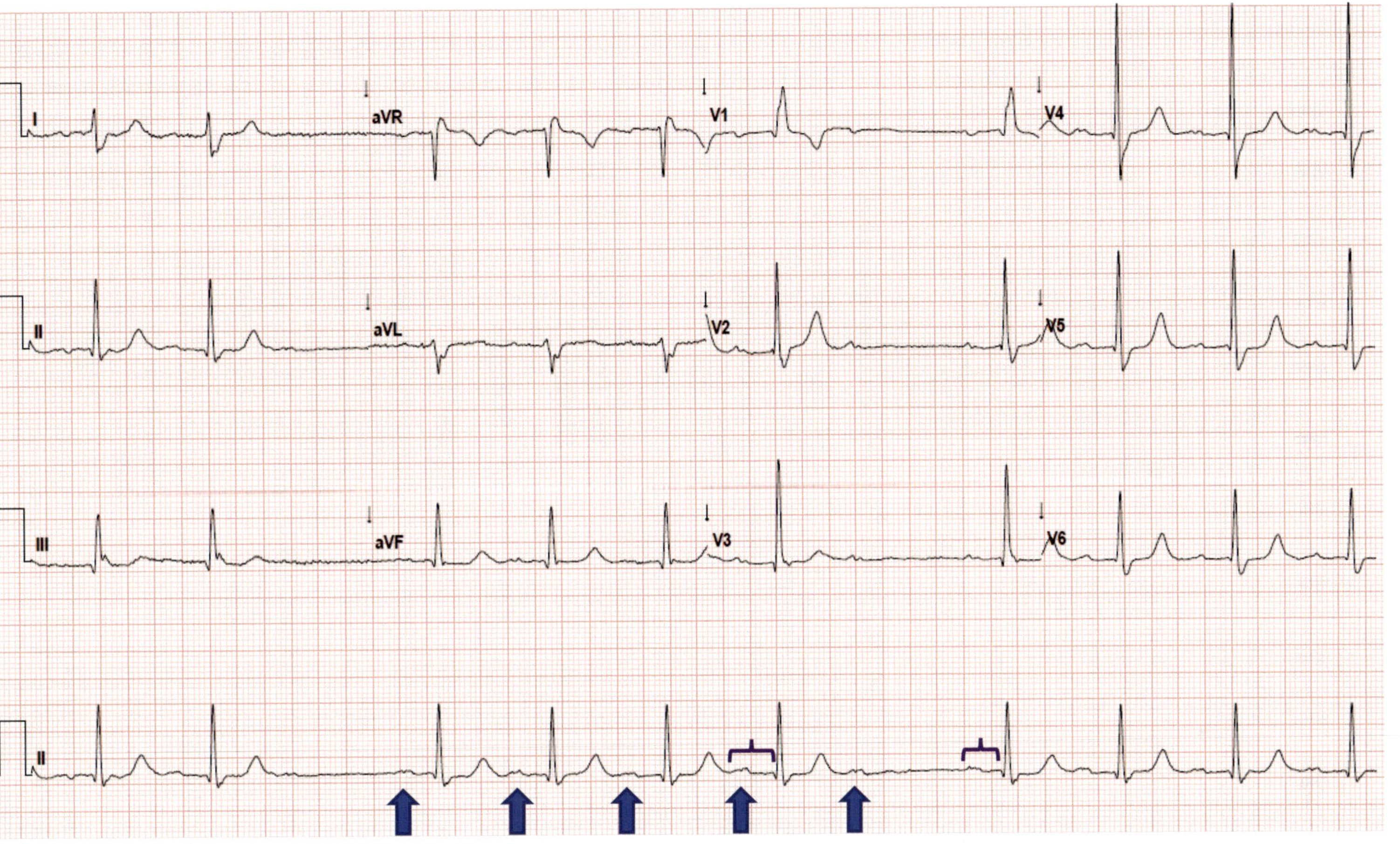

Fig. 23 2nd degree AV block, Mobitz type I. Note Wenkebach phenomenon. This patient also has a right bundle branch block. P waves are marked by blue arrows. Braces show the PR interval following the blocked P wave is shorter than the PR interval preceding the blocked P wave. See text

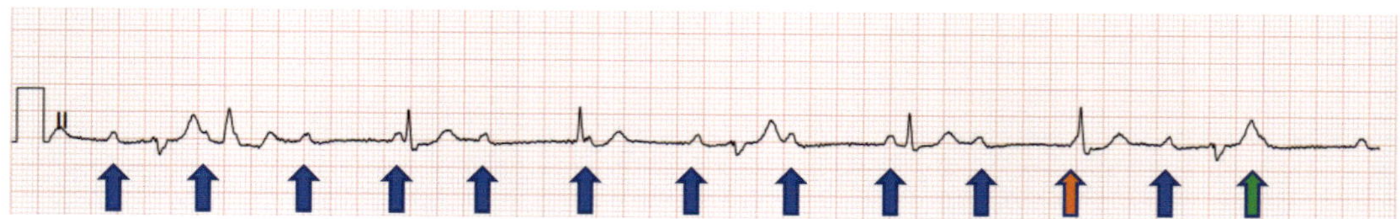

Fig. 24 Complete (3rd degree) AV block. P waves are marked by arrows. The orange arrow points to a change in the QRS complex caused by a 'hidden' p wave. The green arrow shows the same for a T wave

6. Positive T waves in leads with upright QRS may be normal (positive concordance).
7. The appearance of LBBB may change the mean QRS axis in the frontal plane to the right, to the left, or to a superior axis, in some cases in a rate-dependent manner.

Right Bundle Branch Block (Figs. 27, and 28).

1. QRS duration greater than or equal to 120 ms.
2. rsr', rsR', or rSR' in leads V1 or V2. The R' or r' deflection is usually wider than the initial R wave. In a minority of patients, a wide and often notched R wave pattern may be seen in lead V1 and/or V2.
3. S wave of greater duration than R wave or greater than 40 ms in leads I and V6 in adults.
4. Normal R wave peak time in leads V5 and V6 but greater than 50 ms in lead V1.

Of the above criteria, the first 3 should be present to make the diagnosis. When a pure dominant R wave with or without a notch is present in V1, criterion 4 should be satisfied.

Left Anterior Fascicular Block ('hemiblock')

1. Frontal plane axis between − 45° and − 90°. (This is the most common reason for left axis deviation).
2. qR pattern in lead aVL.
3. R-peak time in lead aVL of 45 ms or more.
4. QRS duration less than 120 ms.

Left Posterior Fascicular Block (Fig. 29).
1. Frontal plane axis between 90° and 180°
2. rS pattern in leads I and aVL.

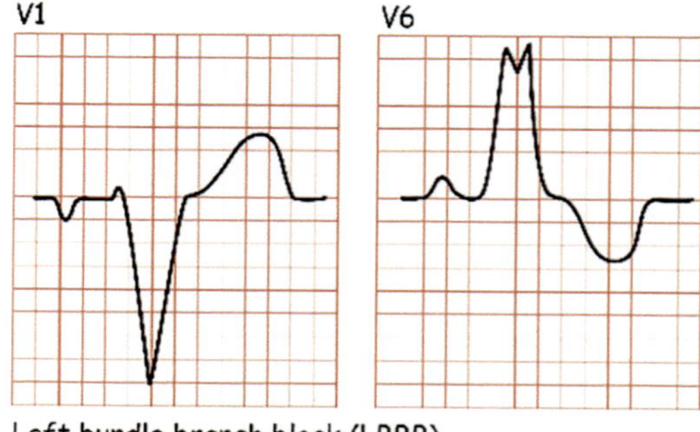

Fig. 25 Diagram of left bundle branch block in leads V1 and V6

3. qR pattern in leads III and aVF.
4. QRS duration less than 120 ms.

6 The ECG in Ischemic Heart Disease

6.1 Ischemia

The hallmark of ischemia on ECG is ST segment depression. There may also be T wave inversion.

ST depressions can be described as upsloping, horizontal or downsloping. Examples are shown in Fig. 30. To be considered specific for ischemia, the ST segment should be horizontal or downsloping. Upsloping ST segment depression is not a specific finding for ischemia.

By definition, the magnitude of ST depression should be measured from the beginning of the Q wave to the beginning of the ST segment (the J point) (Thygesen et al. 2018). ST segment depression is considered a sign of ischemia when it is depressed at least 0.5 mm in two contiguous leads.

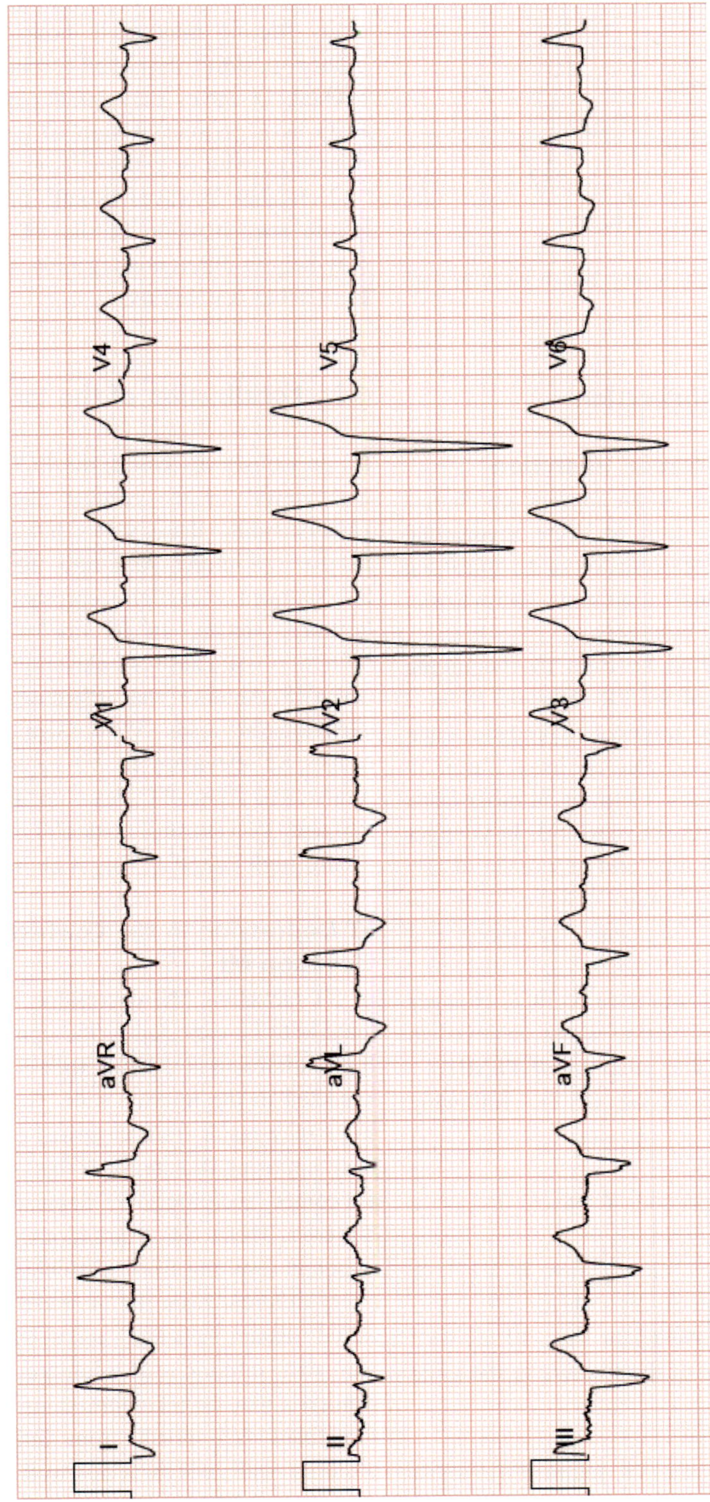

Fig. 26 ECG showing left bundle branch block

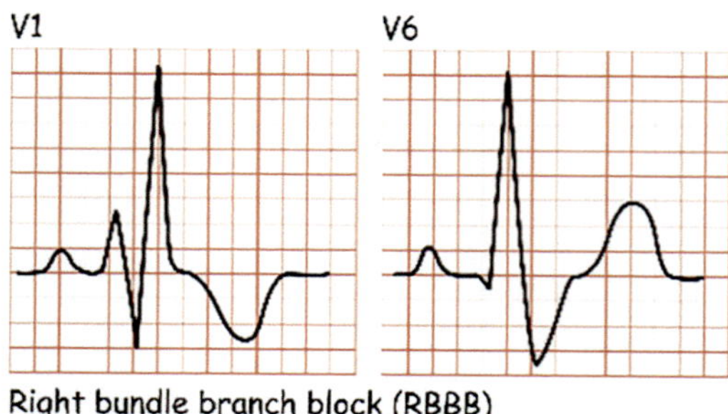

Fig. 27 Diagram of right bundle branch block in leads V1 and V6

6.2 Myocardial Infarction

ST Elevation Myocardial Infarction

ST segment elevation, in an appropriate clinical setting, is usually a sign of acute myocardial injury due to complete occlusion of an epicardial coronary artery and represents *myocardial infarction*, a medical emergency.

Measurement should be from the beginning of the Q wave (end of the PR segment) to the J point. The ECG is considered diagnostic when the ST segment is elevated at least 2 mm in leads V2–V3, or at least 1 mm in all other leads (2 mm is for men over 40 years old. In younger men the cutoff is 2.5 mm, and in women of any age the cutoff is 1.5 mm). Figure 31 is an illustration of ST segment elevation and depression.

There is a natural sequence of ECG changes that take place if reperfusion is not achieved in ST elevation myocardial infarction (STEMI).

This sequence involves, in the following order:

- Hyperacute (tall, peaked) T waves
- ST segment elevation
- Abnormal Q waves (any Q wave in V1-3, or Q wave wider than 30 ms in leads 1,2, AVL, AVF, V4-6. Q wave wider than 40 ms with depth at least 25% of the R wave in the same lead)
- T wave inversion
- Normalization of the ST segment (in most cases).

The development of abnormal Q waves is considered a sign of heart muscle necrosis, generally starting minutes to hours after onset of infarction. If the obstructed coronary artery is not opened, Q waves may remain on the patient's ECG as a permanent sign of prior myocardial infarction, with or without T wave inversion.

Note that T waves usually become inverted before normalization of the ST segment. This may help in differentiating myocardial infarction from acute pericarditis.

6.3 Localization of the Infarct

As previously discussed, the ECG shows different 'views' of the cardiac electrical activity. Understanding these views helps the caregiver localize the infarct. As a rule, the leads showing ST segment elevation represent the infarcted territory. Hence, an inferior wall myocardial infarction will cause ST elevation in leads II, III and aVF. Anterior wall infarction will cause ST elevation in leads V3-4; septal involvement causes ST elevation in V1-2, and lateral wall infarct will cause ST elevation in leads I, aVL, V5 and V6. (Lead I and aVL are sometimes called 'high lateral'). This is shown in Fig. 32.

ST Depression in the Context of ST Elevation MI

In ST elevation MI, depression of the ST segment is to be expected in the opposing territory: If the infarction is anterior, then ST depression is expected in the inferior wall. These ST depressions may result from electrical currents viewed from opposing directions. If this is the case, they are coined 'reciprocal' ST depressions. At times, however, these ST depressions may represent ischemia resulting from narrowing of a coronary artery different from the infarcted artery. This is called 'distant ischemia' and is more commonly seen with inferior wall infarction. Another possibility is that the ST depressions in V1, V2 and sometimes V3, result from infarction of the posterior wall, which is not well represented in the standard 12 lead ECG.

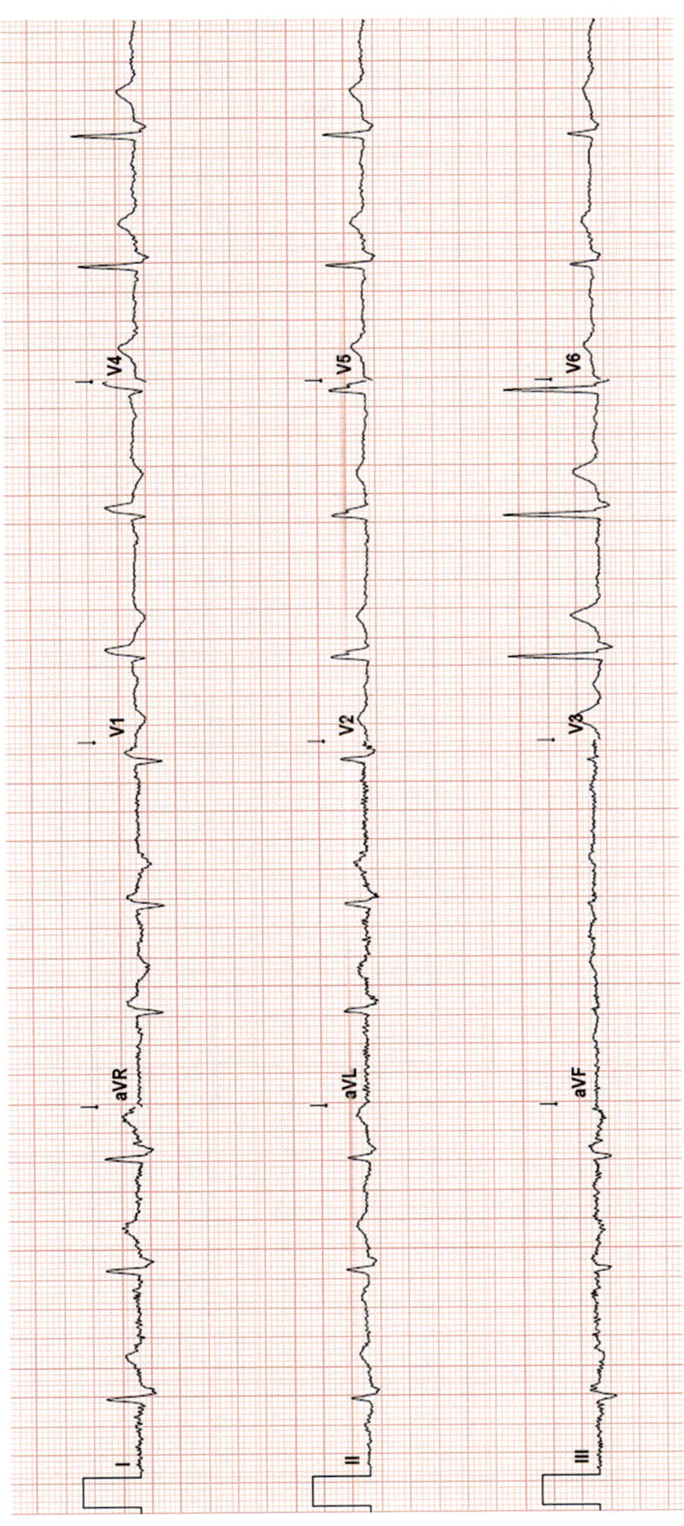

Fig. 28 ECG with right bundle branch block

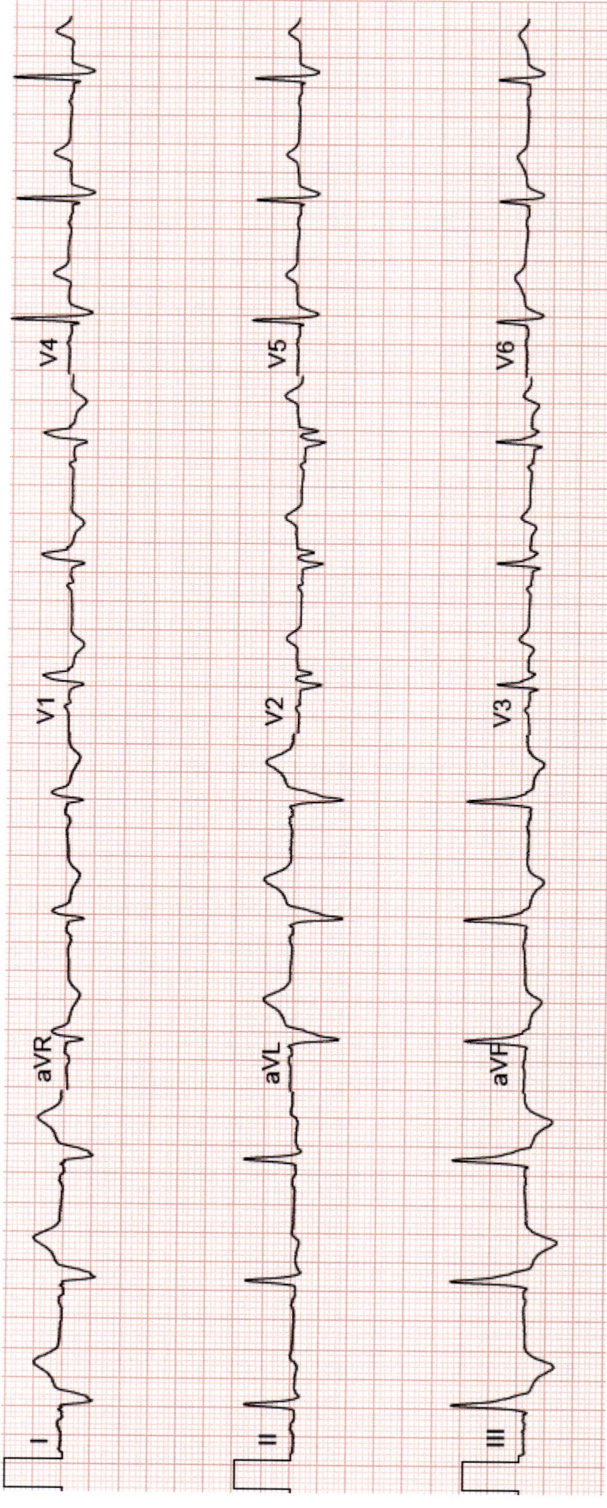

Fig. 29 ECG showing left posterior fascicular block and right bundle branch block. In this case, QRS duration is more than 120 ms due to the right bundle branch block, not the left posterior block

ST segment depression morphology

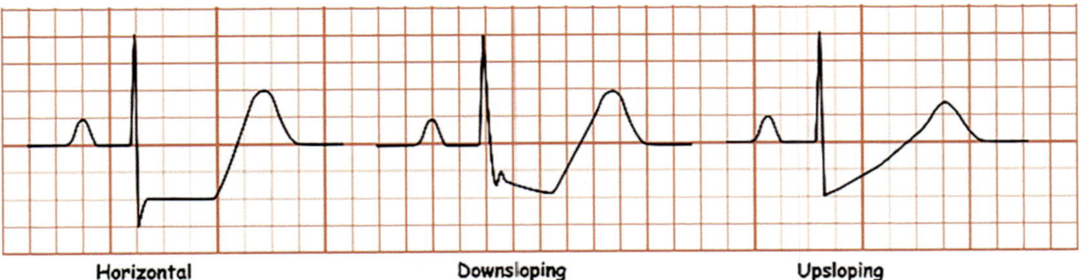

Fig. 30 Diagram showing ST depression morphology

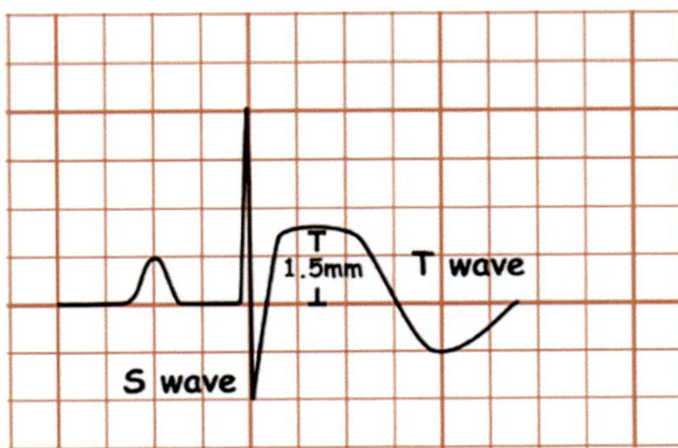

ST Segment elevation

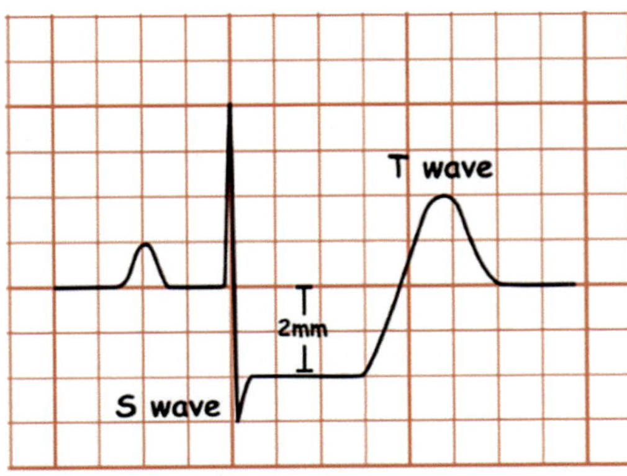

ST Segment depression

Fig. 31 Diagram showing ST elevation and depression

It is important to perform additional ECG tracings with posterior leads (V7, 8, 9) as well as right-sided leads (V4R), especially in inferior wall infarction. In cases of right ventricular ischemia or infarction, one may see ST elevation in right-sided leads, especially in V4R. In case of posterior infarct, ST elevation may be seen in posterior lead positions V7, 8, 9.

Examples of ST elevation myocardial infarction in different locations are seen in Figs. 33, 34 and 35.

7 Pericardial Disease

7.1 Pericardial Effusion

The main ECG sign of a significant pericardial effusion is low voltage. Measurement of QRS complex voltage includes both the positive (R) and negative (S) components. The definition of low voltage is an amplitude of less than 10 mm in all precordial leads and less than 5 mm in all limb leads. In case of a large pericardial effusion, electrical alternans may be evident. This is a cyclic beat to beat change in QRS amplitude.

7.2 Pericarditis

The typical ECG sign of acute pericarditis is ST elevation. Since chest pain is the typical clinical presentation, this must be differentiated from acute myocardial infarction. Early repolarization may also be considered in the differential diagnosis.

In acute pericarditis, ST elevation is typically concave and is almost never convex.

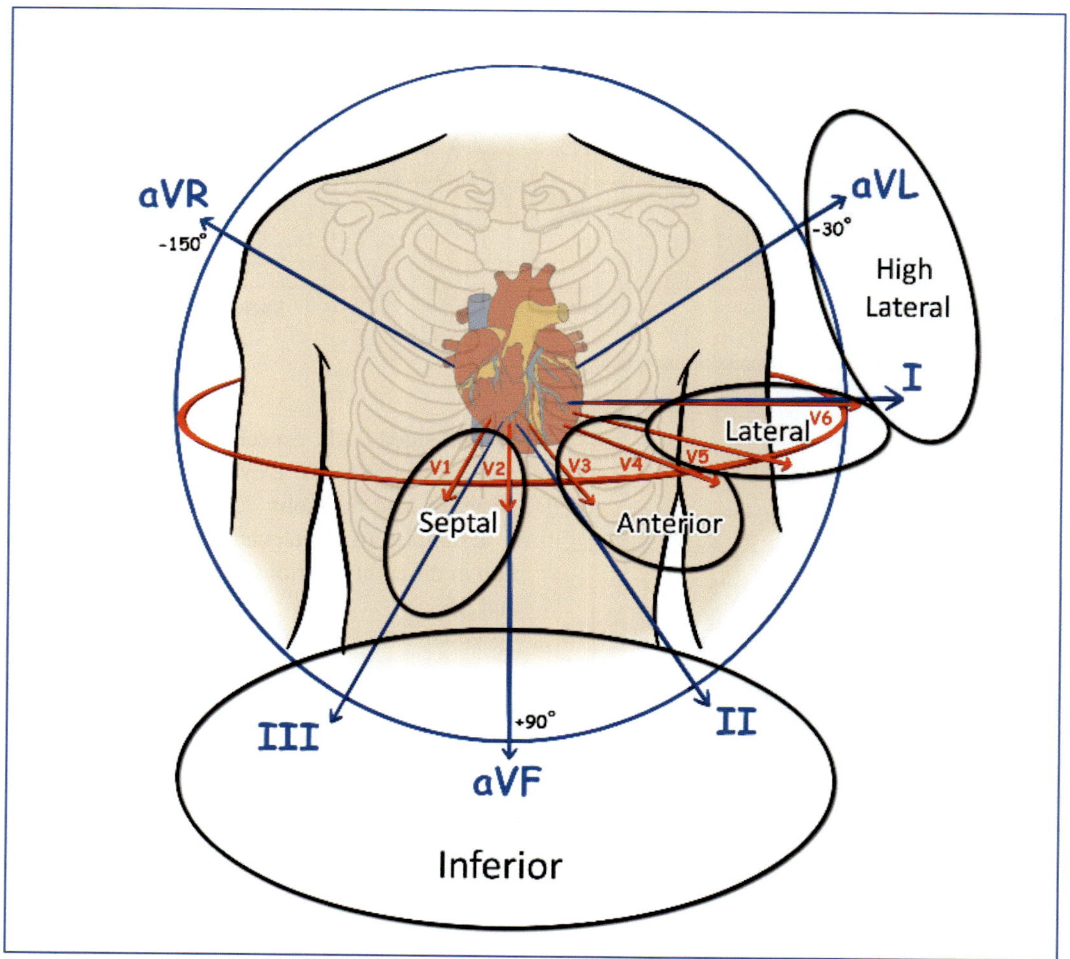

Fig. 32 Diagram showing myocardial territories represented by ECG lead groups. See text

It is commonly diffuse and not associated with a specific coronary anatomic distribution. In aVR, and sometimes in V1—looking at the heart from the right, the reverse pattern is to be expected: ST depression with a negative T wave. However, ST depression should not be present in leads other than aVR or V1, as opposed to myocardial infarction where these changes are usually present.

Another sign of acute pericarditis is PR segment deviation. In aVR, the PR segment will be elevated, while in all other leads the PR segment will be depressed.

Figure 36 is an example of an ECG showing acute pericarditis.

The ECG in pericarditis tends to evolve over several days: The ST elevation usually resolves, followed by flattening or even inversion of T waves. In STEMI, T wave inversions may be seen before resolution of ST elevation.

Pericarditis may present with or without pericardial effusion. If there is significant pericardial effusion, a low voltage complex is to be expected on the ECG. At times electrical alternans may be seen the QRS complex amplitude is alternating from beat to beat. Electrical alternans is presumed to result from the heart 'rocking' within the fluid-filled pericardium. Figure 37 shows an example of electrical alternans.

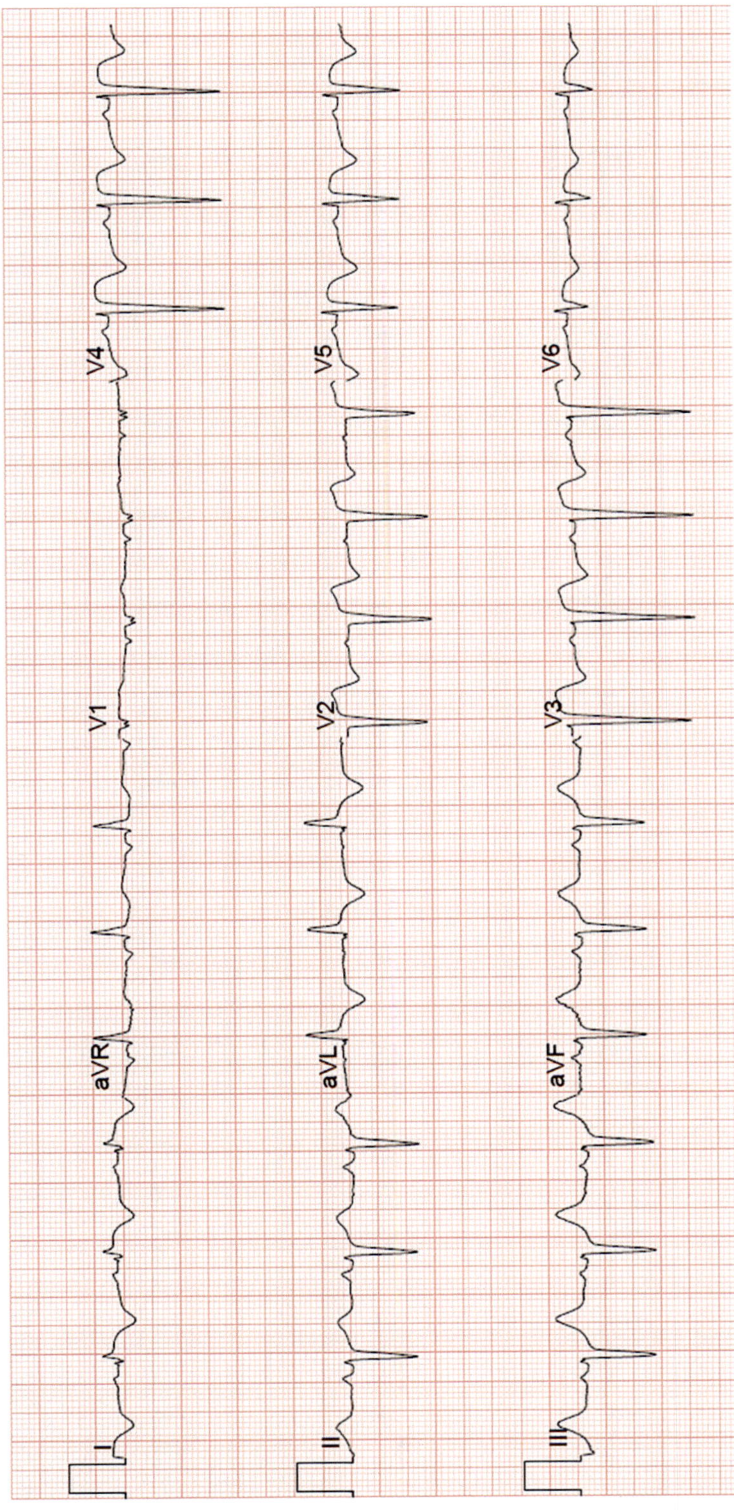

Fig. 33 Extensive anterior wall myocardial infarction. The ECG shows ST segment elevation in leads I, aVL, V2–V6. In leads V2-3 there are abnormal Q waves, signifying anteroseptal myocardial necrosis. There are also T wave inversions in the involved territory

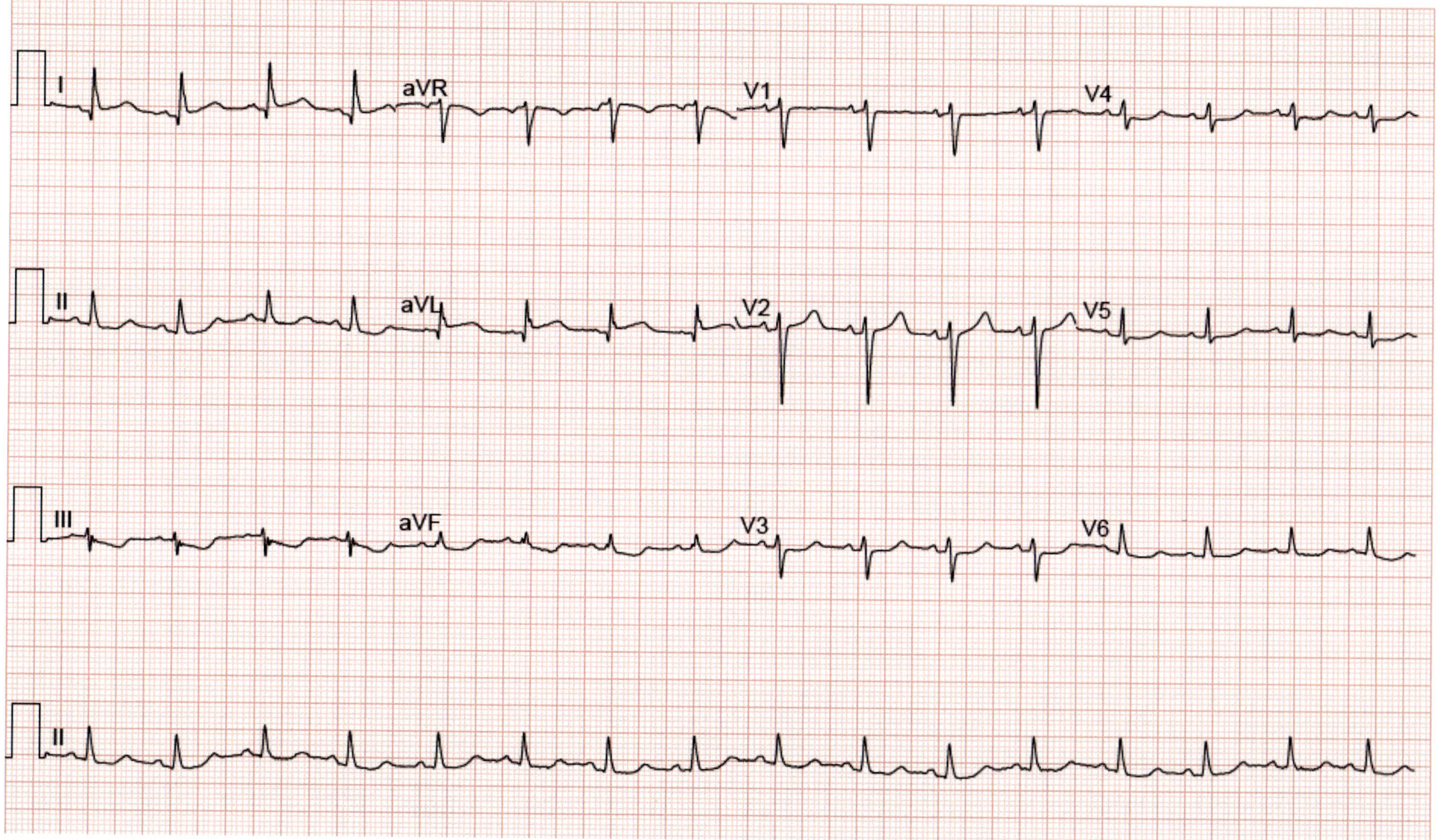

Fig. 34 Acute high lateral mi. There is ST segment elevation in leads I and aVL. There is 'reciprocal' ST depression and T wave inversion in inferior leads II, III and AVF

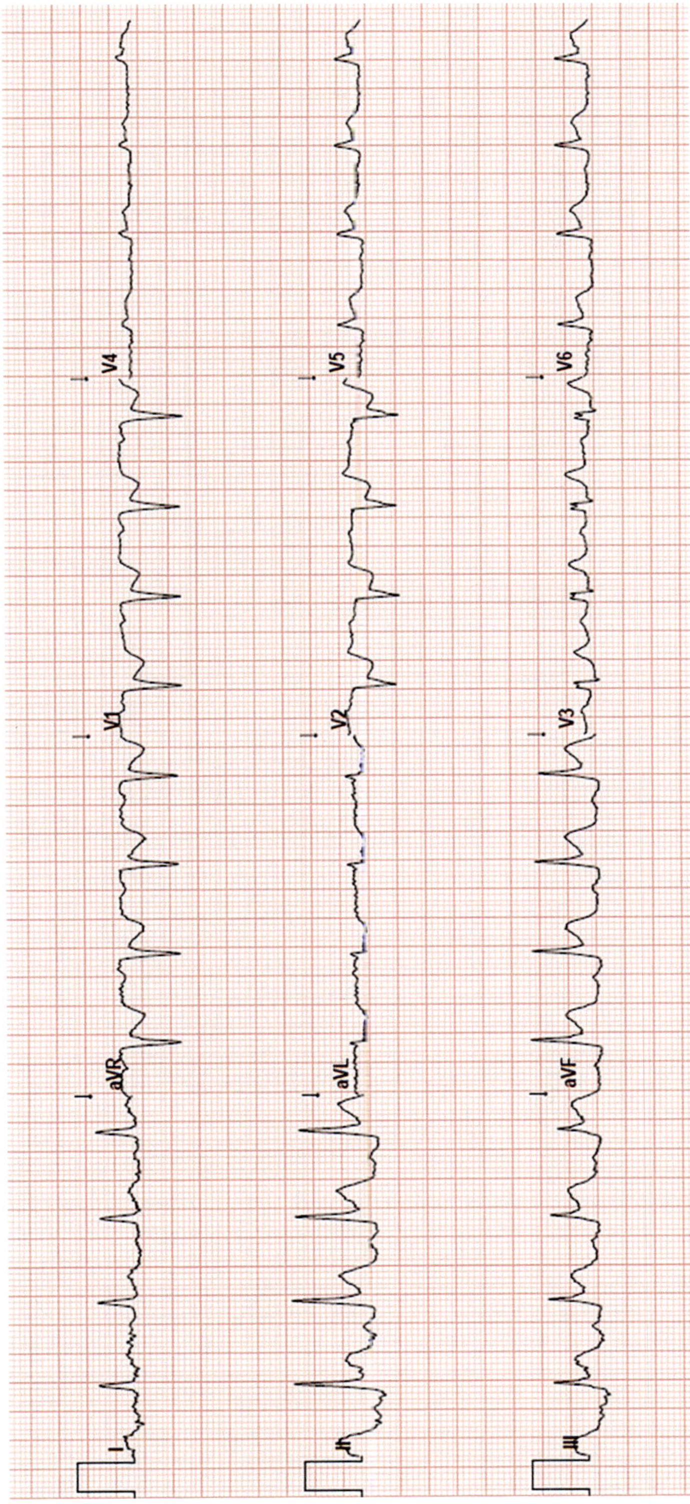

Fig. 35 Acute infero-postero-lateral myocardial infarction. Note ST depression and T wave inversion in leads V1–V2. This has the shape of 'upside down ST elevation', hinting it may be a mirror image of posterior wall infarction

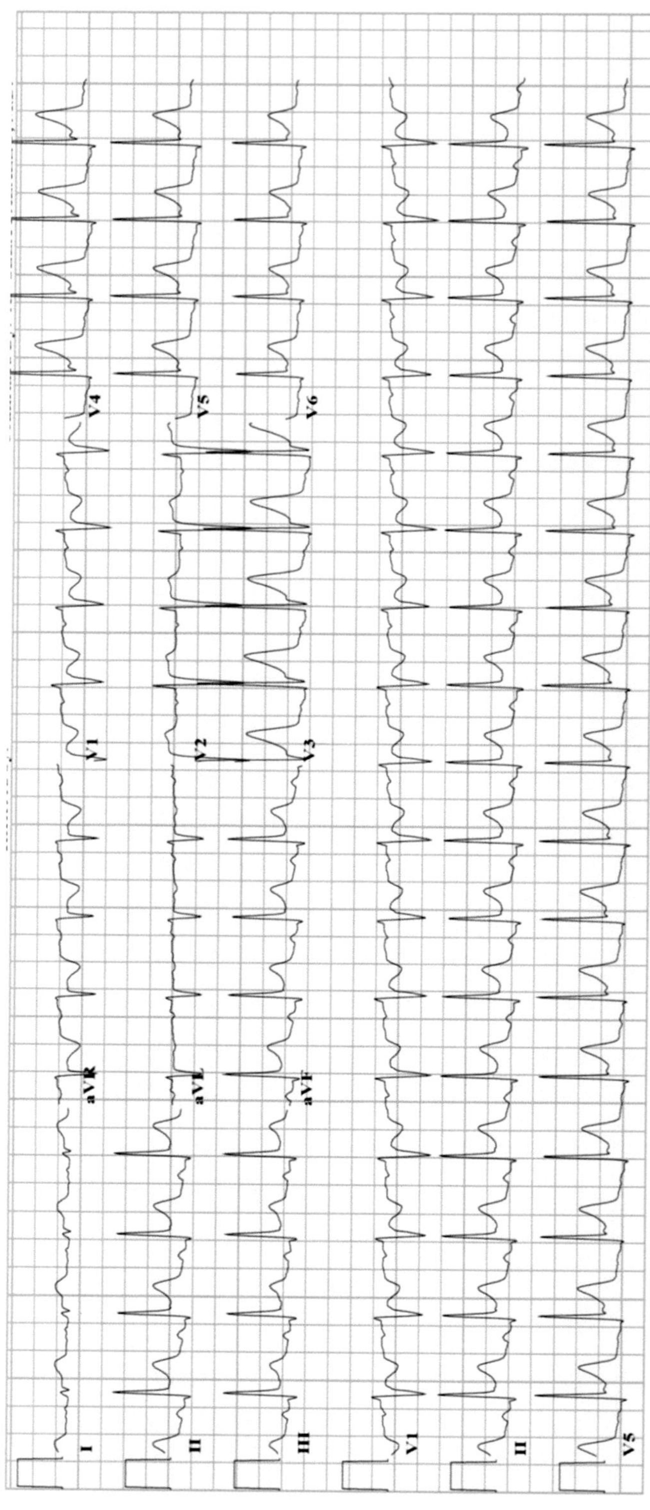

Fig. 36 Acute pericarditis. Note diffuse, concave ST elevation in leads I, II, III, aVF, V3-6. Note also PR segment depression in the same leads. In right-sided leads aVR and V1, PR is elevated and the ST segment is depressed

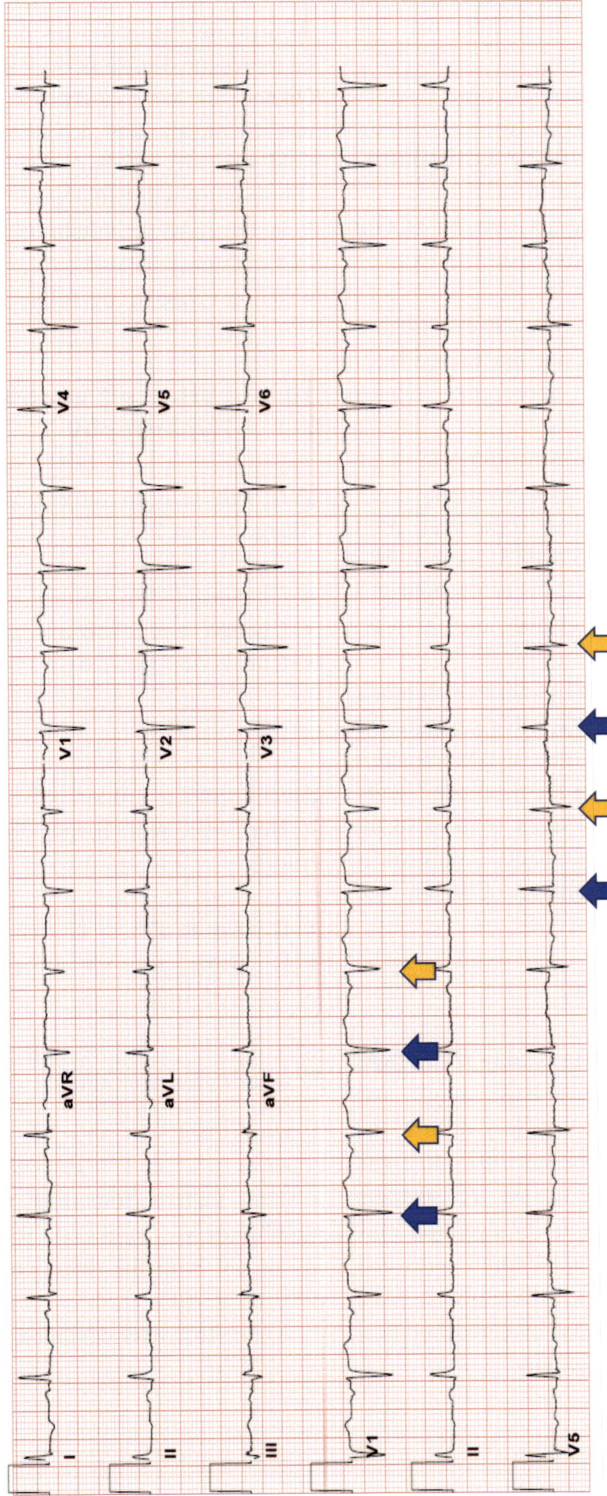

Fig. 37 Electrical alternans in a patient with a large pericardial effusion. Note also low voltage

Echocardiography is of great value in differentiating pericarditis, myocardial infarction and early repolarization, although at times the diagnosis may still be challenging.

8　The ECG in Pulmonary Embolism

Several typical findings characterize the ECG in a patient with pulmonary embolism. An example is shown in Fig. 38.

It is important to note, however, that none of these is specific. Therefore, one must consider all findings together, in the appropriate clinical context.

The most sensitive ECG finding in acute pulmonary embolism is sinus tachycardia.

Other, less sensitive but somewhat more specific ECG signs, are 'S1Q3T3'—meaning a prominent S wave in lead I (if very prominent, a rightward QRS axis), Q wave and T wave inversion in lead III.

Other signs may be right bundle branch block, prominent r waves in V1, T wave inversion in V1-3 and 'clockwise rotation'—a late transition from negative to positive in the precordial leads.

The utility of the ECG signs is to raise the caregiver's suspicion of pulmonary embolism in the patient with sudden shortness of breath.

9　The ECG in Stroke

Stroke, especially hemorrhagic, may show signs on ECG. Intracranial hemorrhage may cause deep T wave inversions, commonly diffuse and symmetric, with a prolonged QT interval. Uncommonly there may also be ST segment elevation or depression. Sinus bradycardia may be a sign of elevated intracranial pressure. The ECG pattern must be differentiated from signs of ischemic heart disease by careful clinical assessment and echocardiography.

10　Structural Abnormalities

Almost any structural anomaly of the heart will be represented in some way in the ECG, as it will change the way electricity spreads throughout cardiac muscle and activates it. Obviously, the gold standard for diagnosis of cardiac structural abnormality will usually be the echocardiogram. It is therefore important to detect hints on the ECG which will lead to a more definitive diagnosis on echocardiography.

10.1　LVH—Left Ventricular Hypertrophy

This will lead to three possible categories of change in the ECG:

- Change in QRS voltage.
- Change in repolarization.
- Change in QRS axis.

Voltage:

Several voltage criteria exist to define LVH.

Here we will focus on relatively simple criteria:

- R wave in aVL > 11 mm
- R wave in V5 or V6 + S wave in V1 > 35 mm.

Repolarization abnormality:

T wave inversion and ST depression, usually concave in V5-6. This is sometimes referred to as a 'strain' pattern. Sometimes mild ST elevation is possible in V1. In general the ST/T changes are discordant with the direction of the QRS complex in the same lead.

Axis—Left axis deviation.

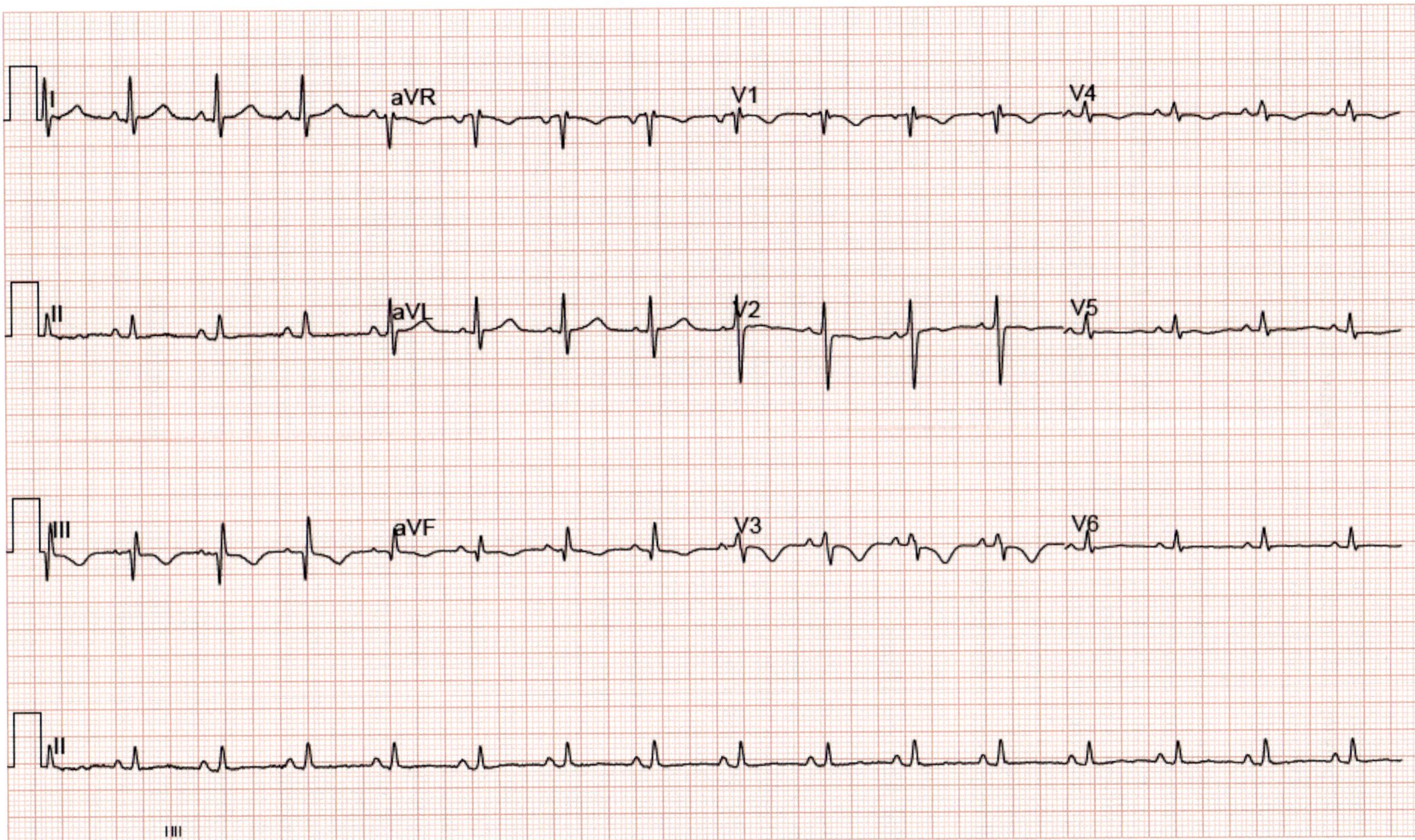

Fig. 38 ECG of a patient with pulmonary embolus. Note sinus tachycardia, 'S1Q3T3', incomplete RBBB and R wave in V2

10.2 RVH—Right Ventricular Hypertrophy

The most common sign is a significant R wave in V1, which is not present on the normal ECG. The diagnosis of RVH requires an R wave amplitude in V1 exceeding 7 mm, or 15 mm in case of RBBB.

Right axis deviation is also possible.

An R wave in V1 may also represent posterior wall infarction of unknown duration. In this case right axis deviation is uncommon. In leads V1-V2, T waves are typically inverted in RVH as opposed to posterior MI. Lastly, posterior MI commonly accompanies inferior wall MI, where q waves will be present in inferior leads.

10.3 Atrial Abnormalities

The P wave represents atrial depolarization. During sinus rhythm the right atrium starts to depolarized before the left; hence, the first (left) portion of the P wave represents right atrial depolarization, whereas the right part represents left atrial depolarization. In lead V1, the first part of the P wave representing right atrial activity is typically positive while the second part may be negative. It is therefore useful to look at the P wave in leads II and V1 to find hints at atrial abnormalities. It is important to note that ECG atrial abnormalities were previously considered to be a specific sign of atrial enlargement. It has since been realized that these signs are not specific for enlargement but may also signify changes in pressure, conduction or atrial wall thickness; therefore, the term 'atrial abnormality' is now preferred over 'enlargement'.

Left atrial abnormality is marked by a P wave that is notched and wider than 120 ms, typically in lead II. This P wave is historically termed 'P mitrale'. In V1, the terminal, negative portion of the P wave would be deep and wide—deeper and wider than one mm.

Right atrial abnormality is signified by a tall P wave in lead II—formally taller than 2.5 mm.

This is historically termed 'P pulmonale'. In V1, the first and positive portion of the P wave would be taller than 1.5 mm.

The two atrial abnormalities may coexist, giving the appearance of 'biatrial abnormality'.

The finding of atrial abnormalities should prompt echocardiographic investigation of the cause of the atrial condition.

10.4 The ECG in Cardiomyopathy

Hypertrophic Cardiomyopathy

Hypertrophic cardiomyopathy is a genetic disorder causing hypertrophy of the heart muscle. This will primarily cause ECG changes that are typical of left ventricular hypertrophy (LVH). These are not specific for hypertrophic cardiomyopathy, and may also be present in concentric hypertrophy which is secondary to chronic pressure overload of the left ventricle, as in long standing hypertension or aortic stenosis. At times, however, the ECG in cardiomyopathy will be different than in secondary hypertrophy, reflecting the fact that thickening of muscle is regional and not concentric.

There are also typical changes in the ST-T segment: ST depression in V5–V6 accompanied by inverted, asymmetrical T waves is common in LVH and is called a 'strain' pattern.

Sarcoidosis

There are no specific ECG signs of cardiac involvement in sarcoidosis. However, patients with cardiac sarcoidosis are at risk for developing conduction disturbances and ventricular tachycardia. For this reason, any young patient with otherwise unexplained atrioventricular conduction disease should be considered for the diagnosis of cardiac sarcoidosis.

Amyloidosis

Cardiac amyloidosis is a condition in which the heart muscle becomes laden with a substance called 'amyloid'. This may cause deterioration of heart function and changes in its structure. The condition is now considered to be much more common than previously thought, especially in the elderly.

The ECG hallmark signs of amyloidosis are low voltage QRS (less than 5 mm in limb leads or 10 mm in precordial leads; in amyloidosis the low voltage is usually in limb leads) and a 'pseudo-infarct' pattern, defined as pathologic Q waves in at least 2 consecutive leads (usually in anterior wall distribution) in the absence of myocardial infarction. Atrial tachy arrhythmias are common. These signs are neither sensitive nor specific, however they should raise suspicion of the disease.

11 Channelopathies and Sudden Cardiac Death

The ECG plays a critical role in the evaluation of patients presenting with cardiac arrest, and should be carefully reviewed for any sign of channelopathy or arrhythmogenic cardiomyopathy in cases of syncope.

The most common causes of cardiac arrest and sudden cardiac death are age dependent. Overall, the most common cause is myocardial infarction. The second most common cause is an arrhythmia. Some arrhythmogenic conditions may be seen on the ECG during sinus rhythm.

11.1 HCM (See Above)

Hypertrophic cardiomyopathy is a relatively common cause of sudden cardiac death amongst young people, especially among athletes arresting during strenuous exercise or competitive sports. The ECG manifestations of this condition (LVH) were previously discussed.

11.2 Long and Short QT

A prolonged QT segment predisposes to a form of polymorphic VT known as Torsades de Pointes, which may deteriorate to ventricular fibrillation. The QT segment varies with heart rate and should be corrected for it. The common formula used for this correction is Bazet's formula, whereby the corrected QT (QTc) is the QT interval divided by the square root of the RR interval, both in milliseconds. Using this formula, the normal QTc interval is 350–450 ms in men and 360–460 ms in women.

Long QT may be a congenital or an acquired condition. An example ECG is shown in Fig. 39. The acquired form of long QT is usually related to use of certain medications or electrolyte disorders.

A prolonged QT interval in a patient presenting with palpitations, dizziness spells, or syncope should prompt further evaluation as this may be a life threatening condition.

A rare condition, also predisposing to sudden cardiac death is the short QT syndrome. It may also present with early and tall peaked T waves.

11.3 Brugada Syndrome

Brugada syndrome is a condition predisposing to sudden cardiac death. It is characterized by a distinct form of QRS-T morphology in leads V1–V2, as seen in Fig. 40. This typically includes an R' component conveying an RBBB shape to the V1–V2 QRS. Additionally, there is ST and J-point elevation of > 2 mm, as well as an inverted T wave. The management and diagnostic workup are quite complex and controversial; therefore, a patient with these findings should be referred to a cardiologist.

11.4 Arrhythmogenic Right Ventricular Cardiomyopathy (ARVC)

Arrhythmogenic Right Ventricular Cardiomyopathy is a genetic form of arrhythmogenic cardiomyopathy, characterized by fatty deposits infiltrating the heart muscle. These may cause electrical abnormalities leading to life threatening arrhythmias. It is now becoming clear that 'right ventricular' may be a misnomer, and that this

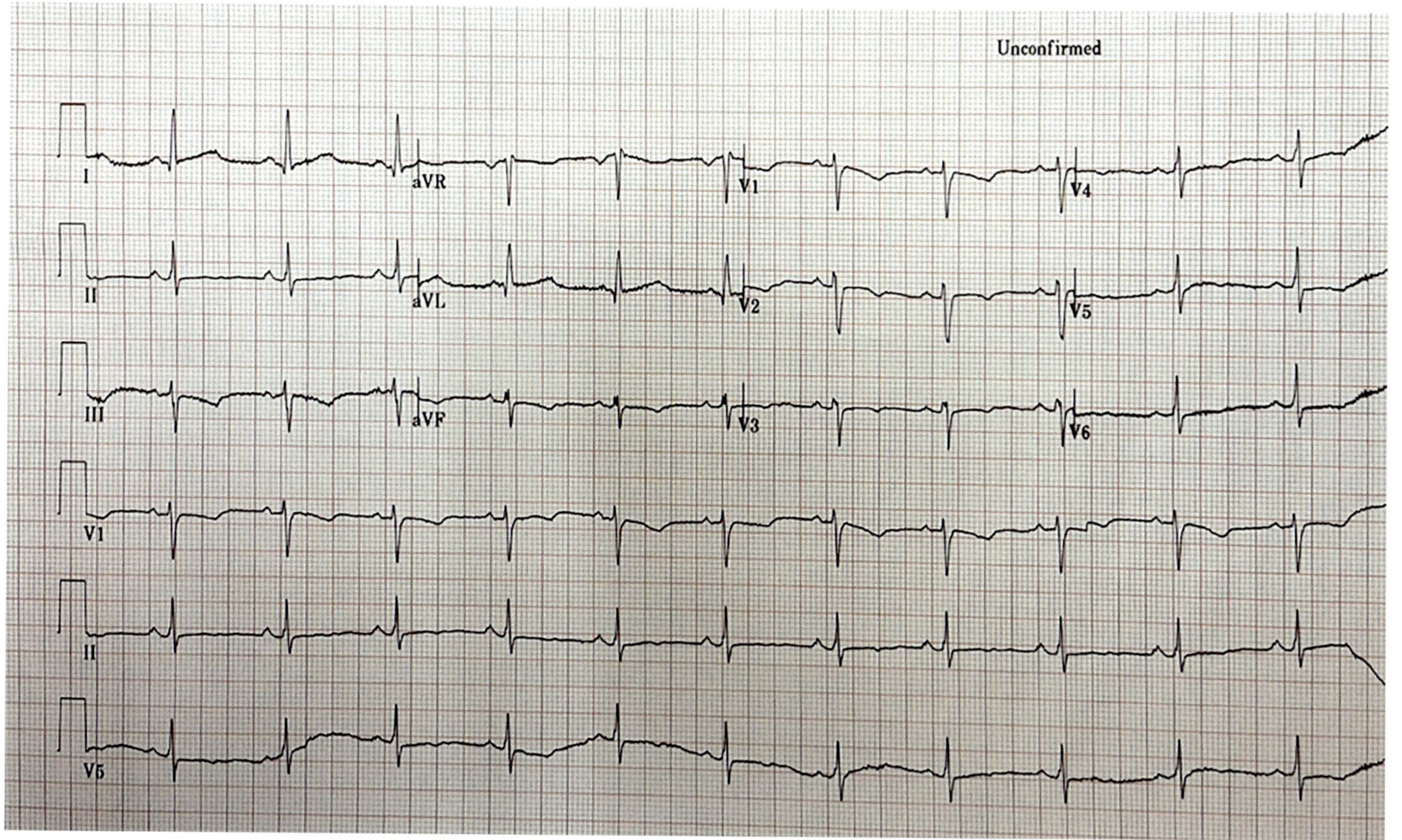

Fig. 39 Congenital long QT syndrome. QTc is 506 ms

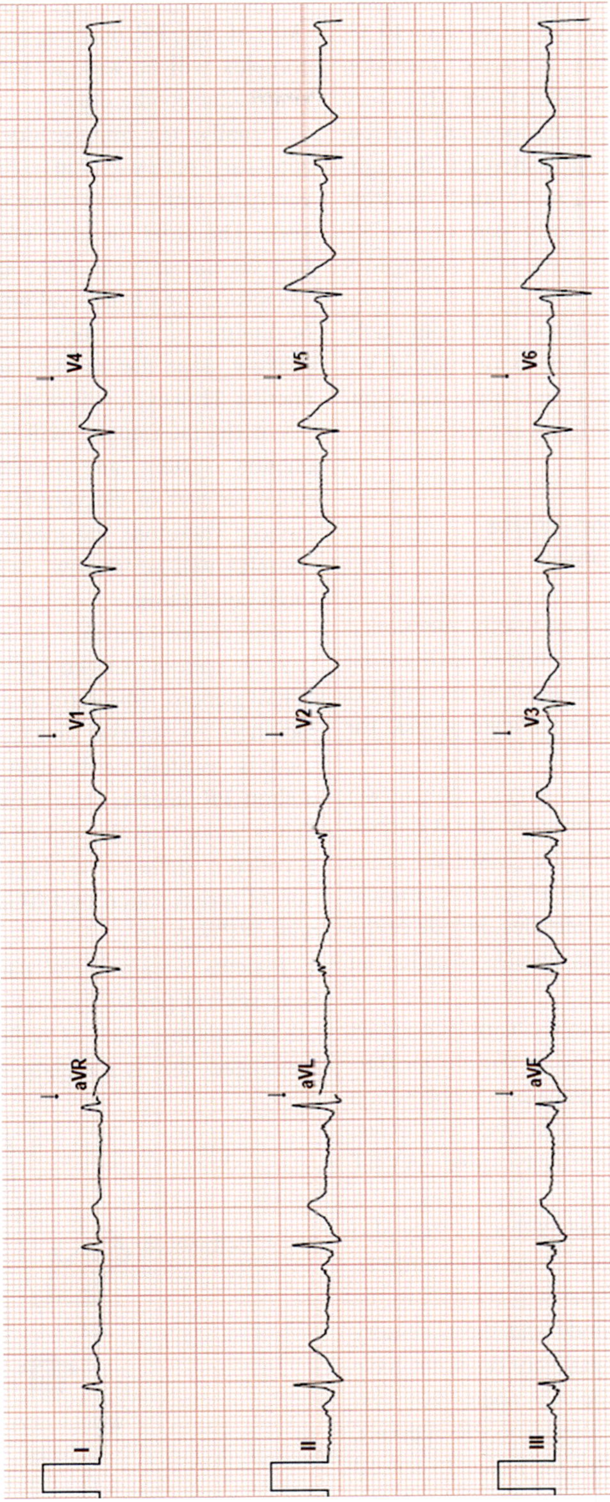

Fig. 40 ECG with Brugada pattern

condition affects the left ventricle and the interventricular septum. Nevertheless, right ventricular involvement may show typical signs on ECG:

QRS widening and/or T wave inversion localized to V1-3, or an epsilon wave. (It is very unusual to have QRS widening localized to a few leads. Usually, QRS width is identical throughout.). The epsilon wave is a small positive deflection present in the early part of the ST segment in V1. Another feature is a prolonged S wave upstroke in V1-3.

Patients with this condition also commonly have premature ventricular beats or runs of VT with an LBBB morphology, indicating the origin of the beats to be in the right ventricle.

11.5 Wolff-Parkinson-White (WPW) Syndrome

(Note: WPW syndrome was briefly mentioned previously in the narrow complex tachycardia section. It is discussed here again in the context of ECG patterns that may indicate a risk for sudden cardiac death.)

Most people have a single connection between the atria and ventricles: the AV node and bundle of His. There are, however, cases where an additional bundle of cardiac muscle fibers connects atria and ventricles outside of the AV node-His system. This bundle is called an accessory pathway.

Some accessory pathways can only conduct electricity from the ventricle to the atrium (retrograde conduction). In this case, a reentry loop may form involving the atria and ventricles, causing a narrow complex tachycardia—AVRT—discussed previously.

However, some accessory pathways may also conduct antegradely—from atrium to ventricle. In this case, every sinus beat will conduct to the ventricles via both AV node and the accessory pathway. The accessory pathway does not have the distinct features of the AV node—His system: there will be no AV delay (no PR interval), and no specialized conduction tissue to spread the electrical impulse rapidly throughout the

ventricle. Hence, a signal that conducts through the accessory pathway **only** will have a very short, if any, PR interval; and the resulting QRS complex will be wide as a result of slow intraventricular conduction.

Usually, the impulse does not use only the accessory pathway, but rather conducts to the ventricles using the both the pathway and the AV node. The atrial impulse will reach the ventricle first via the pathway since it has no AV delay. Therefore, the PR interval will be very short. The beginning of the QRS complex will have a shallow slope due to slow intraventricular conduction. However, following the AV delay at the AV node, the impulse will travel down the conduction system and rapidly spread through whatever part of the ventricle not already depolarized. Therefore, the terminal part of the QRS complex will be 'narrow', with steep slopes and rapid conduction.

The above sequence of events will cause a typical pattern known as 'preexcitation', or WPW pattern. (the term preexcitation refers to the short PR interval and the fact that the ventricle is 'excited' earlier than expected). There is a short PR interval, and a first part of the QRS that is wider than the second part. This widening is called a 'delta wave'. Figure 41 is an illustration of preexcitation on ECG; Fig. 42 is an ECG with WPW pattern.

Patients with a WPW pattern on ECG may have several types of arrhythmias. Most are not life threatening, such as orthodromic AVRT (as mentioned, this is a reentry circuit whereby the

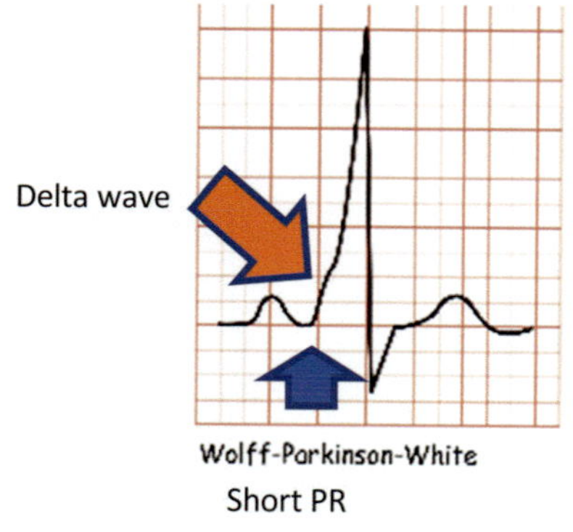

Fig. 41 Diagram of P-QRS with preexcitation

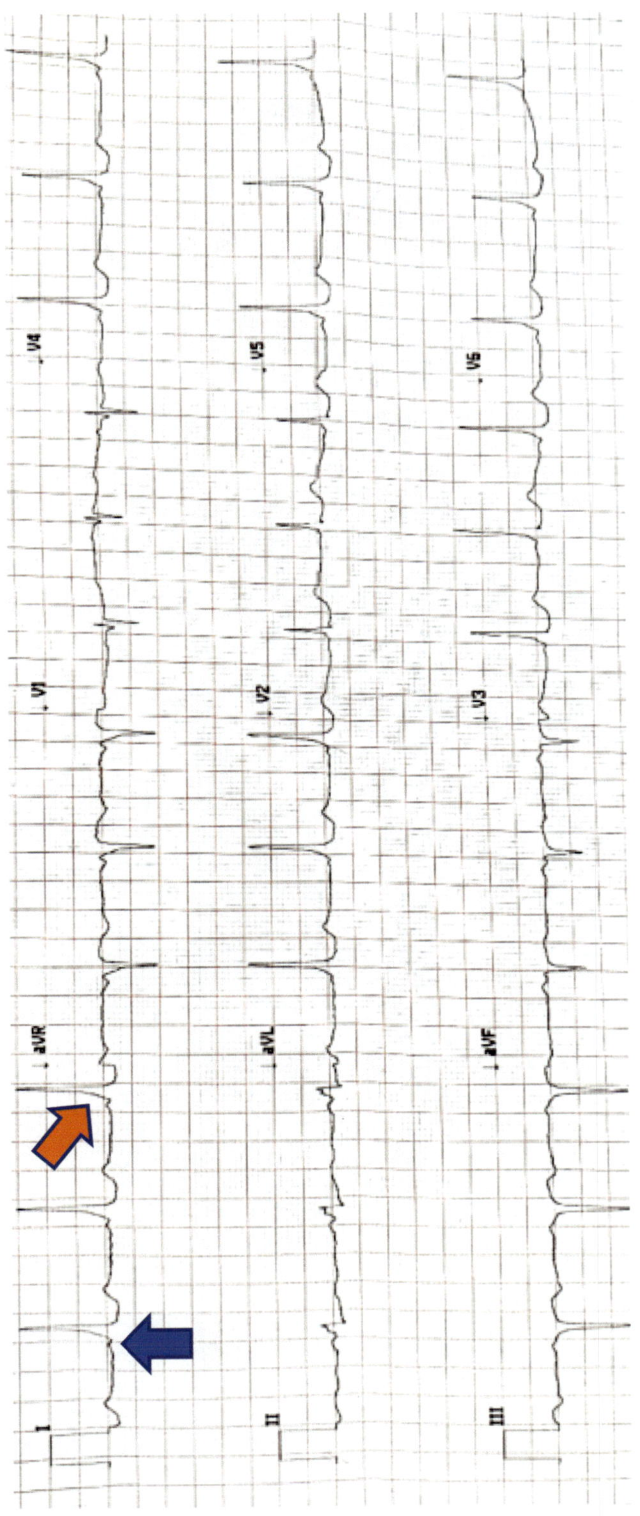

Fig. 42 An example of **WPW pattern**. Blue arrow points to **short PR** interval; orange arrow points to **delta wave**

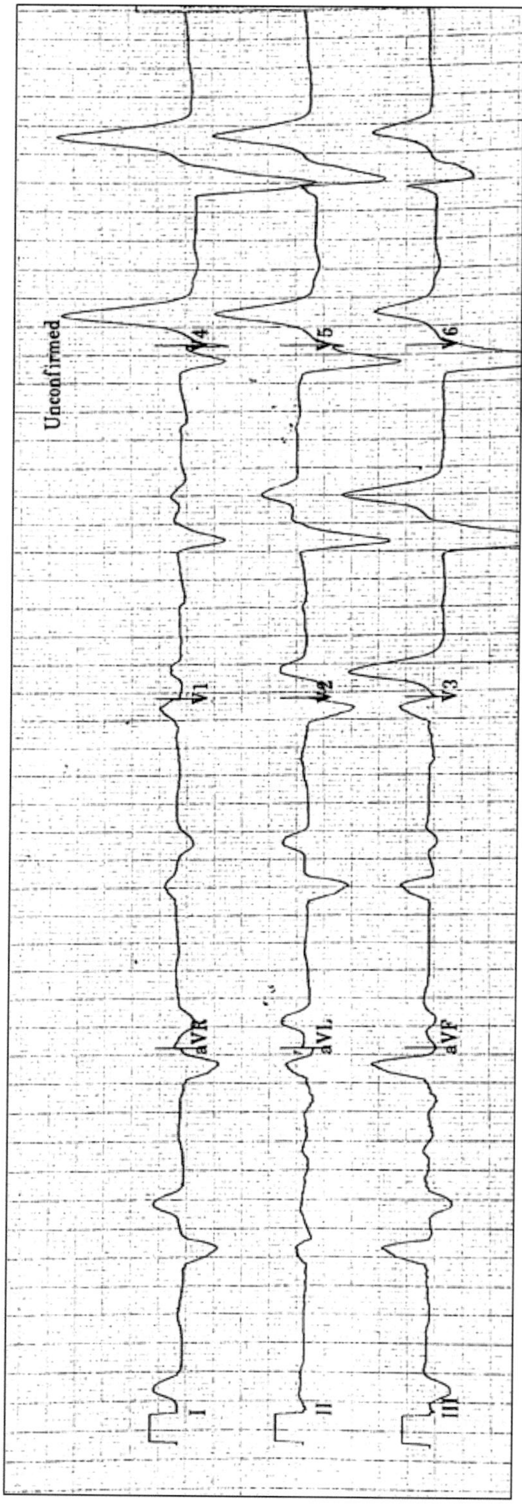

Fig. 43 Hyperkalemia. Tall, peaked T waves, short QT interval, wide QRS and disappearance of P waves

impulse conducts to the ventricles via the AV node, then back up to the atria via the accessory pathway).

An exception to this is atrial fibrillation. Since there is no AV delay in the accessory pathway, atrial fibrillation may cause a very rapid and irregular ventricular rate, that may deteriorate to VT and VF, causing sudden cardiac death. Atrial fibrillation conducting via an accessory pathway is called 'preexcited atrial fibrillation', and has distinct ECG features: it is very rapid, irregular, with QRS complexes that are wide, changing in width from beat to beat. This is an emergency medical condition.

Any patient with WPW pattern on ECG, especially if he or she has suffered syncope or palpitations, should be promptly referred for cardiac consultation.

12 Electrolyte Imbalance

Severe abnormalities of potassium and calcium concentration cause typical ECG patterns.

It is worthwhile to check electrolytes in any patient with an unusual ECG pattern that is not quickly recognized by the caregiver at point of care.

12.1 Potassium

Hyperkalemia

ECG abnormalities in hyperkalemia have been described as a sequence, depending on the severity of hyperkalemia.

Main features are seen in Fig. 43 and include:

Tall, peaked T waves
Short QT interval
PR interval prolongation

Flattening and widening of P waves, progressing to P wave disappearance
Wide QRS, ST segment elevation. In severe cases a 'sine wave pattern' may be seen
Ventricular arrhythmias.

Hypokalemia

- Prominent U waves
- ST segment depression
- T wave flattening
- Prominent P waves (increased amplitude and duration)
- Prolonged QT interval
- Arrhythmias and conduction disturbances.

12.2 Calcium

The main ECG changes to be expected are that hypercalcemia shortens the QTc interval, whereas hypocalcemia prolongs it.

13 Summary

ECG reading is a fundamental skill required for evaluation of patients with various clinical presentations.

Adoption of a systematic approach to reading the ECG is essential for formation of a meaningful differential diagnosis.

This short tutorial is not meant to replace a comprehensive electrocardiography textbook; but rather to provide a concise, algorithmic reference for the point-of-care healthcare professional faced with common acute presentations.

As discussed in Chapter I, the ECG in this book is regarded as one of the two fundamental tools comprising the 'electrosonography' approach.

References

Brugada P, et al. A new approach to the differential diagnosis of a regular tachycardia with a wide QRS complex. Circulation. 1991;83(5):1649–59.

Kindwall KE, Brown J, Josephson ME. Electrocardiographic criteria for ventricular tachycardia in wide complex left bundle branch block morphology tachycardias. Am J Cardiol. 1988;61:1279–83.

Kligfield P, et al. Recommendations for the standardization and interpretation of the electrocardiogram, part I: the electrocardiogram and its technology. Circulation 2007:1306.

Moccetti F, et al. Simplified integrated clinical and electrocardiographic algorithm for differentiation of wide QRS complex tachycardia: the Basel algorithm. JACC Clin Electrophysiol. 2022;8(7):831–9.

Thygesen K, et al. Fourth universal definition of myocardial infarction. Circulation. 2018;138:e618–51.

Tutorial for Transthoracic Echocardiography Performance and Interpretation

David Leibowitz, Donna Zwas, Momen Abassi, Yair Elitzur, and Eyal Herzog

Abstract

Echocardiography has become a widely-used diagnostic test in the practice of medicine. It can diagnose a wide range of cardiovascular pathology in a rapid and efficient manner without the use of radiation or potentially harmful contrast agents. The introduction of high quality, miniature, easily portable machines has enabled the performance of echocardiographic studies by non-cardiologists in varied clinical settings such as emergency rooms, intensive care units and private offices and clinics. This tutorial outlines the performance of the basic echocardiographic examination, and provides a framework for the evaluation of specific cardiac diagnoses in the acute setting.

Keywords

Echocardiography · ECG · Electrosonography · Transducer · Ventricular function · Valvular disease

D. Leibowitz (✉) · D. Zwas · Y. Elitzur · E. Herzog
Department of Cardiology, The Heart Institute, Hadassah Medical Center, Hebrew University of Jerusalem, P.O. Box 12000, Jerusalem, Israel
e-mail: oleibo@hadassah.org.il

M. Abassi
Department of Nephrology Hadassah Medical Center, Hebrew University of Jerusalem, Jerusalem, Israel

1 Introduction

Echocardiography has become a widely-used diagnostic test within the field of cardiology. It has the ability to diagnose a wide range of cardiovascular pathology in a rapid and efficient manner without the use of radiation or potentially harmful contrast agents. The introduction of high quality, miniature, easily portable machines has enabled the performance of echocardiographic studies by non-cardiologists in varied clinical settings such as emergency rooms, intensive care units and private offices and clinics. This tutorial outlines the performance of the basic echocardiographic examination, and provides a framework for the evaluation of specific cardiac diagnoses in the acute setting.

2 The Standard Transthoracic Echocardiogram

2.1 Subject Preparation

It is preferable to perform the study with as little ambient light as possible to ensure adequate study quality and room lighting should be adjusted accordingly. The examiner should be seated comfortably, generally to the left of the patient who should be supine (Fig. 1).

The patient's name and medical record number should be entered, and three ECG electrodes attached. An adequate ECG signal showing a clear

© The Author(s), under exclusive license to Springer Nature Switzerland AG 2023
E. Herzog et al. (eds.), *Cardiac Electrosonography*,
https://doi.org/10.1007/978-3-031-38469-1_3

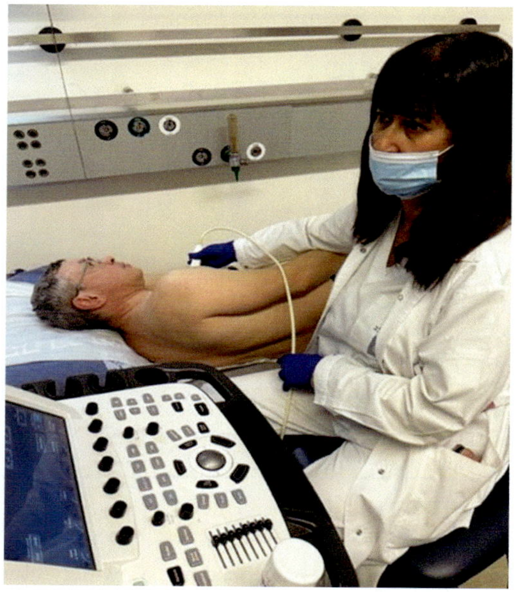

Fig. 1 Appropriate positioning of the technician and subject before beginning standard echo exam

QRS complex on the echo machine monitor must be present throughout the exam. The patients' height and weight should be recorded if possible, and heart rate and blood pressure should be measured and added to the report.

2.2 Image Optimization

One should use the highest frequency cardiac phased array transducer that produces good quality images. The higher the frequency, the better the resolution, but the poorer the penetration (Fig. 2). Particularly in obese patients, it may be necessary to use lower frequencies to achieve adequate visualization.

Bones and lungs obstruct ultrasonic access to the heart, and a large proportion of the technical skill required to perform the examination lies in being able to find a patient position and transducer site from which clear images can be obtained. The best

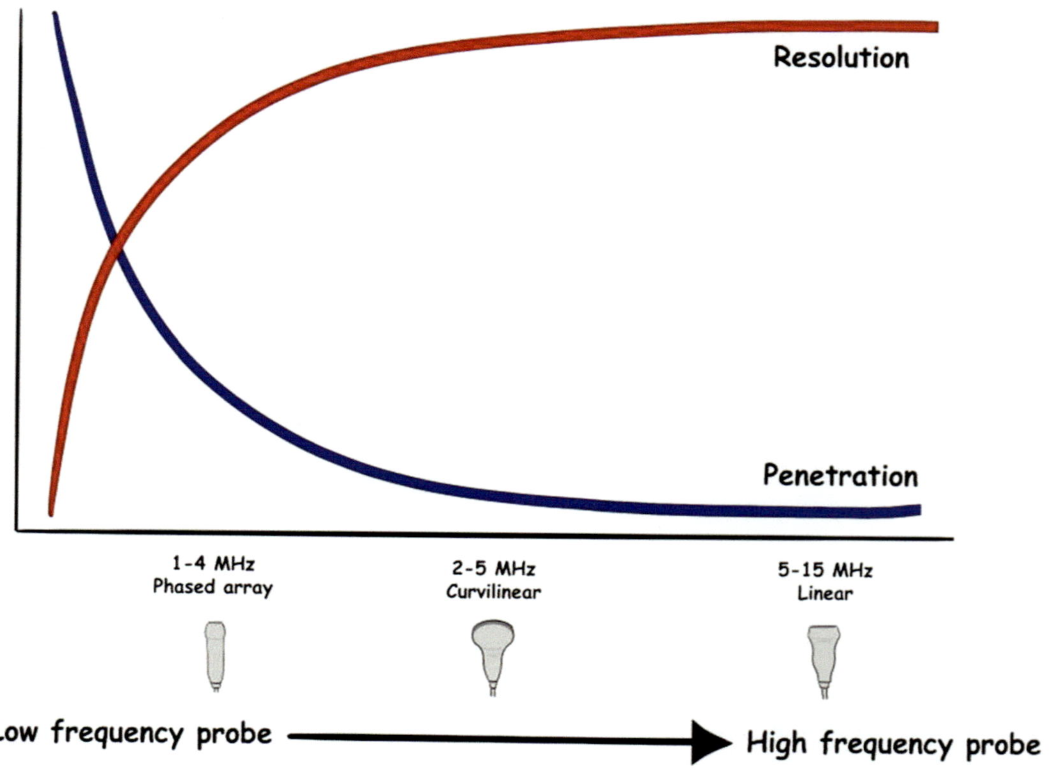

Fig. 2 Relationship between frequency, resolution and penetration

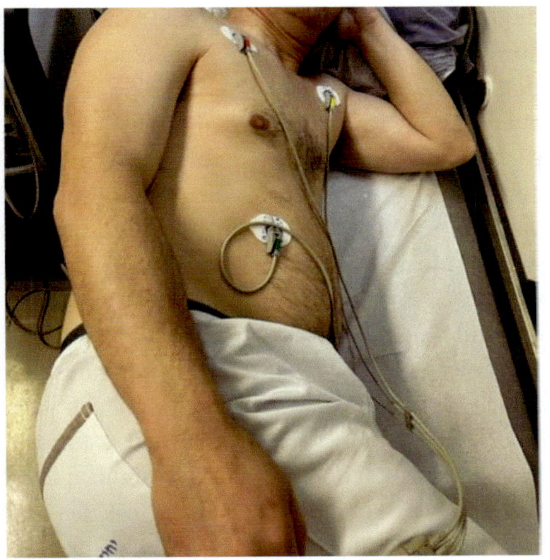

Fig. 3 Patient positioning for optimal imaging

views are usually obtained with the patient in the steep left-lateral decubitus position. The patient's left arm above the head should be raised to spread the ribs and optimize the imaging window (Fig. 3).

Record at least 2–3 beats of each view for digital images in sinus rhythm, and a minimum of 5 beats in atrial fibrillation. Recording should only commence when the view is optimized. Depth should be adjusted so that the cardiac image occupies most, but not all of, the screen. Imaging should be performed using ultrasonic gel between the transducer and the subject to prevent air from interfering with study quality. In each view, it may be necessary to utilize the zoom feature to magnify a particular structure in order to accurately measure, or to better assess pathology. Depending on the particular view, the transducer may need to be tilted or rotated while sliding or rocking motions should be avoided (Fig. 4).

Cardinal transducer manipulation / movement

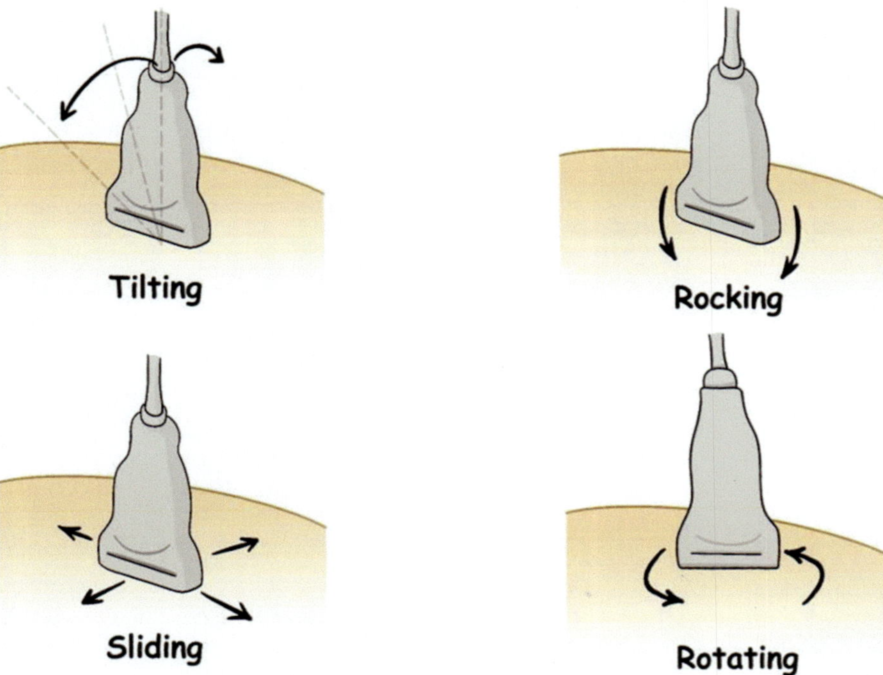

Fig. 4 Figure depicting the various motions of the transducer

2.3 Doppler Examination

Assessment of each valve in each view includes 2D and color flow Doppler, as well as pulse and continuous wave Doppler in parallel with flow to measure flow velocity.

Continuous wave Doppler (CW) can be used to estimate the peak pressure difference across a cardiac valve, using the modified Bernoulli equation:

$$\text{Pressure difference}(\text{mmHg}) = 4 * (\text{Peak}(\text{m/sec}))^2, \text{ or } P = 4V^2$$

This equation is based on the fact that the velocity of blood traveling from one chamber to another is directly related to the pressure difference between the two chambers (Fig. 5). This formula has been shown to be valid for the estimation of gradients across all 4 cardiac valves. The ultrasound beam must be aligned parallel to the blood flow of interest. The cursor should be placed within 20° of the direction of flow, otherwise the pressure difference may be significantly underestimated (Fig. 6). Keep in mind that CW will measure all points along the cursor and display the maximum velocity. It will not be able to precisely localize the position of maximal velocity. Generally the measurement software in the echo machine will translate the velocity measured by Doppler into pressure gradient automatically.

Pulse wave Doppler (PW) measures the velocity at a given point, and is of particular value in calculating aortic valve area and estimating flow across the mitral valve orifice in the apical 4 chamber view in order to help assess diastolic function. The sample volume should be placed in the area of interest. By convention, blood flow towards the probe is a positive deflection and away from the probe is a negative deflection (true for CW as well) (Fig. 7). PW is limited in the maximum velocity that it can detect.

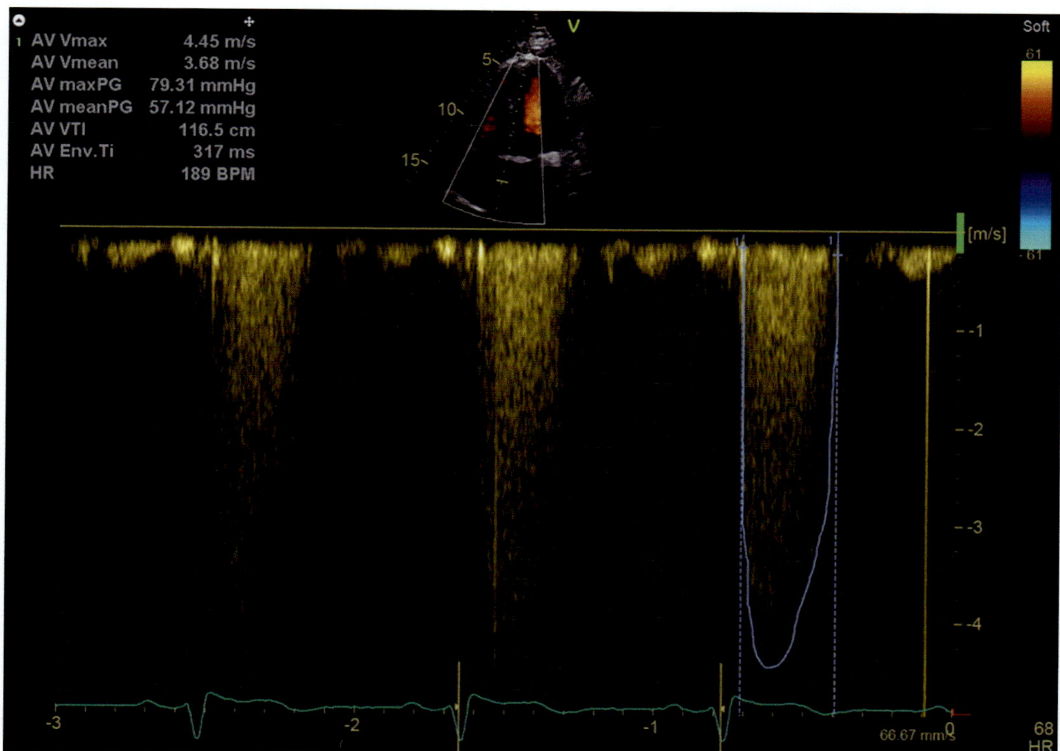

Fig. 5 An example of use of continuous-wave (CW) Doppler imaging. The echo machine automatically translates the velocity information obtained to a pressure gradient (in this case over the aortic valve)

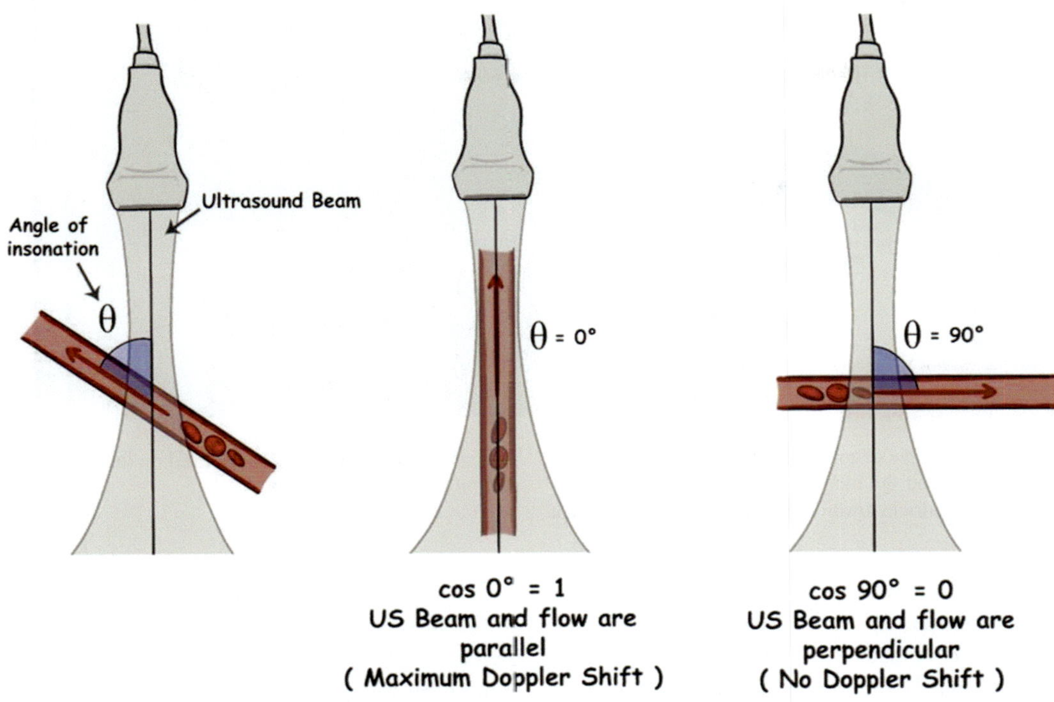

Fig. 6 The relationship between angle of ultrasound beam and Doppler shift

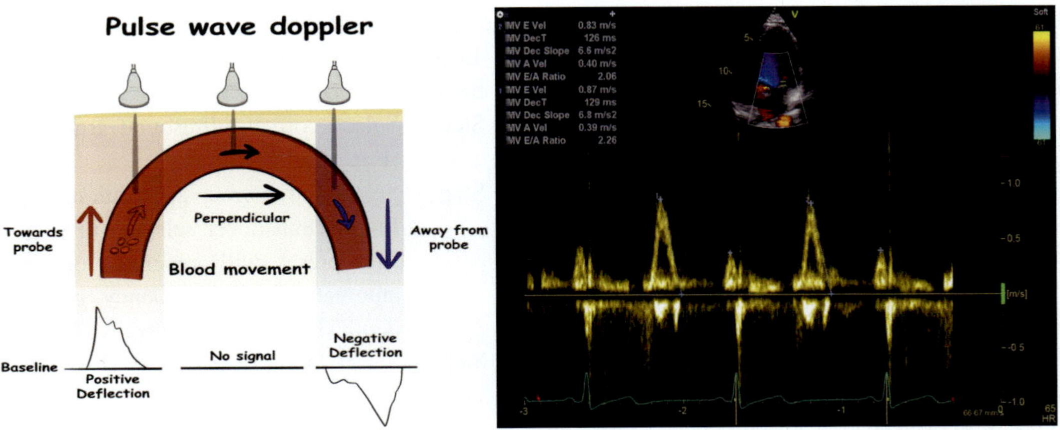

Fig. 7 An example of pulsed-wave (PW) Doppler imaging, in this case of mitral inflow demonstrating early and late filling of the left ventricle during diastole. Note that as opposed to the CW tracing, the PW tracing has a velocity signal only along the outer envelope of the tracing

Color Doppler allows imaging of blood movement. By convention, red flow is flow towards the position of the transducer and blue flow is flow traveling away from the transducer (Fig. 8). High velocity jets (such as regurgitant valvular lesions) will cause turbulent mosaic flow.

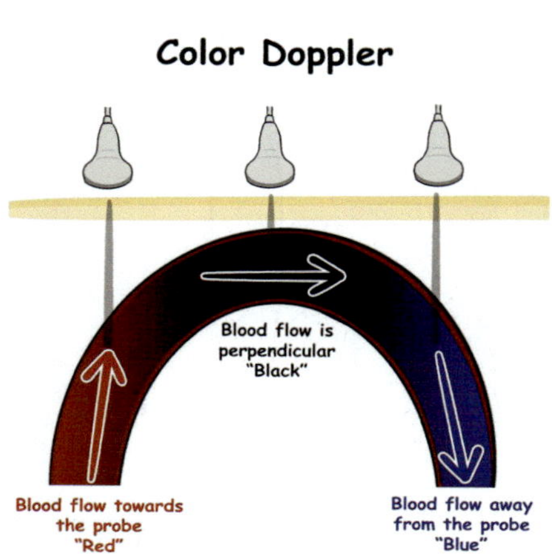

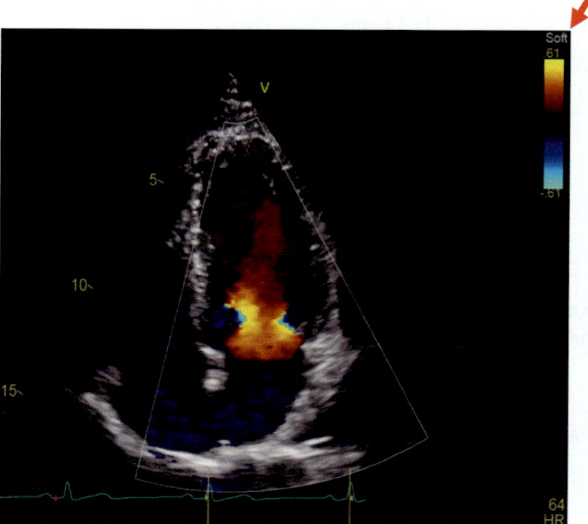

Fig. 8 An example of color Doppler imaging. The mitral valve is open and the blood flow is from the left atrium into the left ventricle towards the transducer. The Nyquist limit of 61 and color scale are depicted on the upper right portion of the image (arrow)

Tissue Doppler imaging (TDI) detects lower velocity frequency shifts in order to calculate myocardial velocity (as opposed to standard Doppler which measures blood flow velocity) (Fig. 9). It is primarily useful in the assessment of LV filling pressures and diastolic dysfunction.

M-mode is a display of motion versus time of the 2D image along a single line corresponding to the placement of the m mode cursor. This imaging technique may be useful in the hemodynamic assessment of pericardial effusions (Fig. 10).

3 Basic Ultrasound Controls (Fig. 11)

Frequency: The higher the frequency the higher the resolution but the lower the penetration (Fig. 2). In obese patients usually need to work at lower frequencies.

Depth: Adjust so that 2D image is displayed across most but not all the screen (Knob A in Fig. 11).

Gain: Increases/decreases the brightness of the image (Knob B in Fig. 11).

Time gain compensation (TGC): Used to adjust the gain regionally should generally be increased from near field to far field (Knobs along C in Fig. 11).

Zoom: Magnifies a particular region of interest (Knob D in Fig. 11).

Focus position: Should be placed alongside the region of interest.

Beginning the 2D exam

Step 1 Turn on power button

Step 2 Select correct ultrasound transducer (Fig. 12).

Step 3 Select the correct application preset for the transducer selected in step 1. The preset will generally optimize automatically the frequency, gain and depth (Fig. 13).

Step 4 Select the correct depth. This should be adjusted so that the image fills most of the screen (Fig. 14).

Step 5 Adjust gain using both overall gain control and the TGC controls (Fig. 15).

Step 6 Adjust the focus position. This maximizes resolution at the level of the region of interest.

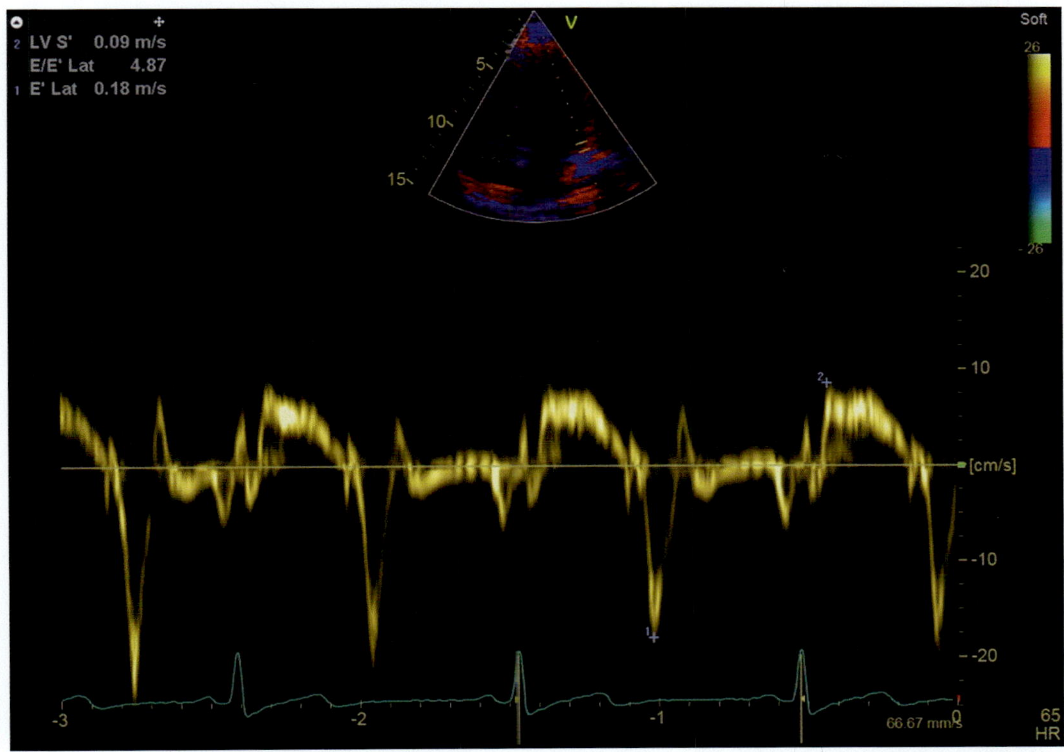

Fig. 9 An example of tissue Doppler imaging (TDI) of the lateral aspect of the mitral annulus with measurement of early diastolic and systolic velocities

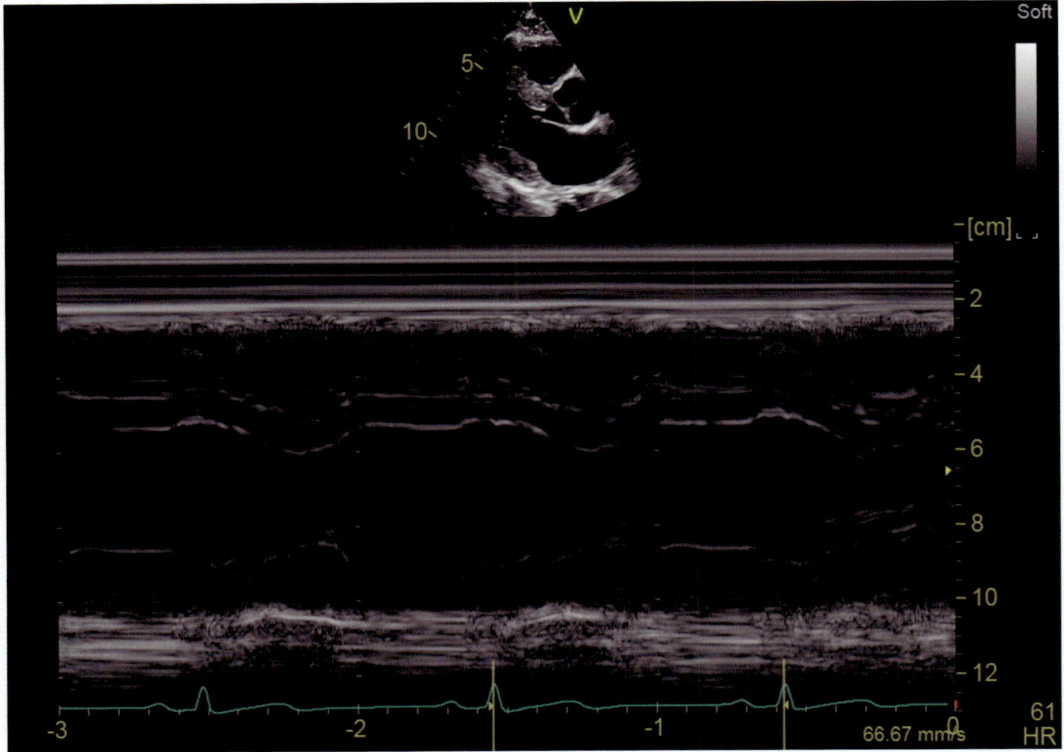

Fig. 10 An example of m-mode imaging through the left ventricle in parasternal long-axis view. Note the position of the cursor in the 2D image above

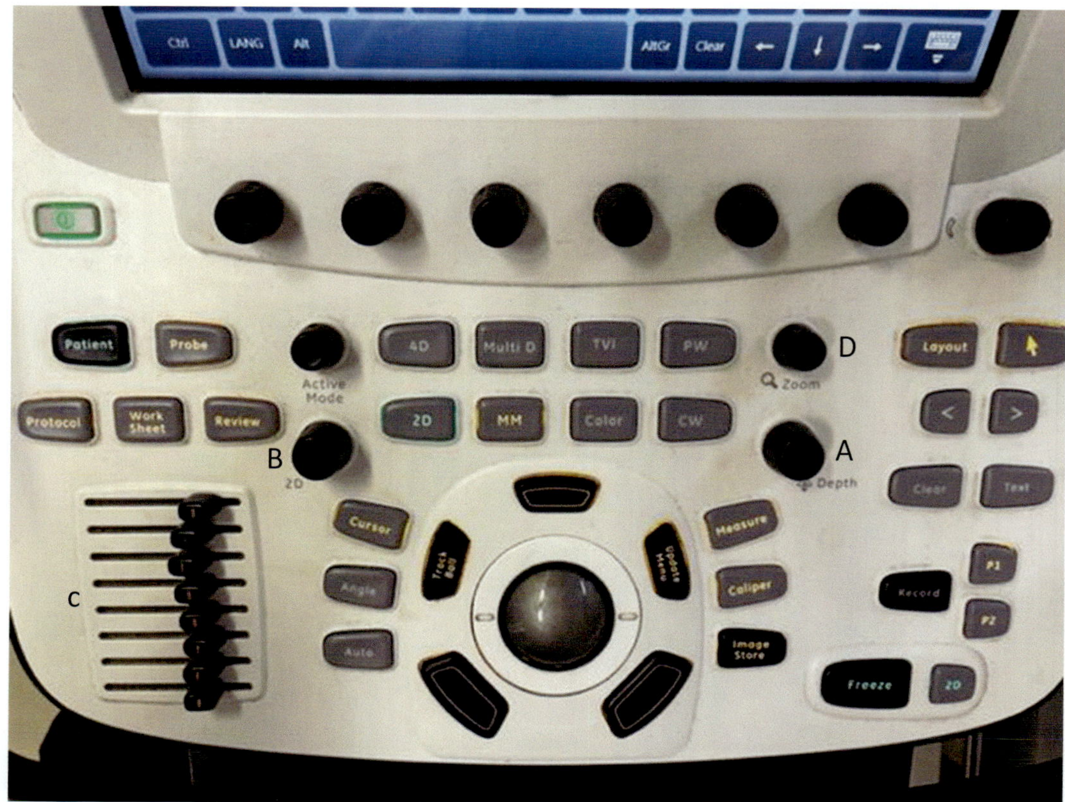

Fig. 11 Typical echo machine dashboard showing the various controls needed for a standard echo exam

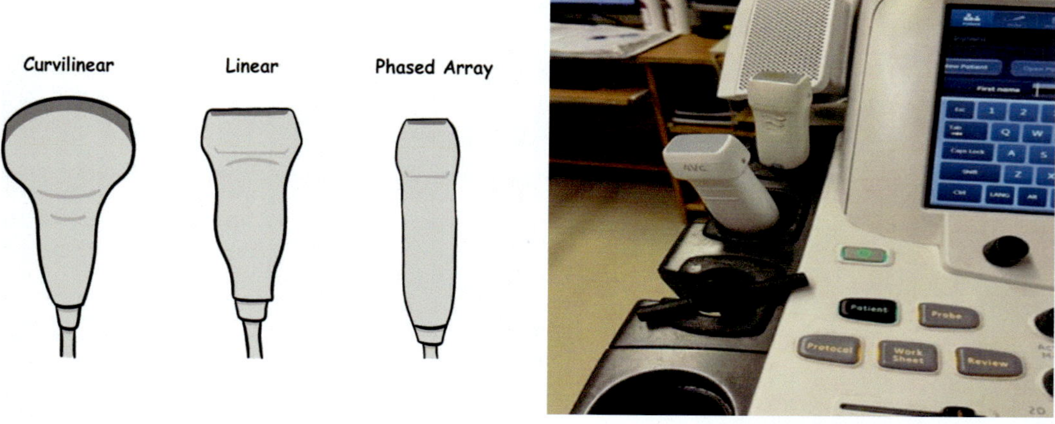

Fig. 12 An example of different probes available. It is critical to choose the appropriate phased array transducer for the performance of adult studies

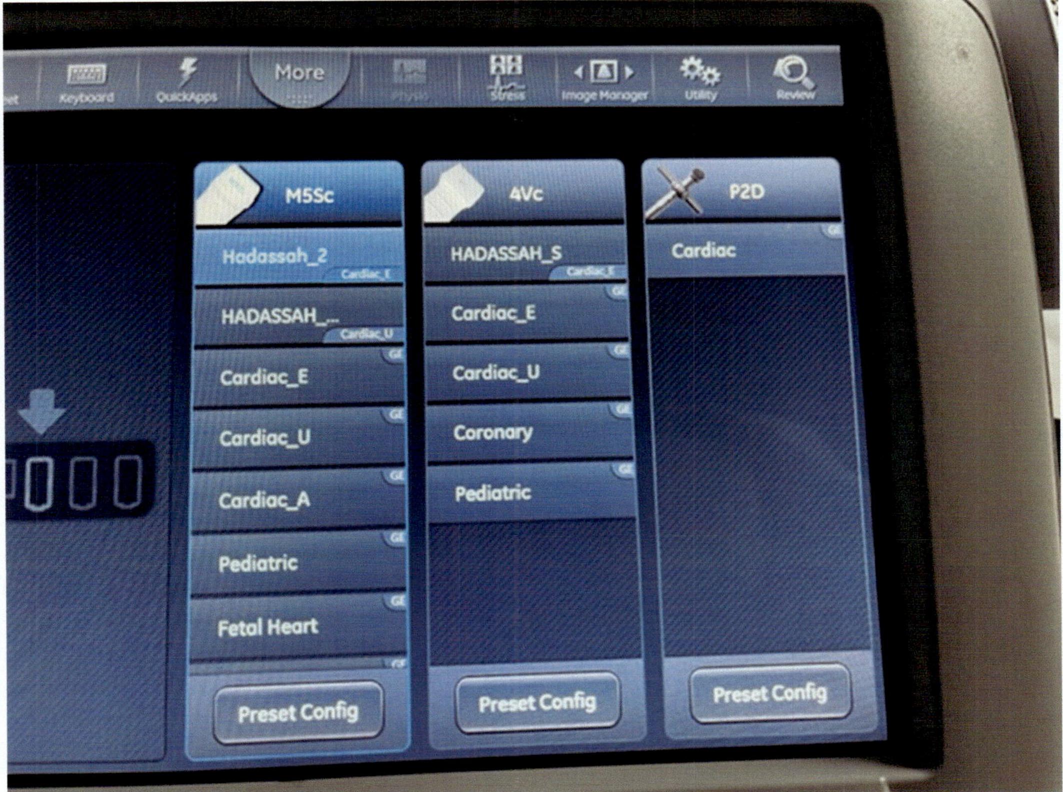

Fig. 13 Touchscreen on the echo machine showing the different probe options and the various presets for each probe. The appropriate probe and preset should be selected prior to beginning any study

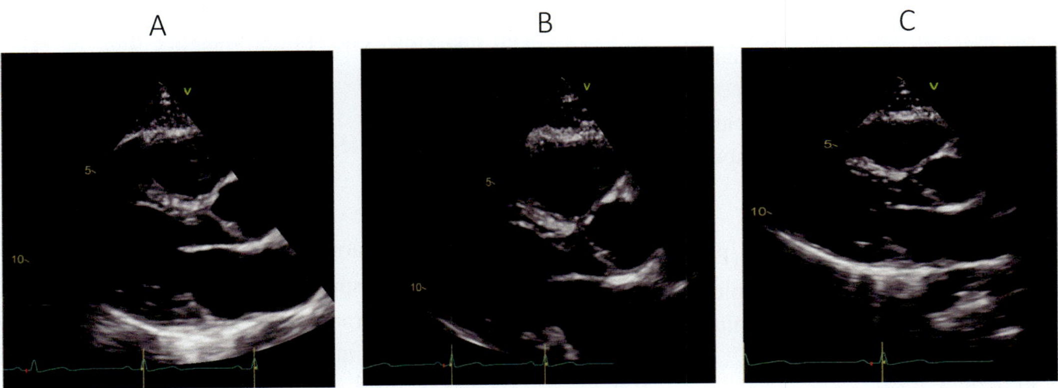

Fig. 14 Examples of proper depth (A), depth too large (B) as the image extends outside the screen and depth too small (C) as the image does not fill enough of the screen

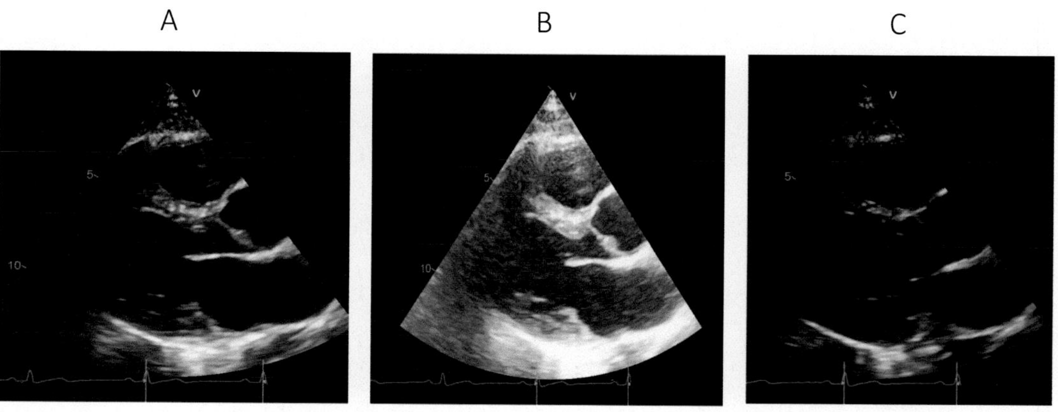

Fig. 15 Examples of optimal 2D gain setting (A), too high gain setting (B) and too low gain setting (C)

Using color Doppler

Step 1 Select the color Doppler button

Step 2 Adjust the region of interest to as to include only the anatomic areas relevant. For example, when evaluating mitral regurgitation, narrow the 2D image sector and place the color sample region over the mitral valve and left atrium only. This will maximize resolution.

Step 3 Adjust scale. This will generally be done automatically by the preset. The authors recommend a Nyquist limit of 55–64 cm/s.

Step 4 Adjust the color gain by increasing until speckles appear outside the region of interest and then slowly reducing until the speckles disappear (Fig. 16).

Using pulse wave Doppler (PW)

Step 1 Select the PW Doppler button

Step 2 Place the sample volume in the position of interest

Step 3 Adjust gain until a well-defined envelope with a lucent center is visible, baseline (either higher or lower depending on the specific measurement), scale, and sweep speed (Fig. 17).

Using continuous wave Doppler (CW)

Step 1 Select the CW Doppler button

Step 2 Place the cursor along the position of interest

Step 3 Adjust gain, baseline (either higher or lower depending on the specific measurement), scale, and sweep speed.

4 The Echocardiographic Views

Parasternal Long Axis, Left Heart

In this view, one should visualize the:

Left atrium

Mitral valve

Left ventricle-the anterior septum and inferolateral wall

Aortic valve

Ascending aorta

Pericardial space

The parasternal views are obtained by placing the transducer in the left parasternal area in the second or third intercostal space (Fig. 18). Care should be taken to avoid placement too medially (over the sternum) or laterally (over the breast tissue). The cursor of the transducer (Fig. 19) should be pointed in the direction of the subject's right shoulder. Initial imaging should focus on the plane of the mitral and aortic valves (Fig. 20).

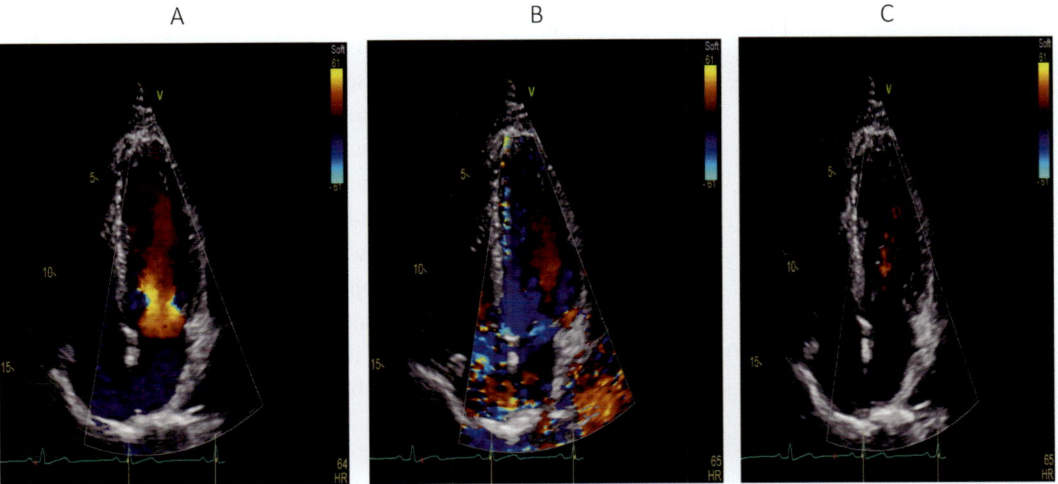

Fig. 16 Examples of optimal color gain (A), too high color gain (B) as speckling can be noted outside of the region of interest, and too low gain (C)

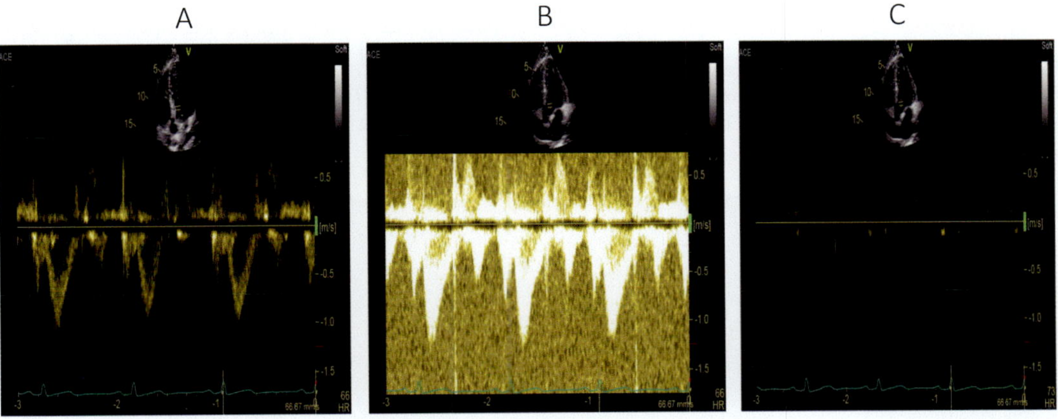

Fig. 17 Examples of optimal PW gain setting (A), too high gain setting (B) and too low gain setting (C)

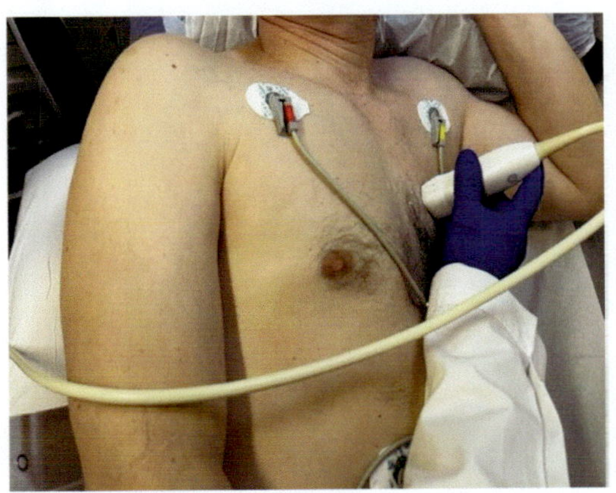

Fig. 18 Approximate position of the transducer on the chest wall for parasternal imaging

Parasternal Long Axis, Right Heart

Inflow view: Tricuspid valve and right atrium

Outflow view: Pulmonic valve and pulmonary artery

To obtain these views, the transducer should be tilted inferiorly (for inflow view) and then superiorly (for the outflow view) (Fig. 21).

Parasternal Short Axis

The main objective of this view is to adequately visualize the left ventricle to assess overall function and regional wall motion abnormalities.

In addition, the following structures may be imaged:

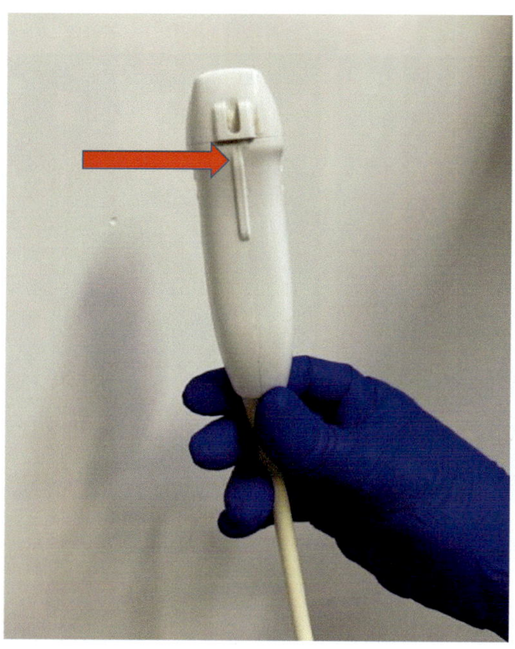

Fig. 19 Example of transducer cursor to guide imaging. For example, in parasternal long-axis view this cursor should be pointed in the direction of the subjects right shoulder

Aortic valve

Left atrium

Interatrial septum

Right atrium

Tricuspid valve

Pulmonic valve

Pulmonary artery

These views are obtained by rotating the transducer approximately 90 degrees from the parasternal long axis view so that the cursor is now directed to the subject's left shoulder. The transducer should be gradually angulated from a superior-medial position (to image the aortic, pulmonic and tricuspid valves) to an infero-lateral position tilting towards the apex to visualize regional left ventricular wall motion at the base, papillary muscle and apical levels. The operator may need to scan from a lower interspace to adequately image the apex. In general, the LV should have a circular shape, an elliptical shape usually reflects a tangential cut and should be adjusted as necessary (Fig. 22).

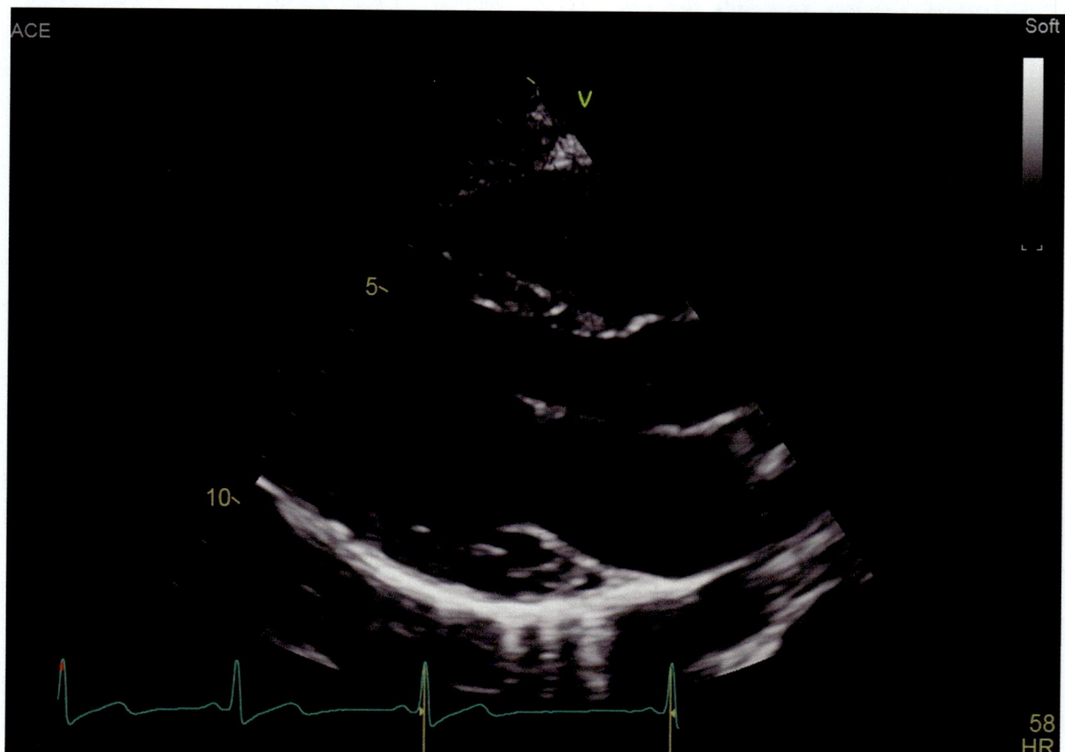

Fig. 20 Example of parasternal long axis image. Note the mitral and aortic valve leaflets are visible. The left ventricular apex is generally not imaged in this view

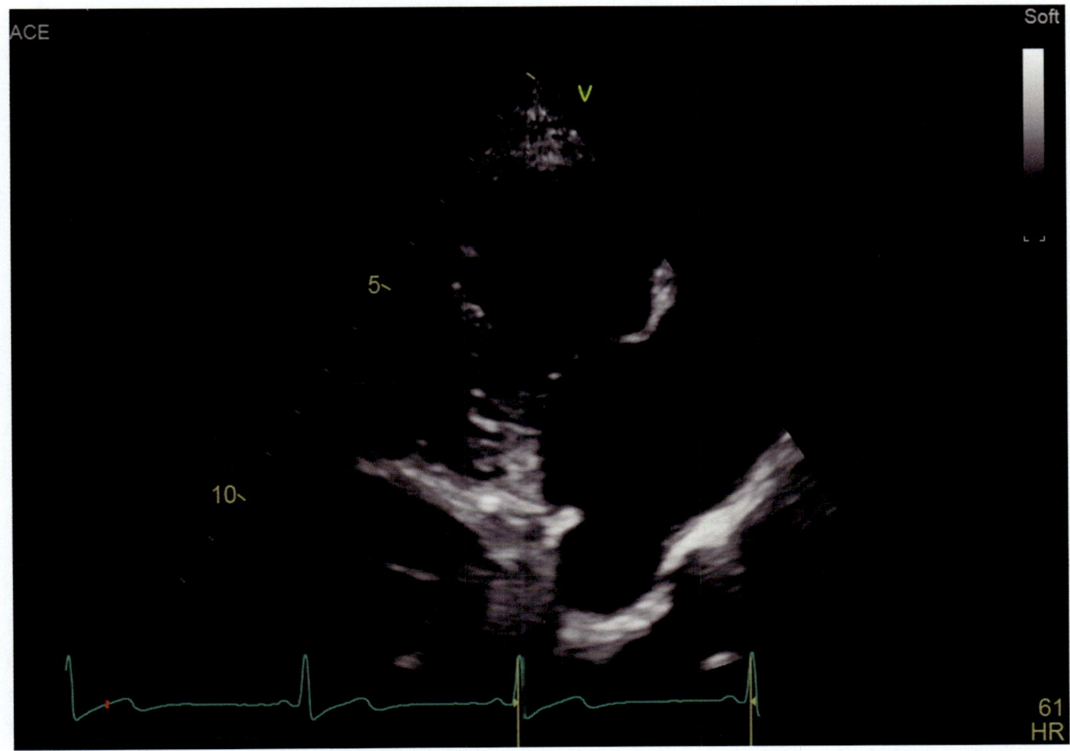

Fig. 21 Image of the right heart in parasternal long axis view obtained by tilting the transducer inferiorly

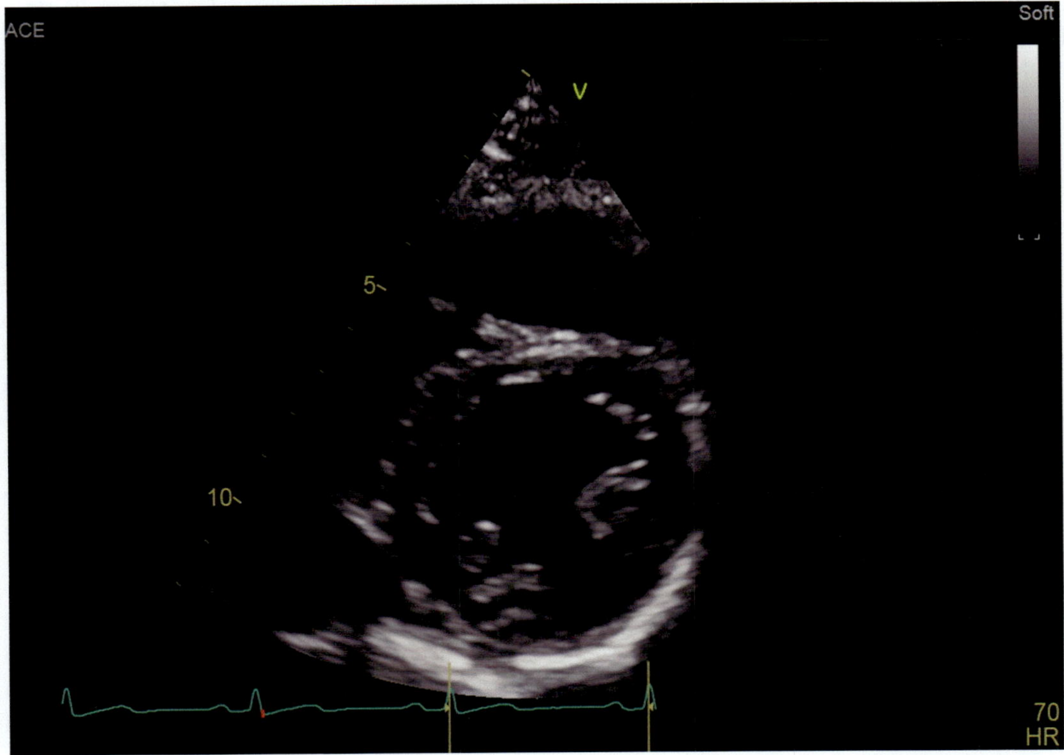

Fig. 22 Parasternal short axis view at papillary muscle level. Note the circular shape of the left ventricle

Apical 4/5 Chamber

The apical views are important to assess the LV and RV, valvular regurgitation/stenosis, diastolic dysfunction

Left ventricle (septal and lateral walls)

Right ventricle

Left/right atria

Interatrial/interventricular septum

Mitral valve/Tricuspid valve

Aortic valve/LVOT

Mitral valve inflow Doppler/Tissue Doppler of the basal septum and lateral wall (if utilizing a machine with these capabilities)

To obtain the apical views, the transducer is moved from the left parasternal space to the area of the maximal apical impulse which is usually slightly inferior and lateral to the left nipple (Fig. 23). It is important to angulate the transducer in direct apposition to the cardiac apex to avoid off-axis images. The transducer cursor should be directed laterally (to the patient's left). By convention in adult echocardiography the images are recorded with the apex at the top of the screen and with left ventricle on right side of the screen and the right ventricle on the left. In rare cases where the distinction between the LV and RV is unclear it should be noted that the insertion of the tricuspid septal leaflet is always apical to the insertion of the anterior mitral leaflet.

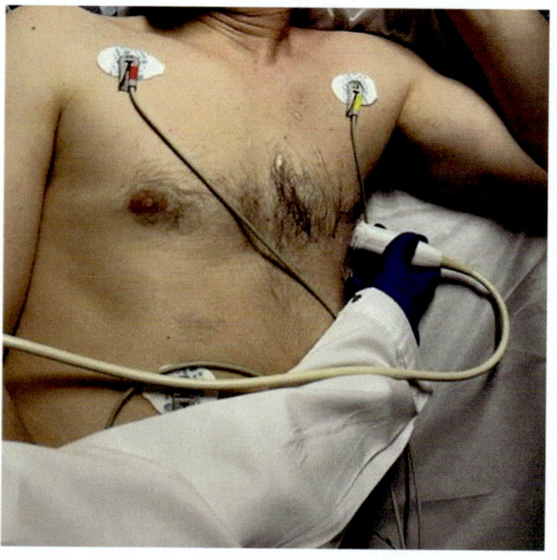

Fig. 23 Approximate position of the transducer on the chest wall for apical imaging

Once adequate 4 chamber imaging has been obtained, the transducer should be tilted slightly superiorly (tail of probe towards the patient's feet) to image the LV outflow tract and the aortic valve (5 chamber view) (Fig. 24).

Apical 2/3 Chamber

Left ventricle (anterior and inferior walls)

Left atrium

Mitral valve

Aortic valve/LVOT

These views are obtained from the apical 4 chamber view by rotating the transducer in a counter clockwise direction until the right ventricle disappears from the image (Fig. 25).

Subcostal View

This view utilizes the liver as an acoustic window and is most useful for the assessment of pericardial fluid and of the inferior vena cava (IVC) to evaluate central venous pressure. In patients with significant chronic lung disease or in intubated patients, it may be the only satisfactory imaging window available.

This view is most useful in imaging:

Pericardial space

Interatrial septum

Inferior vena cava (width and respiratory changes).

The subcostal view should be obtained with the patient supine and the knees bent. The transducer should be positioned underneath the xiphoid process with the cursor pointing laterally with gentle downward pressure applied on the transducer (Fig. 26). Generally an overhand grip on the probe is necessary. The plane of the heart is relatively superficial and care should be taken to avoid excessive tilting downwards. Once initial imaging of the cardiac chambers and the pericardial space in this view is complete, imaging of the IVC is performed (Fig. 27). The IVC is imaged by rotating the transducer counterclockwise until the IVC is imaged entering the right atrium. The IVC width at rest and with inspiration should be assessed 1–2 cm proximal to its entry into the right atrium. In spontaneously breathing patients with normal

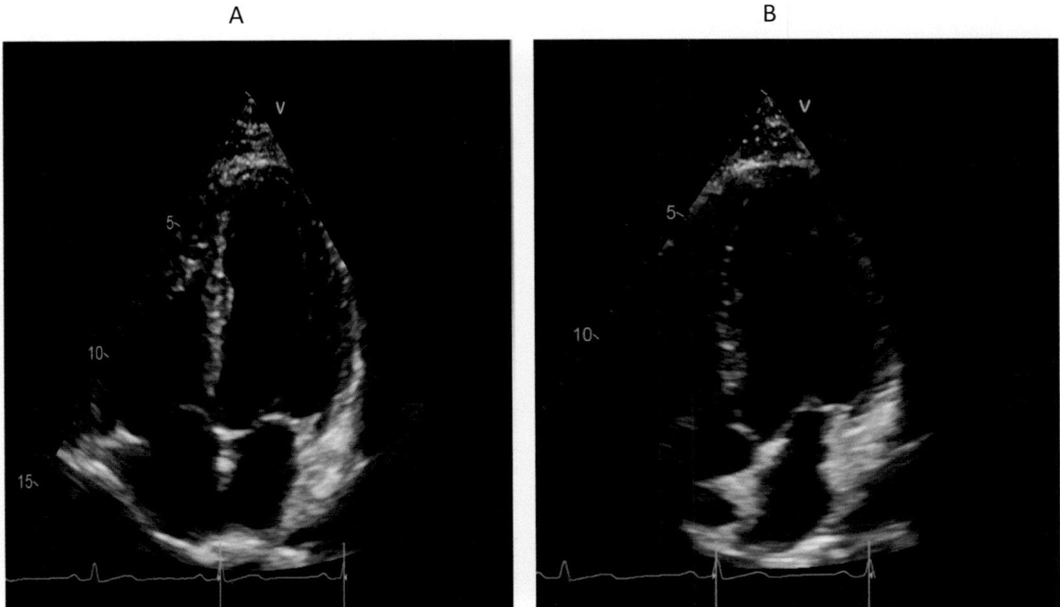

Fig. 24 Apical 4 chamber (A) and 5 chamber (B) images. Note the lack of foreshortening of the images

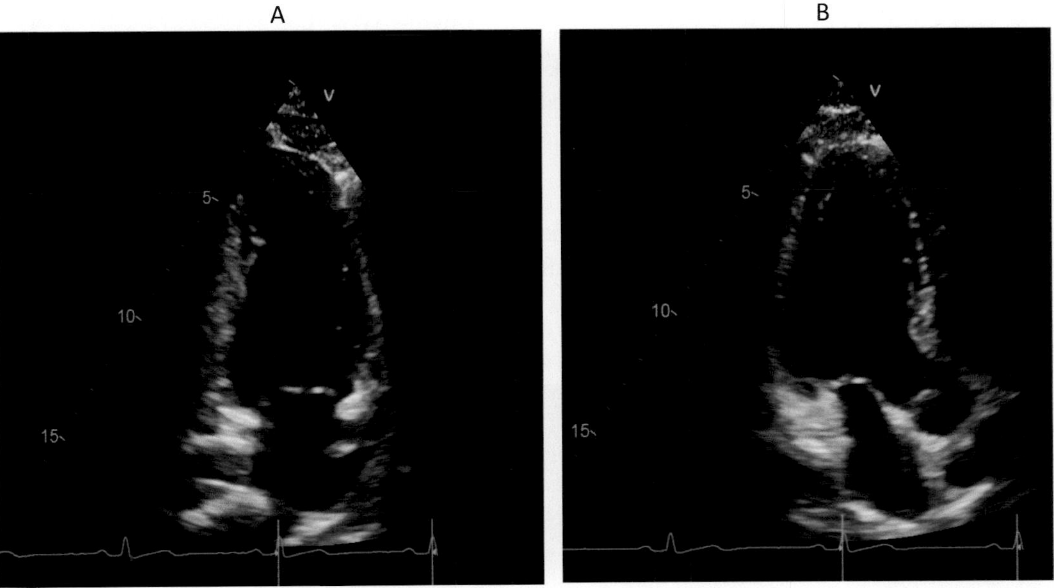

Fig. 25 Apical 2 chamber (A) and 3 chamber (B) images

central venous pressures, inspiration should cause increased venous return to the right heart and at least a 50% decrease in the width of the IVC. In ventilated patients, the positive pressure from the ventilator will cause the opposite effect.

Suprasternal View

This view allows visualization of the ascending aorta, the aortic arch and the descending thoracic aortic. It is important in cases of suspected aortic disease such as dissection.

This view is most useful in imaging:

Ascending aorta

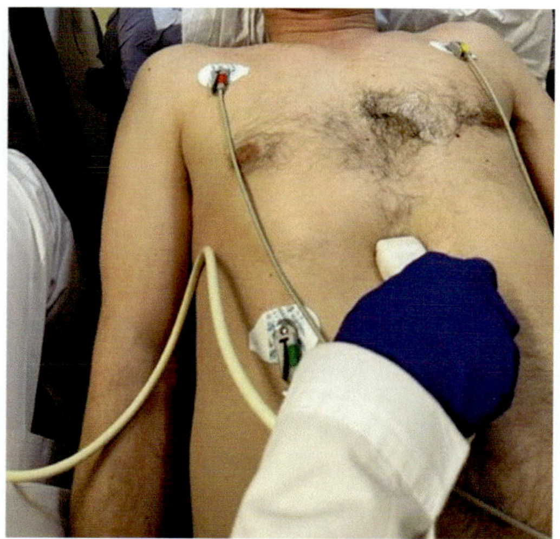

Fig. 26 Approximate position of the transducer for subcostal imaging. Note the superficial angulation of the transducer

Aortic arch

Origins of the great vessels

This view should be obtained with the patient lying supine with the head tilting slightly backwards (Fig. 28). The cursor should be pointed superiorly with gradual clockwise rotation.

Assessment of LV Systolic Function

Left ventricular ejection fraction (EF) is the accepted form for assessment of overall left ventricular systolic function. Ejection fraction is defined as a percentage using the formula: (End-Diastolic Volume) − (End-Systolic Volume)/End-Diastolic Volume × 100

The recommended method for calculating ejection fraction is the "biplane Simpson's method of disks." (1) Packages for this calculation exist in commercially available echocardiography systems and reporting systems. The left ventricle is traced in the apical 4 chamber and apical 2 chamber long axis views, in both diastole and systole, and end-diastolic volume and end-systolic volume are calculated (Fig. 29).

Grading ejection fraction:

Ejection fraction

Normal	≥ 50%
Mildly reduced	40–49%
Moderately reduced	30–39%
Severely reduced	< 30%

Alternatively, LV systolic function can be assessed visually and reported semi-quantitatively as normal, mildly, moderately, or severely reduced. This assessment should be performed using multiple echocardiographic views. Impaired function should be described as diffuse or global such as seen in dilated cardiomyopathy or regional with description of

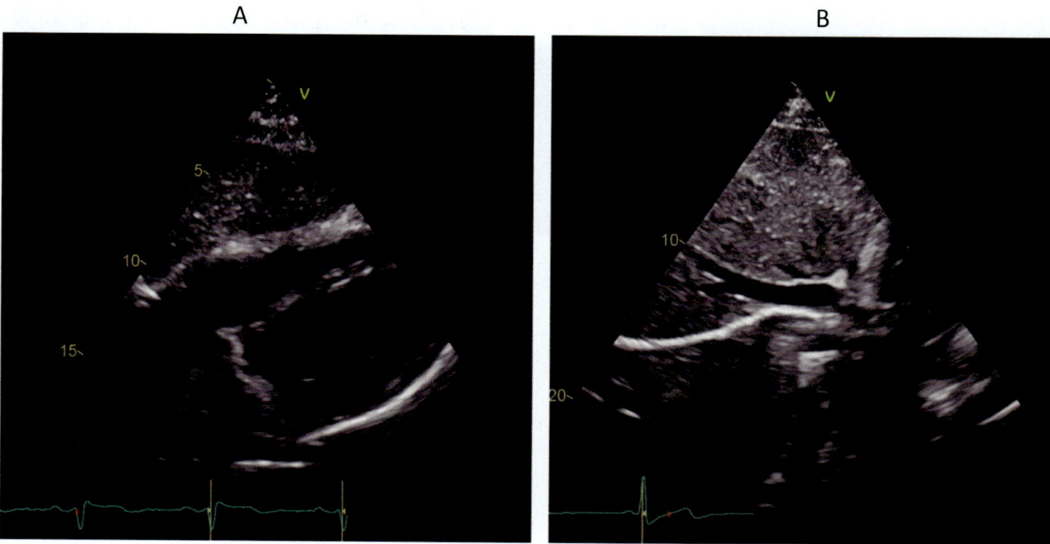

Fig. 27 Subcostal images of the cardiac chambers (A) and inferior vena cava (B)

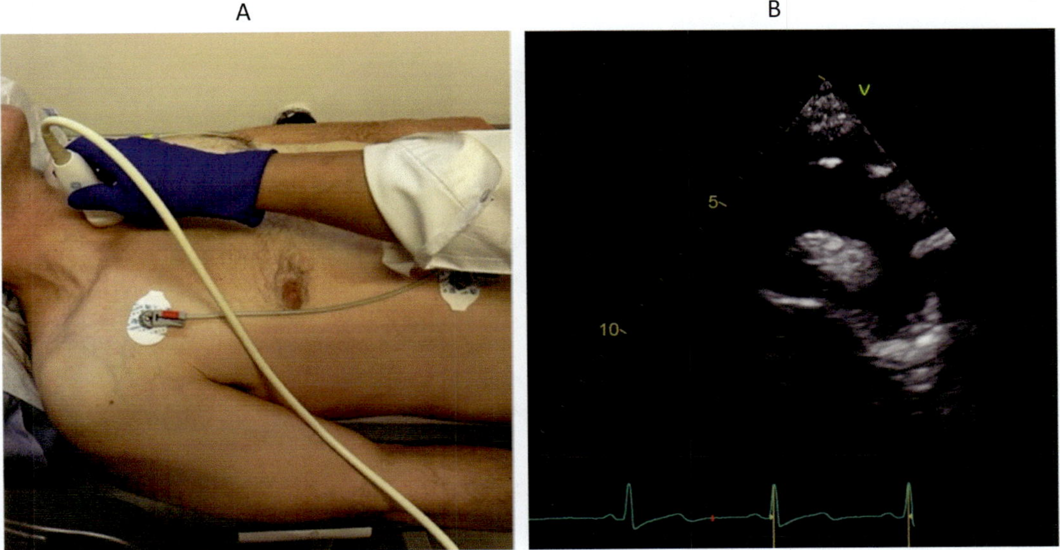

Fig. 28 Approximate position of the transducer for suprasternal imaging. (A) Suprasternal imaging showing the aortic arch and proximal great vessels (B)

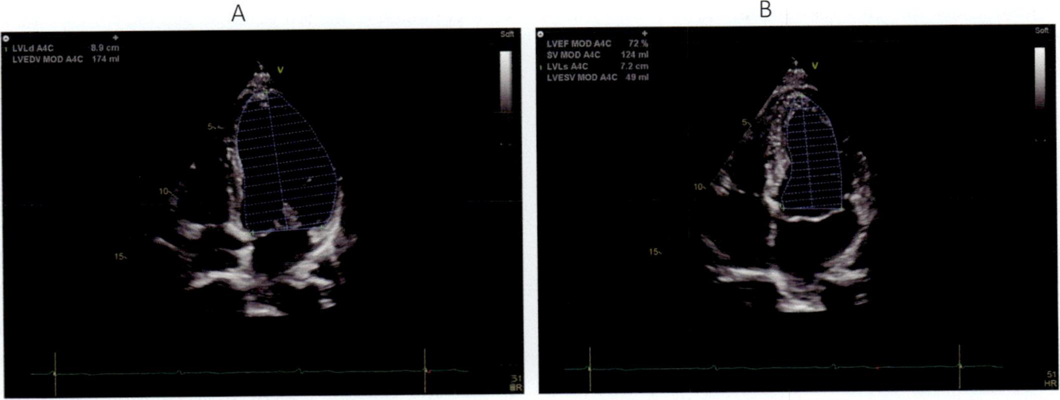

Fig. 29 Calculation of ejection fraction using the Simpson's formula in apical 4 chamber view at end-diastole (panel A) and end-systole (panel B)

regional wall motion abnormalities as in ischemic heart disease.

Assessment of LV Regional Wall Motion

Coronary artery disease leads to segmental ischemia and infarction which can be seen as abnormalities of motion of the left ventricular walls. (2) Significant disease in an epicardial coronary artery leads to a loss of contractile function in the myocardial segments supplied by that vessel. The magnitude and duration of the wall motion abnormalities depends on the severity, extent and duration of the coronary occlusion. The American Society of Echocardiography has adopted the 17 segment model for depiction of segmental wall motion (Fig. 30). Wall motion is traditionally described as normal, hypokinetic, akinetic, dyskinetic or aneurysmal. The wall motion score is an index of cardiac dysfunction wherein each visualized segment is given a score: 1 = normal; 2 = hypokinetic; 3 = akinetic; 4 = dyskinetic; 5 = aneurysmal. The

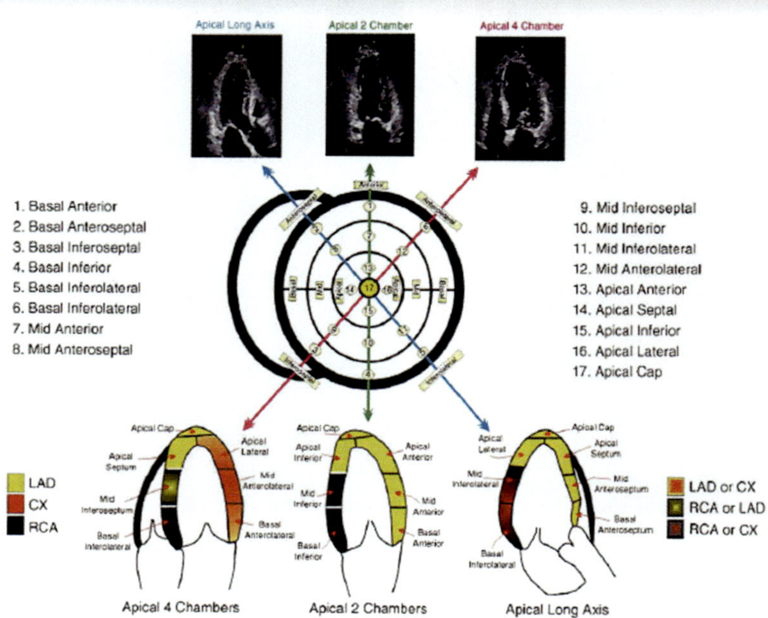

Fig. 30 Standard echocardiographic views showing segmental wall motion of the left ventricle and the corresponding distribution of coronary artery perfusion

score is the total of all scores divided by the number of segments. Care should be taken to assess wall thickening/endocardial motion rather than motion of the segment as a whole. Optimal visualization of endocardial borders is critical in assessment of regional wall motion. In the setting of left bundle branch block or post-operative paradoxical motion, the septum may move away from the center of the ventricle, but as it thickens normally, this should not be considered a hypokinetic segment. Similarly, akinetic or hypokinetic segments may be dragged by neighboring hypercontractile segments, leading to the appearance of motion, but without thickening. It is important to note that while regional wall motion abnormalities are usually due to coronary artery disease, other myocardial pathologies such as myocarditis or takutsubo syndrome can present with acute wall motion abnormalities.

Assessment of LV Filling Pressures and Diastolic Function

The assessment of diastolic function is an important part of the echocardiographic examination, in particular in patients with shortness of breath or heart failure. The assessment of left ventricular filling pressure and diastolic function is complex, however, a series of basic measurements can lead to a general assessment of these parameters.

First, in the apical 4 chamber view, the pulse Doppler sample volume should be placed at the tips of the open mitral leaflets in order to assess peak early diastolic flow (E wave) and peak late or atrial contraction velocity (A wave) (Fig. 7). In patients with significant tachycardia there may be fusion of the E and A waves. As the presence of an A wave is dependent on atrial contraction, this wave will not be present in patients with atrial fibrillation. Measurements should be performed on three consecutive beats. Measurements of mitral inflow velocities are very dependent on hemodynamic loading conditions and must be supplemented by measurements of myocardial tissue velocities of the mitral annulus. These are performed by placing the Doppler sample volume on the lateral aspect of the mitral valve annulus and switching filters from PW to TDI imaging (Fig. 9). As with mitral inflow, three consecutive measurements should be performed. The presence of significant mitral annular calcification or a mitral valve prosthesis may affect diagnostic accuracy. The ratio of mitral inflow E wave divided by the average of the medial and lateral annular velocity e' waves provides a rough estimate of LV filling pressures with values over 13 generally being associated with elevated LV filling pressures. In addition to this somewhat non-specific hemodynamic finding, significant diastolic dysfunction may be associated with structural changes such as LV hypertrophy and left atrial dilatation as well as pulmonary hypertension.

Assessment of Right Ventricular Function

The right ventricle is the most anteriorly situated cardiac chamber located immediately behind the sternum. Echocardiographic assessment of RV function is challenging given the crescent-shaped geometry of the RV. In addition, the heavily trabeculated myocardium limits the delineation of the RV endocardial surface. Most of the RV contraction occurs longitudinally from base to apex along with radial thickening/inward motion. To accurately assess RV structure and function a complete set of standardized views should be obtained including the parasternal long-axis, parasternal RV inflow, apical 4-chamber, right ventricle–focused apical 4-chamber, and subcostal views.

RV size is best assessed from the apical four-chamber view at end-diastole and should appear about two-thirds of the width of the LV on qualitative assessment. To best assess RV function the right ventricular chamber focused view enables the most accurate assessment of RV function although RV size may be overestimated.

To obtain this view the transducer should be moved slightly laterally with mild rotation to maximize the diameter of the RV base. RV systolic function can be assessed by measuring fractional area change (FAC) from the apical 4 chamber view. FAC is the percent change in RV area from diastole to systole. [(end-diastolic RV area − end-systolic RV area)/end-diastolic RV area] × 100. Another relatively simple method to assess RV function is measuring tricuspid annulus systolic plane excursion (TAPSE). TAPSE is assessed in an apical four-chamber view by placing the M-mode cursor on the lateral tricuspid annulus. Maximum systolic excursion of the lateral annulus along its longitudinal plane toward the apex is then recorded and measured (Fig. 31).

In the setting of acute pulmonary embolism a regional pattern of RV dysfunction has been described with akinesis of the RV free wall but normal or even hyperdynamic function of the apex. If noted, this pattern is highly suggestive of the diagnosis of acute pulmonary embolus.

Assessment of Pulmonary Hypertension

The peak velocity of the tricuspid regurgitant jet should be measured in multiple views (primarily apical 4 chamber and parasternal long axis inlet views) to determine the peak gradient across the tricuspid valve utilizing the Bernoulli equation as described above (Fig. 32). Assuming that right atrial pressure is equal to the RV diastolic pressure, adding right atrial pressure to the gradient provides the right ventricular peak systolic pressure. Assuming there is no pulmonic stenosis, PA systolic pressure is assumed to be identical to right ventricular systolic pressure. In the setting of "free" tricuspid regurgitation with non restricted flow between the right atrium and right ventricle, peak regurgitant velocities are very low, as there is near equalization of pressure between atrium and ventricle, and the TR velocity may understate the severity of pulmonary hypertension. Right atrial pressure may be estimated in most instances from the subcostal view based on the size of the inferior vena cava and the degree of collapse of the inferior vena

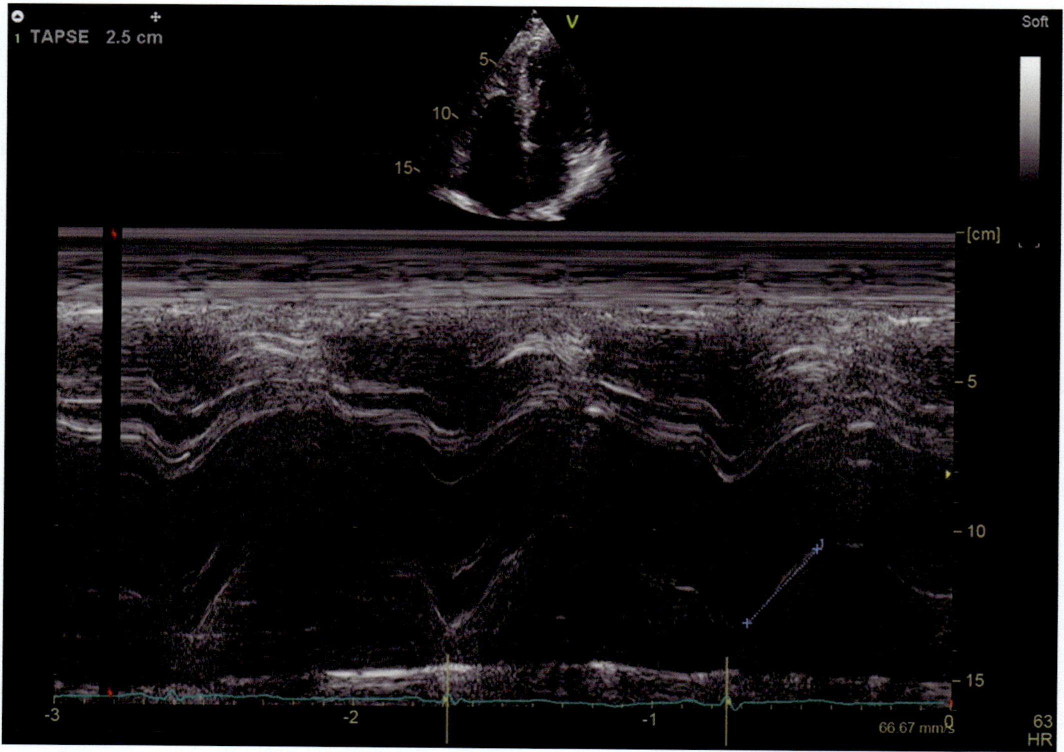

Fig. 31 Example of TAPSE with a m-mode cursor placed through the lateral tricuspid valve annulus in the apical 4 chamber view

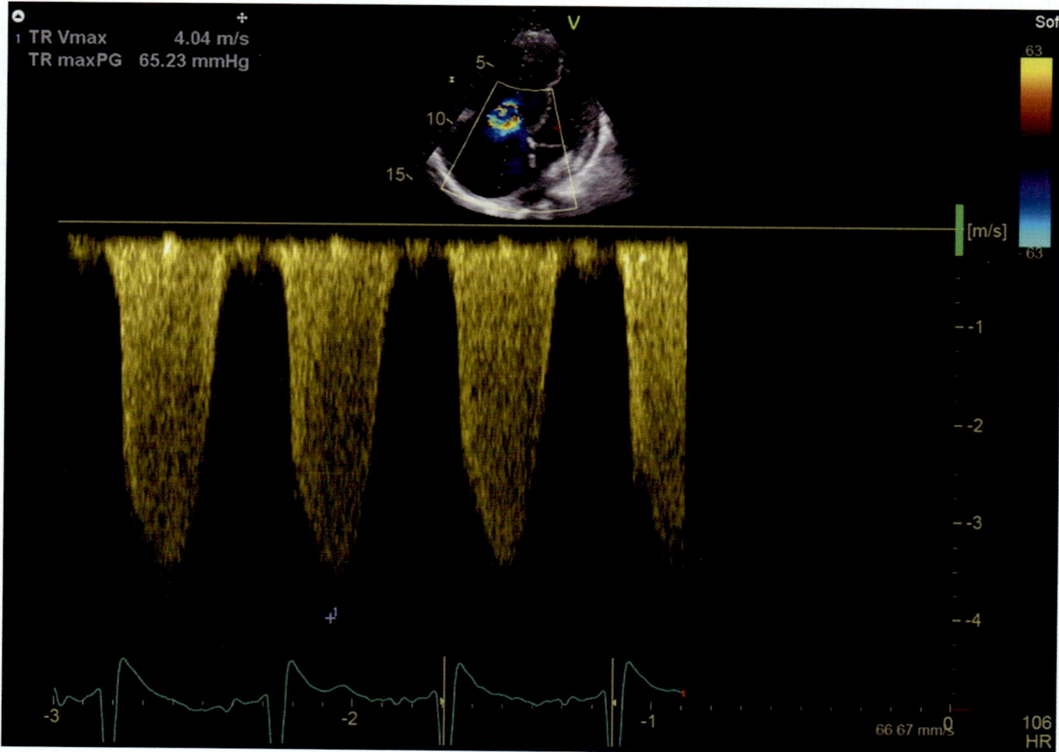

Fig. 32 Continuous wave Doppler of the jet of tricuspid regurgitation showing calculation of RV-RA pressure gradient

cava collapse with inspiration as described earlier.

Assessment of Pericardial Effusions and Cardiac Tamponade

Assessment of pericardial fluid is one of the common reasons for performing emergent, focused echocardiography. The exam should first evaluate anatomically the location and severity of the pericardial effusion and then assess the hemodynamic significance of the fluid.

2D Imaging

Image from all views to assess the amount of fluid anteriorly and posteriorly around heart. The subcostal view is particularly important given the acoustic window provided by the liver in this view (Fig. 33, panel A). Measure the diameter of the effusion at end diastole anteriorly and posteriorly in the parasternal and subcostal views.

Hemodynamic evaluation of tamponade physiology by echocardiography

Tamponade physiology occurs when the pressure in the pericardial space exceeds the pressure within the cardiac chambers, leading to decreased cardiac filling, and decreased cardiac output. As the right atrial pressure is usually lowest, prolonged collapse or inversion of the right atrium is the most sensitive (but least specific) sign, followed by right ventricular collapse during diastole. Left atrial or left ventricular collapse are rare but highly specific for tamponade physiology. These occur most frequently with loculated pericardial effusions for example following cardiac surgery that exert pressure specifically on those chambers.

1. Evaluate right atrium for signs of collapse. The subcostal and apical views are the best. M-mode assists in the assessment of timing. Right atrial collapse is defined as inversion of the atrium for more than 30% of the cardiac cycle. Collapse normally begins at end-diastole, and persists into systole. This is a highly sensitive but less specific sign of tamponade physiology.

2. Evaluate right ventricle for evidence of diastolic collapse (Fig. 33, panel B). It may be useful to place the M-mode cursor through the right ventricle in the parasternal long axis and subcostal views to assist in the assessment of timing. Any inversion in the setting of an open mitral valve is consistent

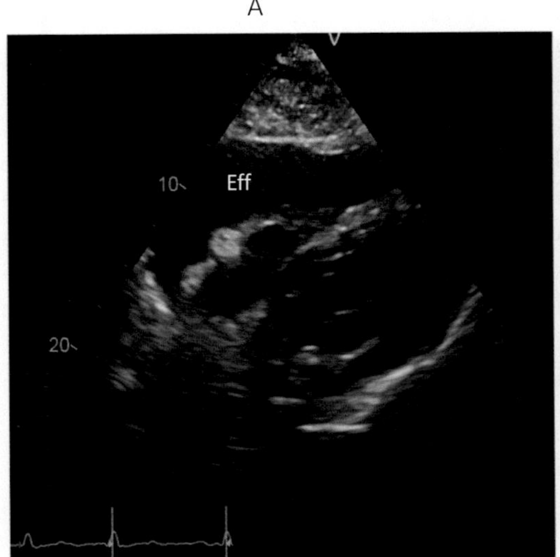
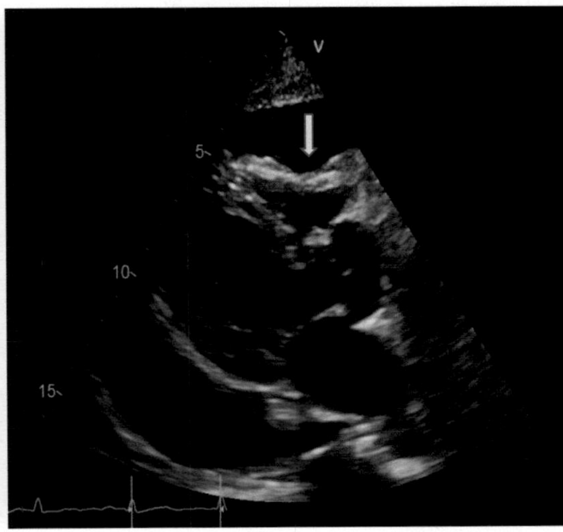

Fig. 33 Subcostal view showing echo free space between the liver and the right ventricular wall consistent with pericardial effusion (panel A, Eff). In parasternal long-axis view invagination of the RV free wall in diastole consistent with diastolic collapse is noted (panel B, yellow arrow)

with collapse. This sign is very specific but less sensitive for tamponade physiology

3. Assess the inferior vena cava. A dilated IVC (> 2.1 cm) with lack of collapse during inspiration is suggestive of elevated right sided pressures which in the presence of pericardial fluid supports tamponade physiology.

Doppler imaging and measurement: Perform pulse Doppler of MV and TV inflow velocities recorded at 25 cm/s speed to assess for e wave velocity changes during respiration. Respiratory variation of greater than 60% across the tricuspid or 30% across the aortic or mitral is suggestive of tamponade physiology. This sign is highly sensitive, but not specific, and can be seen in the setting of respiratory distress from pulmonary causes.

Two important notes: 1. The hemodynamic effects of pericardial effusion are independent of its size. Even a small effusion which accumulates quickly can cause tamponade physiology.

2. Cardiac tamponade is a clinical and not echocardiographic diagnosis and the absence of the signs described above do not rule out the presence of cardiac tamponade. Conversely the signs described may be present in a clinically stable or even asymptomatic patient.

Cardiac output

Noninvasive Doppler measurement of stroke volume can be made through the left or right ventricular outflow tracts by measuring the time velocity integral using pulsed wave Doppler at that orifice, which is a measure of flow, and multiplying by the cross-sectional area of the outflow tract (Fig. 34). This can only be used to measure stroke volume if there is not significant regurgitation across the orifice, and if the patient is in a regular rhythm. The cross sectional area is estimated by measuring the diameter at the level of the annulus, and, assuming circular symmetry, using the equation cross-sectional area = πr^2, whereas r = diameter/2, or 0.785* (diameter)^2 and multiplying

by the time-velocity integral derived from pulsed Doppler tracings with the sample volume also at the valve annulus. In the absence of significant mitral regurgitation, stroke volume can also be estimated by the modified Simpson method, by subtracting LV volume at end systole from that at end diastole. If one multiplies stroke volume by heart rate, one obtains the cardiac output.

5 Evaluation of Common Valvular Heart Disease

Aortic Stenosis

Make sure to

(a) Measure peak and mean pressure gradients
(b) Calculate aortic valve area (AVA) using continuity equation
(c) Correlate measurements with 2D appearance of the aortic valve.

2D Imaging

Carefully image the valve in the parasternal long axis and short axis views, so as to determine the number of leaflets, the extent of calcification, and the degree of restriction of leaflet motion (Fig. 35). The bicuspid valve exhibits doming and asymmetric closure in the long axis view, and a fish-mouth opening in the short axis view. Frequently there are 3 sinuses, even if the valve is bicuspid, and a pseudoraphae can mimic a commisure. In rheumatic aortic stenosis, there is commissural fusion with scarring and calcification. In degenerative stenosis, there is diffuse calcification and restriction of all leaflets. If imaging quality permits, aortic valve area can be planimetered in the short axis view.

2D Measurements

The left ventricular outflow tract should be measured in the parasternal long axis view, at high magnification adjacent to the aortic valve

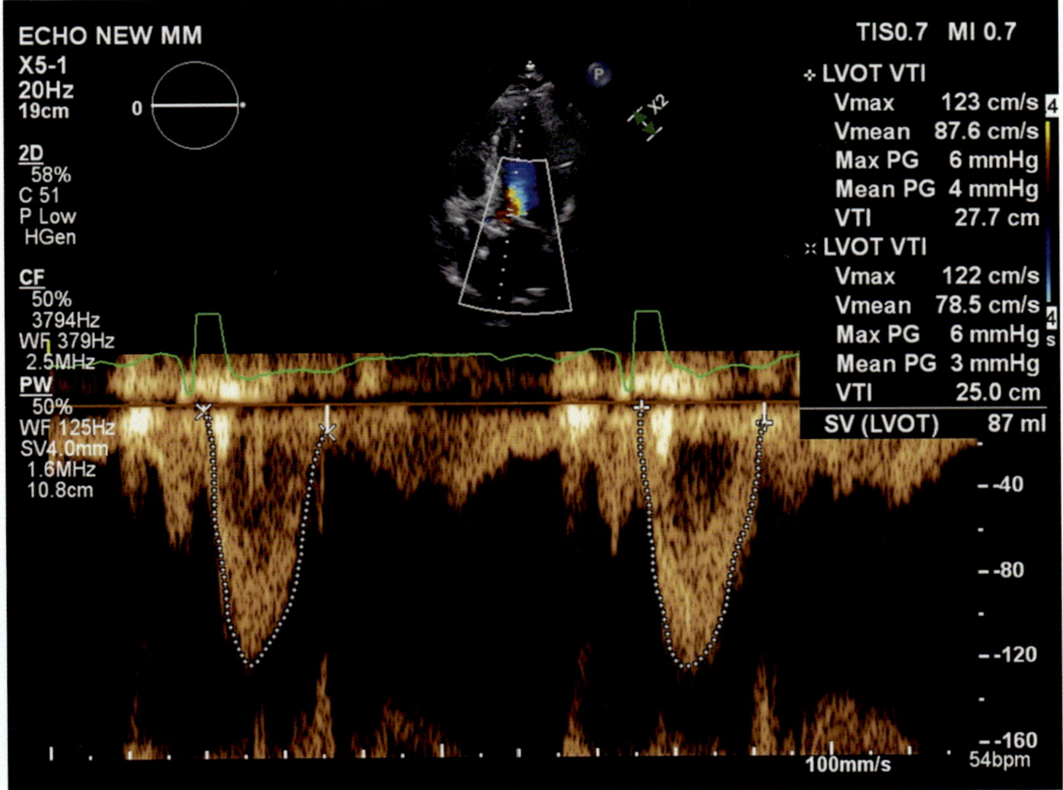

Fig. 34 Demonstration of calculation of LV stroke volume using pulse wave Doppler placed in the LVOT in apical 5 chamber view

annulus. It is usually between 1.8 and 2.2 cm. An underestimation of LVOT diameter will lead to significant underestimation of aortic valve area.

Doppler Measurements

Peak and mean gradients across the aortic valve should be obtained utilizing continuous wave Doppler generally from apical views (Fig. 36).

Time velocity integral should be measured in the left ventricular outflow tract utilizing pulse wave Doppler, in the apical 5 or apical 3 chamber view (whichever is higher). The cursor should be placed as close to the aortic valve as possible, as long as a smooth profile is present.

Calculations

The continuity equation is used to estimate the aortic valve area. The continuity equation is based on the conservation of mass, which requires that within a closed system, the amount of fluid (or flow) going through the different segments of the system must be the same. Thus, the stroke volume going through the left ventricular outflow tract must be the same as the stroke volume going through the narrowest part of the valve. In order to achieve that, the flow through the narrowest portion is significantly faster than the flow in the wider portions. Thus:

$$\text{LVOT flow} * \text{LVOT area} = \text{Aortic Valve flow} * \text{Aortic valve area}$$

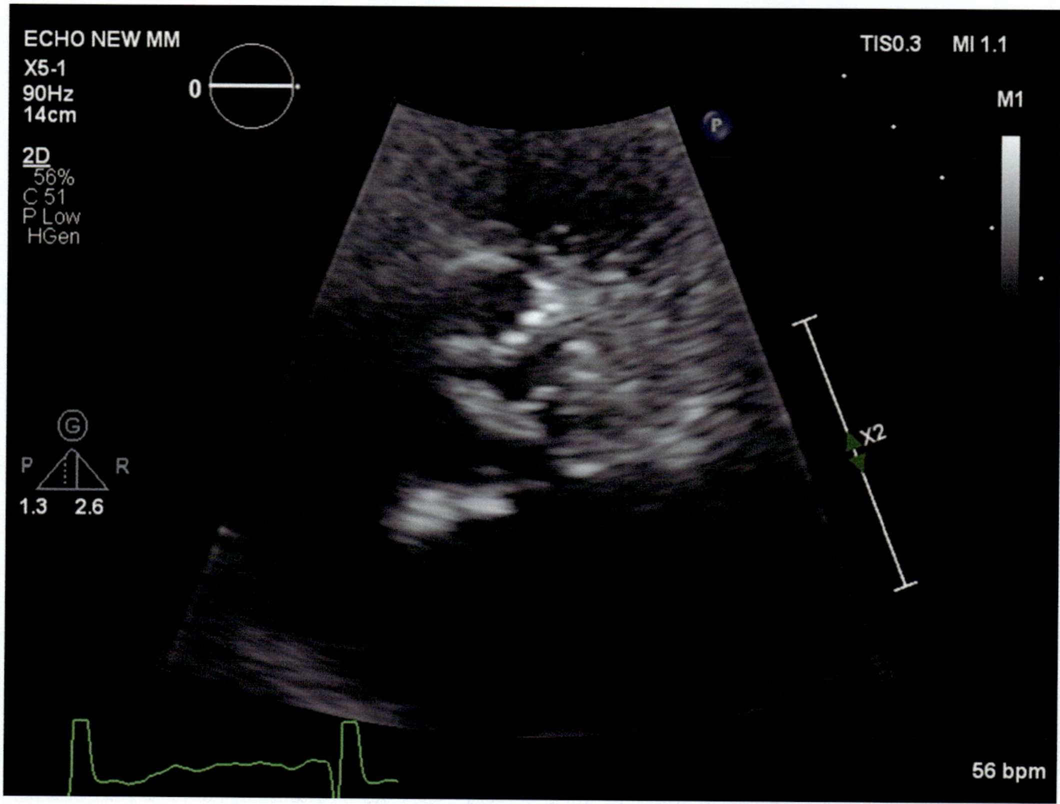

Fig. 35 Parasternal short axis view showing diffuse thickening and calcification of the aortic valve

Rearranging this equation, Aortic valve area $= (\text{LVOT flow} * \text{LVOT area}) / \text{Aortic valve flow}$.

LVOT flow = The time − velocity integral across the left ventricular outflow tract (measured from pulse Doppler)

$$\text{LVOT area} = \pi * (\text{LVOT diameter}/2)^2$$

Aortic valve flow = time velocity integral across the aortic valve (measured from the continuous wave Doppler across the aortic valve.)

Grading aortic stenosis: Native valve (3)

	Peak gradient (mmHg)	Mean gradient (mmHg)	Valve area (cm^2)
Normal	< 8		> 2
Mild	< 36	< 25	> 1.5
Moderate	36–64	25–40	1.0–1.5
Severe	> 64	> 40	< 1.0 (index < 0.6/m^2)

In the setting of low cardiac output, the valve gradients may underestimate the degree of aortic stenosis.

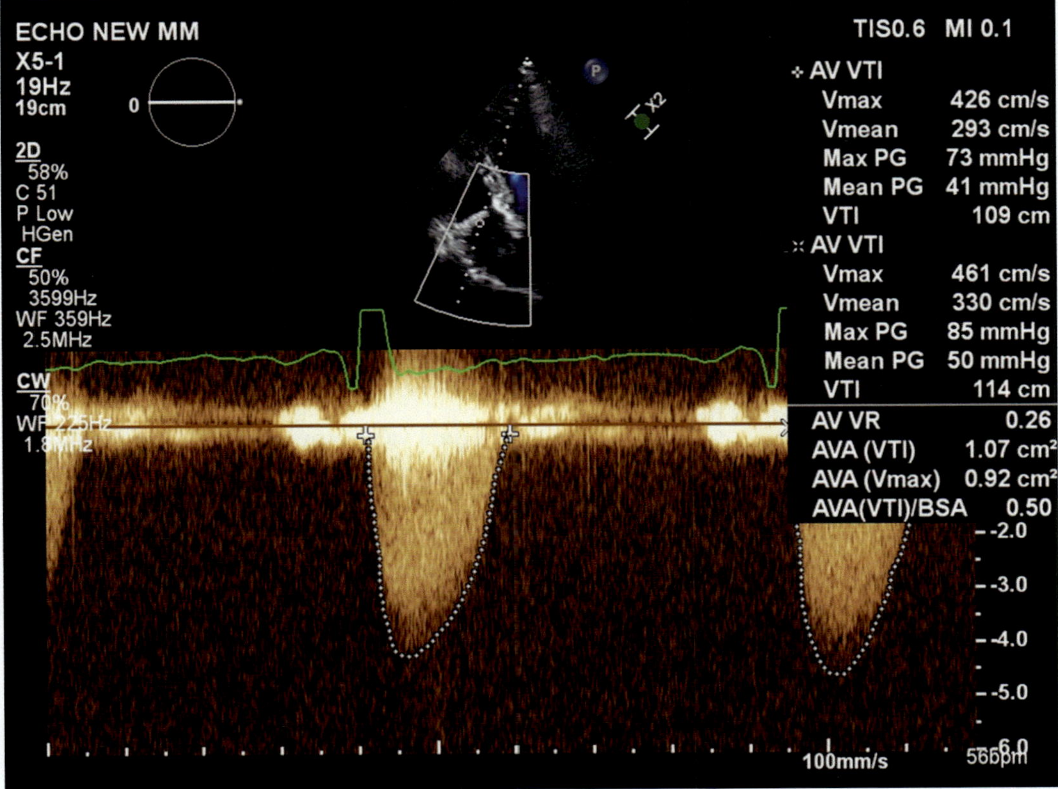

Fig. 36 Continuous wave Doppler over the aortic valve in apical 5 chamber view showing calculation of RV-RA pressure gradient

Note: *the calculated valve area should correlate with the visual estimate of valve opening.* Underestimation of the LVOT diameter will lead to a significant underestimation of valve area, and should be reviewed when the calculated valve area is less than would be expected. Similarly, if the pulse Doppler measurement is taken above the actual left ventricular outflow tract, a low velocity may also lead to an artificially low valve area calculation. There is also a phenomenon described as "pressure recovery", wherein a small (< 3.0 cm) stiff aorta may magnify the measured peak velocity, but the measurement does not reflect the hemodynamic stress on the heart.

Mitral stenosis

Make sure to

(a) Planimeter the mitral valve area
(b) Obtain the pressure half time across the mitral valve
(c) Measure peak and mean MV pressure gradients
(d) Determine if rheumatic deformity is present
(e) Correlate measurements with the 2D appearance of the valve.

2D imaging

Careful imaging of the mitral valve (primarily in the parasternal long axis view) to assess for rheumatic changes. One should assess the morphological appearance of the MV apparatus, including leaflet mobility and flexibility, leaflet thickness, leaflet calcification, subvalvular fusion, and the appearance of commissures.

2D measurement

Planimeter the mitral valve area at the tips of the MV leaflets. Sweep down to chordal level then up just into the MV leaflets to find the smallest mitral orifice for planimetry.

Doppler measurement

- Place the continuous wave Doppler across the MV from apical view, and measure the pressure half time. The pressure half time is the amount of time it takes for the LA-LV pressure gradient to be reduced by half during diastole. (note, this is not the *gradient* half time, but the *pressure* half time) The longer the pressure half time, the smaller the mitral valve orifice (Fig. 37).

CW Doppler across the MV from apical view and trace for peak and mean pressure gradients. If the patient is in atrial fibrillation average 5–10 beats.

- Mitral valve area is calculated by the pressure half time formula as

Calculations $\boxed{\text{MVA} = 220/\text{PHT}}$

This formula was empirically derived, and should not be used when there is moderate or

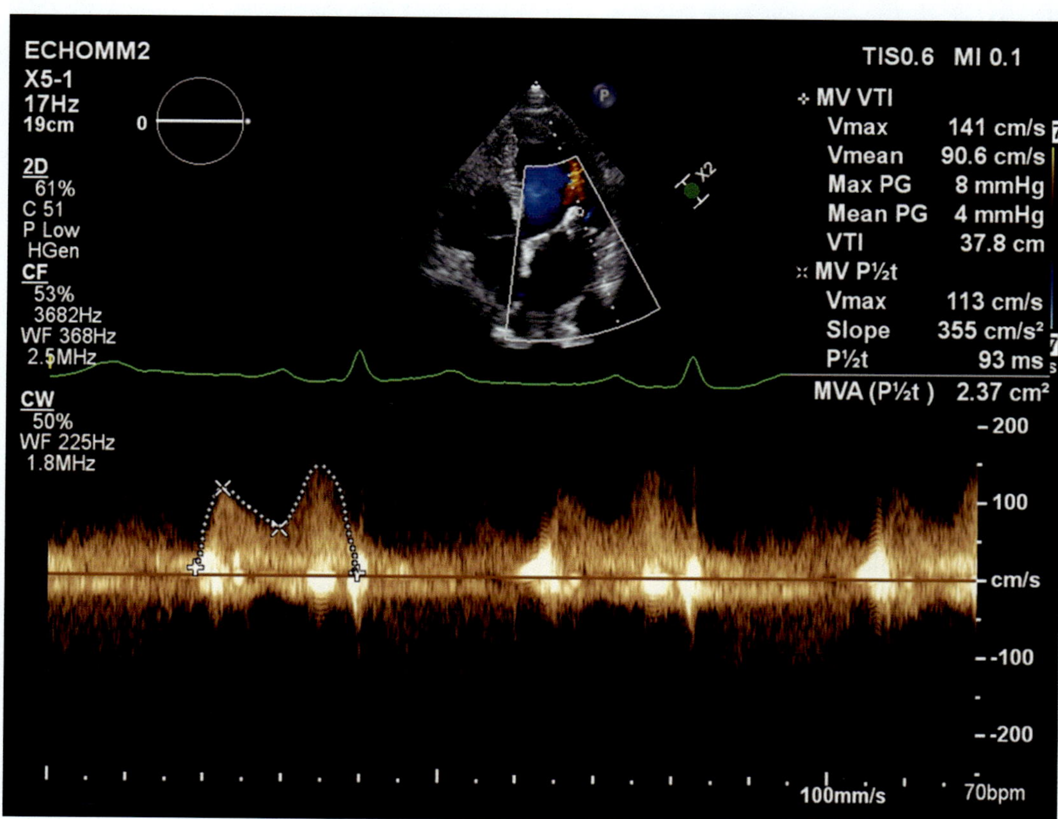

Fig. 37 Continuous wave Doppler over the mitral valve in apical 4 chamber view showing calculation of mitral valve gradient and pressure halftime

severe aortic regurgitation, or within 48 hours of balloon valvuloplasty. Abnormalities of LA or LV compliance may also adversely affect the calculation of mitral valve area.

Grading mitral stenosis (native valve)

	Mean gradient (mmHg)	Valve area (cm^2)
Normal	< 2	> 4
Mild	< 5	2.0–3.0
Moderate	5–10	1.5–2.0
Severe	> 10	< 1.5

Mitral Regurgitation

Make sure to

1. Assess the morphology of the mitral leaflets and mitral apparatus
2. Assess regurgitation in multiple views
3. Measure the vena contracta
4. Doppler the pulmonary veins
5. Assess pulmonary artery pressure
6. Assess LV size and function.

The assessment of the severity of mitral regurgitation requires multiple components, including (a) the evaluation of the structure of the MV and its supporting structures (b) color flow Doppler, (c) MV inflow and regurgitant velocities (d) indirect signs of severe MR such as increased LA size and hyperdynamic or decreased LV function.

2D imaging

Mitral regurgitation can be caused by abnormalities of the valve leaflets themselves (primary or organic MR) or by geometric changes in surrounding structures such as the left ventricle (secondary or functional MR). The mitral leaflets should be evaluated for abnormalities such as prolapse, and the systolic and diastolic excursion of each leaflet should be assessed. In secondary MR the leaflets may be tented or tethered leading to central malcoaptation. Myocardial remodeling

beneath just one of the papillary muscles may lead to restriction of one leaflet, with malcoaptation and eccentric mitral regurgitation.

Doppler imaging and measurement

(a) Color Doppler should be done in all views looking for eccentric jets and jet width. Jet area may be planimetered if the jet is central.

(b) Pulse Doppler flow in the pulmonary veins to assess for flow reversal in systole

(c) Measure the vena contracta of the MR jet in orthogonal planes. Vena contracta width $\geq$ 7 mm is suggestive of severe MR.

What is the vena contracta?

The vena contracta is the smallest, highest velocity region of a flow jet and is typically located at or just downstream from the regurgitant orifice (Fig. 38). Vena contracta should be measured in a long axis view, prefererably perpendicular to the flow of the jet. In mitral regurgitation, a vena contracta of 7 mm or above is consistent with severe mitral regurgitation.

Overall assessment

There is a poor correlation between jet area and severity of MR due to technical and hemodynamic factors, and jet area alone should not be used to determine the severity of MR. Central jets may appear larger but be of little hemodynamic significance, whereas a wall jet may appear smaller

The following table can be used to assist in determining the severity of mitral regurgitation:

	Vena contracta (mm)	Jet area (cm^2)
Mild	< 4	> 4
Moderate	4–6	4–6 mod 6–8 mod-severe
Severe	$\geq$ 7	< 8

SUMMARY: Integration of multiple parameters, including valve anatomy, left atrial and left ventricular size, the appearance, size, location,

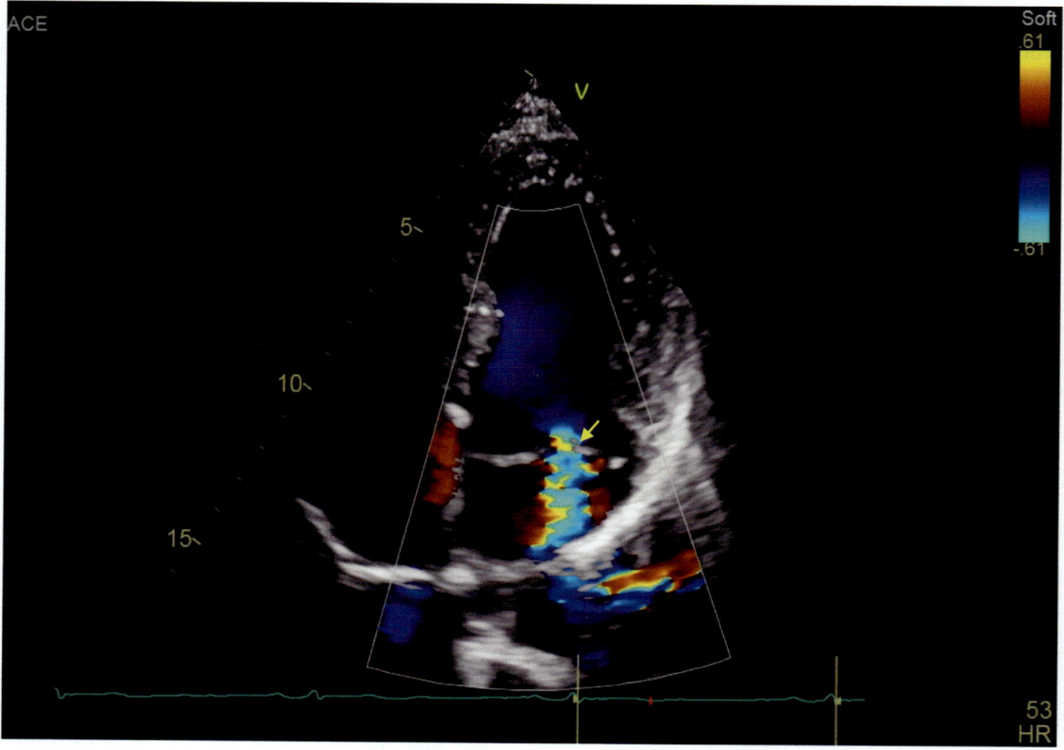

Fig. 38 Apical 4 chamber view showing color flow jet over the mitral valve with area of vena contracta indicated (yellow arrow)

intensity and timing of the jet, vena contracta width, quantitation of regurgitant volume and fraction, pulmonary artery pressure and flow reversal in the pulmonary vein, are all important for accurate assessment of MR severity.

Aortic Regurgitation

Make sure to

1. Assess the morphology of the aortic leaflets and ascending aorta
2. Assess regurgitation in multiple views
3. Measure the jet height to LVOT ratio
4. Measure the vena contracta
5. Continuous wave across the aortic regurgitant jet, with measurement of deceleration time.
6. Assess LV size and function.

2D Imaging

Carefully examine the aortic valve and the proximal ascending aorta in the parasternal long axis view. The aorta should be measured at the level of the sinuses of Valsalva, the sinotubular junction, and the ascending aorta, as frequently aortic dilatation can lead to malcoaptation of leaflets. In the short axis view, assess the number of aortic valve leaflets, the degree of thickening, calcification and restriction, and the nature of coaptation. LV internal diameter should be measured during systole and diastole, as severe aortic regurgitation is accompanied by ventricular dilatation, and LV size is critical in the decision to pursue surgical repair.

Doppler imaging and measurement

Color flow mapping should be performed in the parasternal long axis, parasternal short axis, and the apical 5 chamber and apical 3 chamber views.

One should assess the width of the jet and the depth of penetration into the left ventricle. Continuous wave Doppler of the regurgitant jet should be performed. A pulse Doppler should be placed in the proximal descending thoracic aorta and abdominal aorta, to assess the degree of flow reversal during diastole.

Quantification:

A: The most robust method of quantification of aortic regurgitation is the **jet height ratio**:

In the parasternal long axis view (with magnification to improve accuracy) measure the height of the regurgitant jet in mid diastole, at the level of the left ventricular outflow tract. This is not the vena contracta, which is narrower than this measurement. Measure the diameter of the left ventricular outflow tract.

Grading is as follows:

Mild (1+)	1–24%
Mild-moderate (2+)	25–46%
Moderate (3+)	47–64%
Severe (4+)	≥ 65%

Other methods of quantification include:

B. Measurement of the **vena contracta**:

Mild	< 0.3 cm
Moderate	0.3–0.6 cm
Severe	> 0.6 cm

C. Measurement of **jet cross-sectional area/cross-sectional area of the LVOT** (Fig. 39). This can be of benefit with eccentric jets, where the single-dimensional measurement in the LVOT understates the severity of regurgitation.

Mild (1+)	1–5%
Mild-moderate (2+)	5–20%
Moderate (3+)	21–59%
Severe (4+)	≥ 60%

Supporting measures include:

Jet Density and Deceleration Time

Use CW Doppler from apical, view to obtain a complete signal of the regurgitant jet. The denser the signal, compared to outflow, the greater the severity of the regurgitation. To measure deceleration time, measure the slope of the jet. Both pressure half time and deceleration should be reported. A shorter deceleration time reflects a faster equalization of pressures, which suggests that the regurgitant orifice area is larger. The jet should be uniform and dense, and the peak velocity should be at least 3.5 m/s to be in the flow correctly.

Mild	> 500 msec
Moderate	200–500 msec
Severe	< 200 msec

Flow Reversal in the Descending Aorta

Place the pulse Doppler parallel to flow in the descending thoracic aorta and the abdominal aorta. There is normally a brief period of flow reversal in the aorta, due to elastic recoil (Fig. 40). The presence of holodiastolic flow reversal in the thoracic aorta is sensitive for at least moderate regurgitation, and if seen in the abdominal aorta, is suggestive of severe regurgitation. The higher the diastolic flow velocities, the greater the likelihood of severe regurgitation. If there is an aortic aneurysm or a severely calcified aorta, this measure should not be used.

Tricuspid Regurgitation

Make sure to

1. Assess the morphology of the tricuspid leaflets
2. Assess regurgitation in multiple views
3. Measure the vena contracta
4. Assess the density and contour of the trans-tricuspid spectral Doppler
5. Measure pulmonary artery pressure
6. Doppler the hepatic vein
7. Assess RA and RV size and function.

2D imaging: Examine the tricuspid valve leaflets in multiple planes, including the right ventricular inflow view, the short axis view, the 4 chamber and

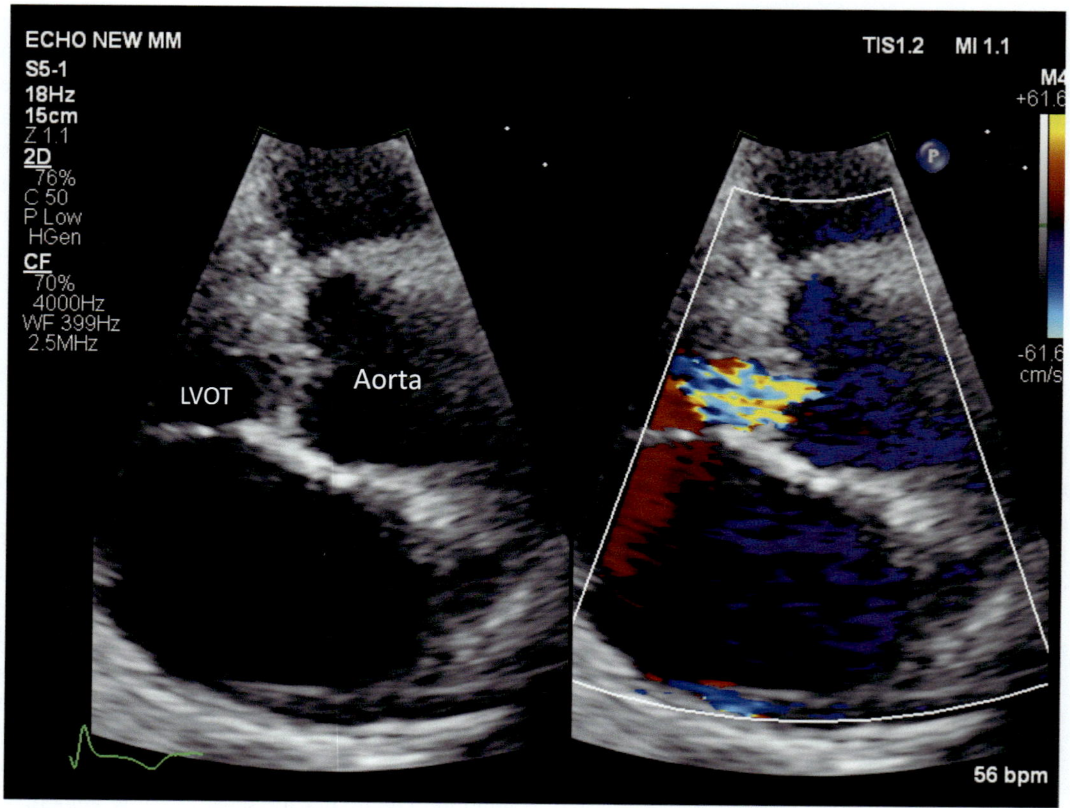

Fig. 39 Parasternal long axis view showing a jet of severe aortic regurgitation extending throughout the left ventricular outflow tract (LVOT)

the subcostal views. Remember that the insertion of tricuspid valve leaflets are more apical than the insertion of the mitral valve leaflets. The RV inflow view is the only view in which the posterior leaflet is seen, otherwise, one sees the anterior and septal leaflets. Abnormalities in leaflet morphology may be due to endocarditis, prolapse, Ebstein's anomaly (with apical displacement of the attachment of the septal and posterior tricuspid leaflets, and malformation and displacement of the anterior leaflet), rheumatic heart disease (with thickening and doming of leaflets), or carcinoid syndrome (with thickening, retraction and immobilization of the tricuspid leaflets). Annular dilatation leading to leaflet malcoaptation due to right ventricular or right atrial enlargement is the most common cause of tricuspid regurgitation, and leads to a vicious cycle of further chamber enlargement and further regurgitation.

In the setting of severe tricuspid regurgitation, right atrial and right ventricular enlargement are seen (Fig. 41). One should assess the interventricular septum for flattening of the septum, which is a sign of volume (during diastole) and pressure (during systole) overload. One should also assess the size and collapse of the inferior vena cava, to assess right atrial pressure.

Doppler imaging and measurement: The evaluation of the severity of tricuspid regurgitation is similar to mitral regurgitation. One should evaluate the size and direction of the regurgitant jet in multiple imaging planes, and jet area of $5–10 \text{ cm}^2$ is consistent with moderate regurgitation, and $> 10 \text{ cm}^2$ (in central jets) is suggestive of severe regurgitation. Vena contracta of 7 mm or above is sensitive and specific for severe regurgitation. In the setting of "free" tricuspid

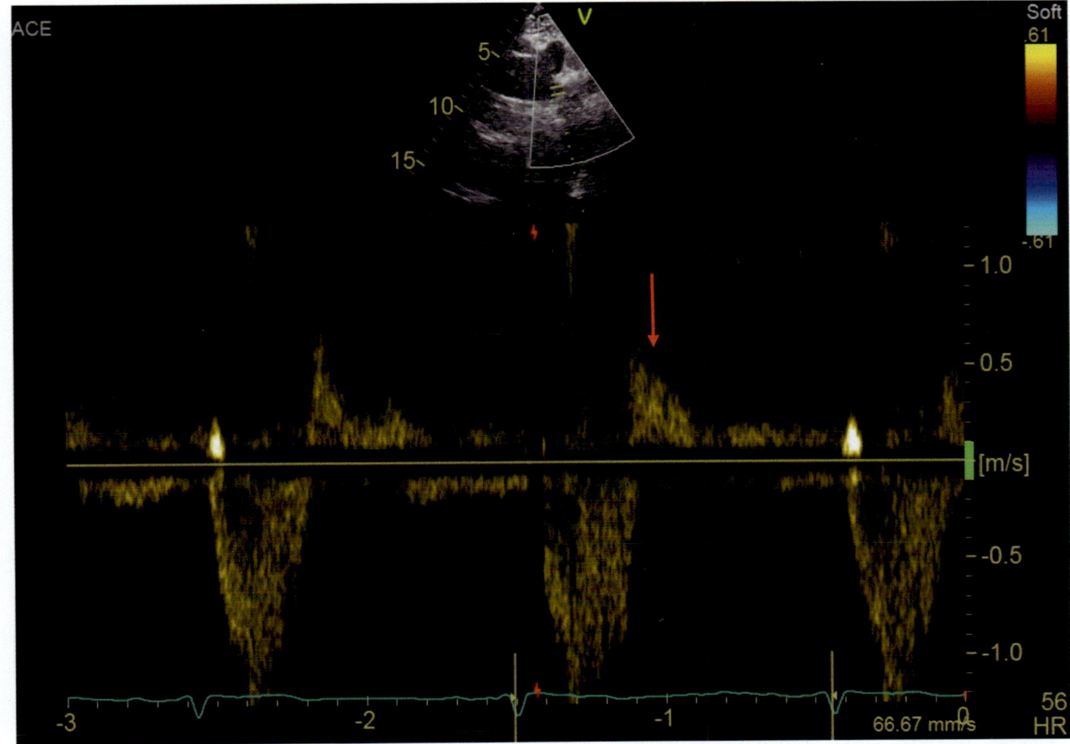

Fig. 40 Suprasternal view showing diastolic flow reversal in the descending thoracic aorta (arrow)

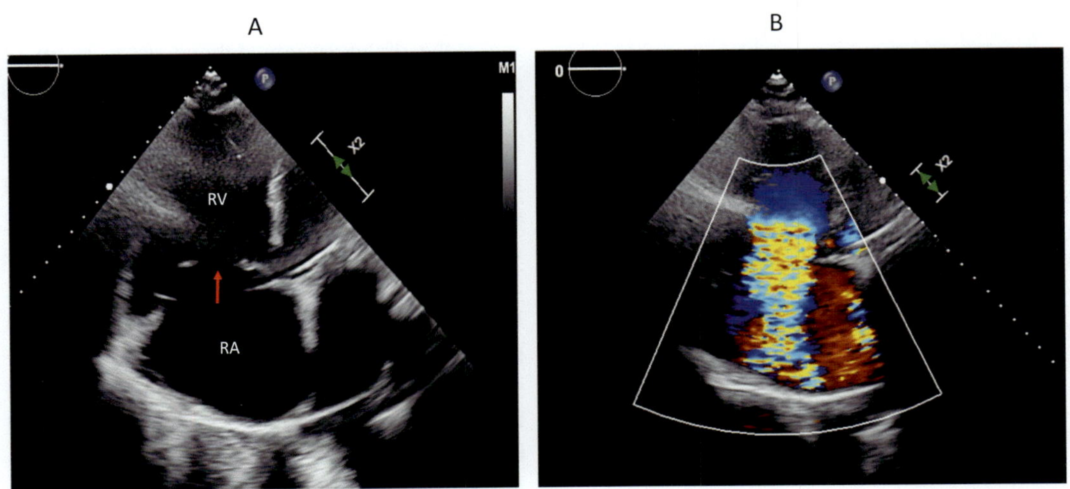

Fig. 41 Apical 4 chamber views with panel A showing dilated right atrium (RA) and right ventricle (RV) with malcoaptation of the tricuspid valve leaflets (arrow). Panel B shows the resultant extensive color Doppler jet consistent with very severe tricuspid regurgitation

A

B

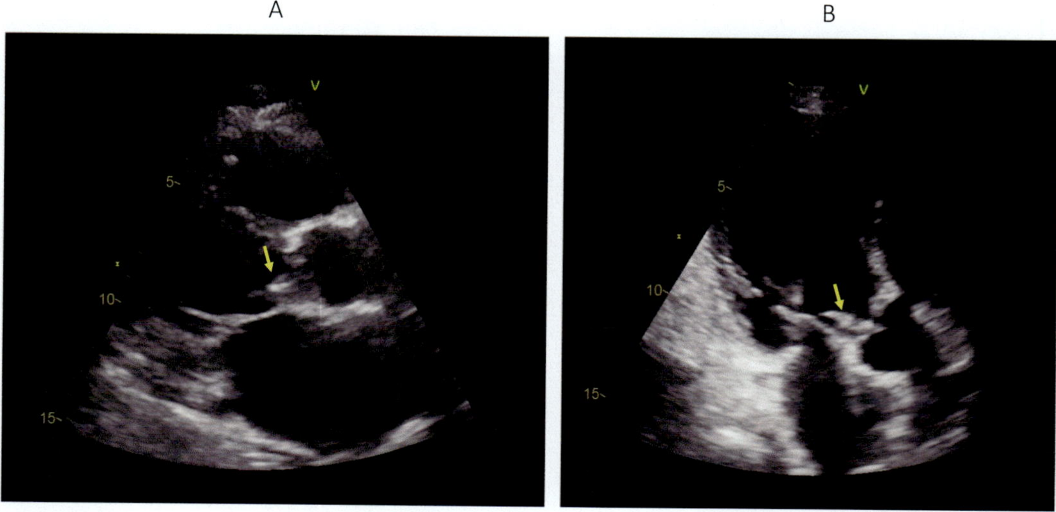

Fig. 42 Parasternal long axis (panel A) and apical 3 chamber (panel B) views show a large long, echodensity attached to the aortic valve (yellow arrows) representing a vegetation

regurgitation, peak regurgitant velocities are very low, as there is near equalization of pressure between atrium and ventricle, and the TR velocity may understate the severity of pulmonary hypertension.

Endocarditis (Vegetations)

Examine all four valves and chordae from as many views as possible for evidence of vegetations suggestive of endocarditis. The classic vegetation is a tissue-density mass with independent, chaotic motion adherent to the upstream surface of the valve (e.g. atrial surface of the mitral valve, ventricular surface of the aortic valve.) (Fig. 42). Unusual thickening of a valve or unexplained regurgitation may also be a sign of endocarditis. An abscess or fistula may form due to bacterial invasion of the tissue surrounding the valve. The infection may track into other structures. Foreign bodies within the heart (prosthetic valves, pacemakers, ICDs) are a frequent focus for endocarditis and pose significant challenges to diagnosis due to the acoustic shadowing of the device. In the setting of high clinical suspicion, trans-esophageal echocardiography should be performed.

Mitral Valve Prolapse

Mitral valve prolapse consists of billowing of one or both of the mitral leaflets into the atrium during systole. It is seen in 2–4% of the population, and is associated with progressive mitral regurgitation, chordal rupture, and increased risk of endocarditis. The echocardiographic criteria to make the diagnosis are defined as > 2 mm of displacement of one or both of the mitral leaflets below the plane of the mitral annulus during systole. Because the mitral annulus is saddle-shaped, rather than planar, it is recommended that one use the parasternal long axis or apical 2 chamber for diagnosis (Fig. 43). One should see asymmetric, buckled appearance of the leaflets. In "classic" mitral valve prolapse there is leaflet thickening, and frequently prolapse of multiple segments. One also sees thinning, elongation and in advanced cases rupture of chordae. Mitral regurgitation results from malcoaptation of leaflets, which occurs as the increasing pressure during systole pushes the leaflets apart. Because of the leaflet formation, regurgitation is usually directed away from the prolapsing leaflet. Eccentrically-directed mitral regurgitation may

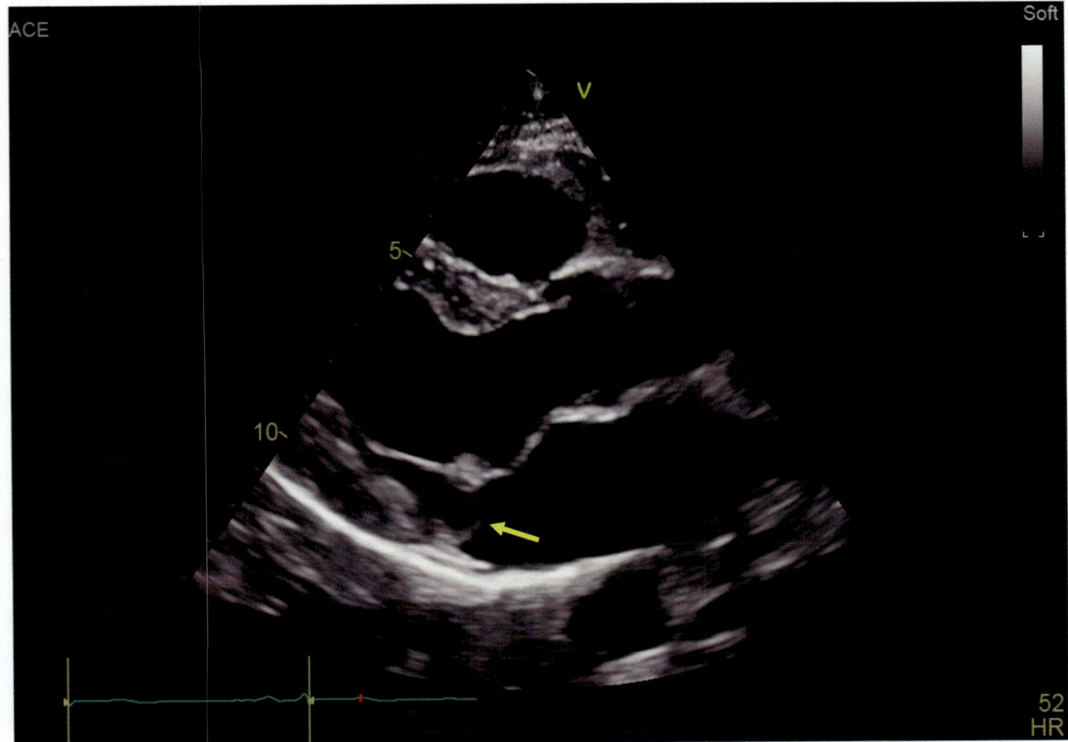

Fig. 43 Parasternal long axis view showing clear prolapse of the posterior mitral leaflet (yellow arrow)

be a clue to prolapse that is not easily seen on the transthoracic echocardiogram.

Evaluation of the prosthetic heart valve

Make sure to

1. Determine if valve is bioprosthetic or mechanical
2. Assess leaflet motion
3. Measure peak and mean pressure gradients

2D imaging: Evaluation of the prosthetic valve is challenging due to the acoustic shadowing of the valve prosthesis. The major complications of prosthetic valves include structural deterioration, pannus formation, thrombus formation, endocarditis, and valvular and paravalvular regurgitation. Each prosthesis should be viewed in multiple planes, and one should report whether the valve is a bioprosthesis or a mechanical prosthesis (Fig. 44). With the increasing use of transcatheter mitral valve repair techniques, prosthetic material may be noted on native valve leaflets. The presence of thrombus or vegetation may lead to limitation of motion. If bioprosthetic, one can often visualize the leaflets, and one can assess the motion and integrity of the leaflets.

Doppler imaging and measurement: Peak and mean gradients should be obtained. Tables exist for comparison of these values to the acceptable values for a given prosthesis. Elevated gradients are suggestive of valvular obstruction, which may result from leaflet dysfunction (due to thrombus or vegetation) or pannus formation. The valve should be interrogated for evidence of intrinsic or paravalvular regurgitation. Regurgitation is usually visible in the aortic prosthesis in standard echocardiographic views. It is often difficult to image mitral regurgitation in the

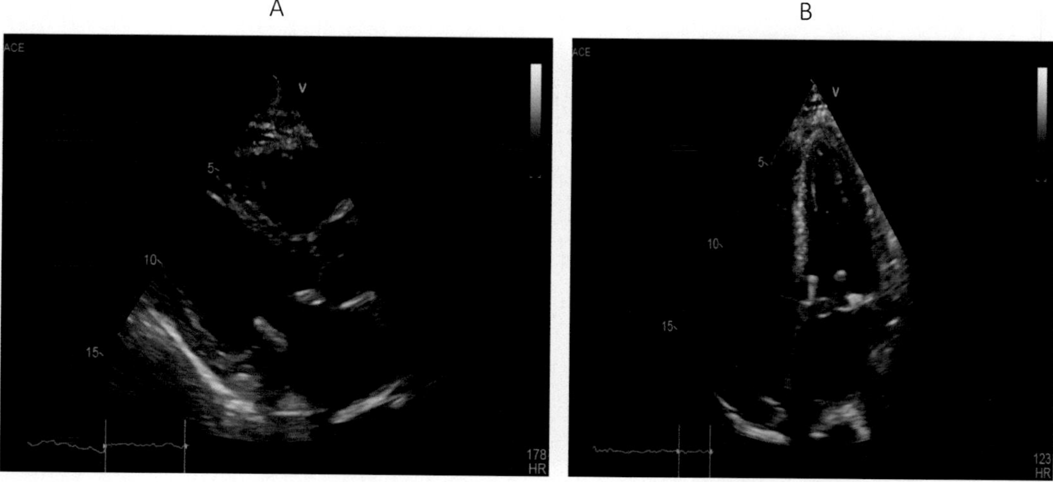

Fig. 44 Parasternal long axis (panel A) and apical 4 chamber (panel B) views showing a mitral valve bioprosthesis (note the elongated struts on both sides of the annulus)

setting of a mechanical valve due to acoustic shadowing of the prosthesis.

Notes:

Prosthetic aortic valve: Peak gradient is usually less than 45 mmHg, and should be compared to previous gradients measured across the prosthesis. It is also of value to compare the peak velocity to the peak LVOT velocity. If the ratio is greater than or equal to 4:1, this is highly suggestive of significant valvular stenosis/obstruction.

Prosthetic mitral valve: The mean gradient across the mitral valve prosthesis is usually less than 5 mmHg. The presence of elevated transvalvular gradients or a jet consistent with mitral regurgitation on continuous wave may suggest the presence of unseen regurgitation.

Hypertrophic Cardiomyopathy

Hypertrophic cardiomyopathy is defined as left ventricular hypertrophy LVH in the absence of another cardiac, systemic, or metabolic disease that explains this hypertrophy, and the diagnosis is established by imaging.

2D imaging and measurement: Measure anterior septal and posterior wall thickness and LV chamber size in systole and diastole. Carefully measure the septum, avoiding trabeculae, and measure any other regions that are abnormally thick. Although asymmetric septal hypertrophy is the most common pattern, one may see concentric hypertrophy, or hypertrophy of the apex or free wall of the heart. In apical hypertrophy, one sees thickening of the apical walls and obliteration of the apex during systole. When assessing concentric hypertrophy, one should keep in mind the clinical context, as the differential diagnosis includes hypertensive heart disease, athlete's heart, and infiltrative diseases such as amyloid.

One should assess the left ventricular outflow tract for evidence of obstruction due to septal morphology. The mitral leaflets and chordal structures should be carefully examined, looking for evidence of systolic anterior motion (SAM). The best view to assess SAM is usually the apical 5 chamber or apical 3 chamber view (Fig. 45).

Doppler imaging and measurement

Doppler gradient of the left ventricular outflow tract (LVOT) should be performed. Measurement should begin from the apex to the valve using PW Doppler, to ascertain where the maximum velocity occurs. At the area of maximum velocity, the signal should also be obtained with the Valsalva maneuver. If the velocities alias, the CW imaging probe should be used taking care to

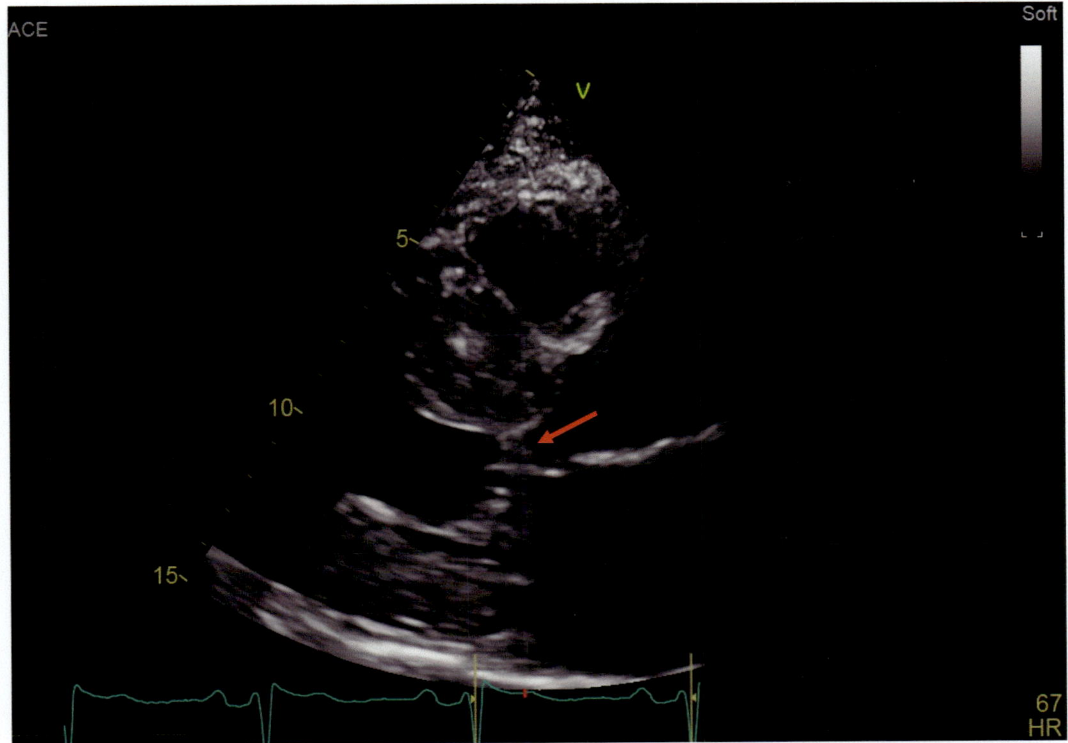

Fig. 45 Parasternal long-axis view showing an hypertrophied septum with LVOT obstruction (arrow) caused by systolic anterior motion of the mitral valve leaflet

try and avoid having the signal line go directly across the aortic valve. The dynamic nature of the obstruction in the setting of systolic anterior motion leads to a characteristic high-velocity, late-peaking continuous-wave Doppler signal, described as "dagger-shaped"). The late-peaking nature may help differentiate this from aortic stenosis, which increases velocity with a more symmetric appearance.

Diseases of the Aorta

Examination of the aorta should be part of the standard echocardiographic examination. Although transesophageal echocardiography allows for more complete imaging of the aorta, most of the thoracic aorta can be imaged on transthoracic echocardiography utilizing primarily the parasternal long axis and suprasternal views. Assessment of acute aortic disease such as aortic aneurysm or dissection should be made using these views. Dimensions of the ascending aorta should be performed in the parasternal long-axis view measuring from inner edge to inner edge. A dissection membrane can be identified as a linear echodensity transecting the lumen of the aorta (Fig. 46). To distinguish this finding from artifact, color Doppler can be utilized. If the linear finding seen in the aorta interferes with color flow it is more likely to be a true finding. In addition, the linear finding should respect the boundaries of the aorta in multiple imaging planes. Imaging of intramural hematoma on transthoracic echocardiography is challenging. The parasternal high short axis view may image the classic crescent shaped echodensity in the area of the aortic root.

Contrast Echocardiography

Contrast echocardiography encompasses techniques for improving resolution of the left ventricular endocardial borders and for providing real-time assessment of intracardiac blood flow.

Agitated saline solution administered via intravenous injection provides air microbubble

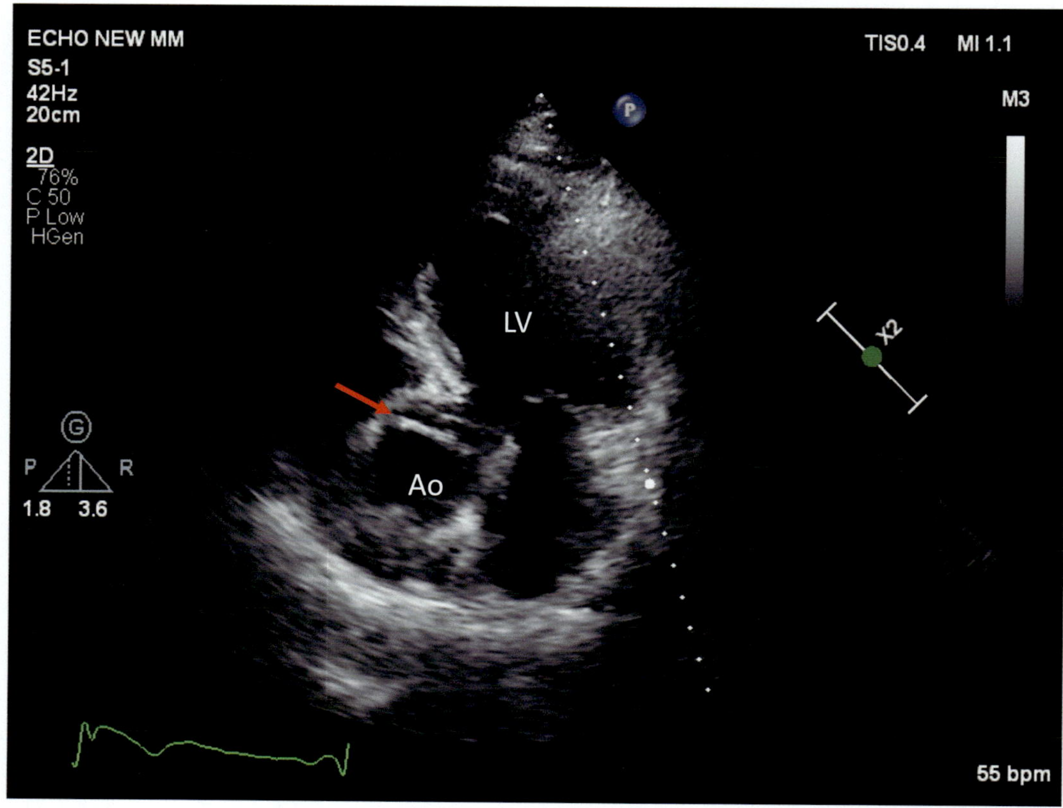

Fig. 46 Apical 5 chamber view showing a dissection membrane (arrow) in the ascending aorta

contrast in the right heart. The air microbubbles are short-lived and are filtered by the lungs when traversing the pulmonary circulation. Therefore the microbubbles enter the left heart only in the presence of a right to left intracardiac or extracardiac (pulmonic) shunt (Fig. 47). Saline microbubbles are therefore helpful in examining the right heart and identifying right to left shunts. This technique is used most often for the detection of patent foramen ovale and atrial septal defects primarily in the clinical setting of suspected paradoxical embolism or unexplained hypoxia. The appearance of bubbles in the left heart early (within three to five beats) after right chamber opacification suggests an intracardiac shunt. Later appearance of bubbles in the left heart (> 5 beats after first seeing bubbles in the right atrium) suggests an extracardiac shunt such as pulmonary arteriovenous malformations.

To perform an agitated saline study, fill a 10 cc syringe with 9 cc of saline and attach to a three way stopcock. Take a second syringe with 0.5–1 cc of air and agitate the saline by mixing it vigorously at least 10 times between the two syringes through the stopcock. The optimal echocardiographic views for assessing intracardiac shunt are the apical 4 chamber or subcostal views. Once adequate imaging has been obtained the agitated saline should be forcefully injected in an antecubital vein and imaging performed. If the resting study is negative than repeat injection using a Valsalva maneuver to increase right sided pressures and increase sensitivity of the exam should be performed. The patient should strain for 10 s, the agitated saline should be injected and imaging performed with release of Valsalva by the patient. If the patient is unable to adequately perform a Valsalva maneuver, abdominal

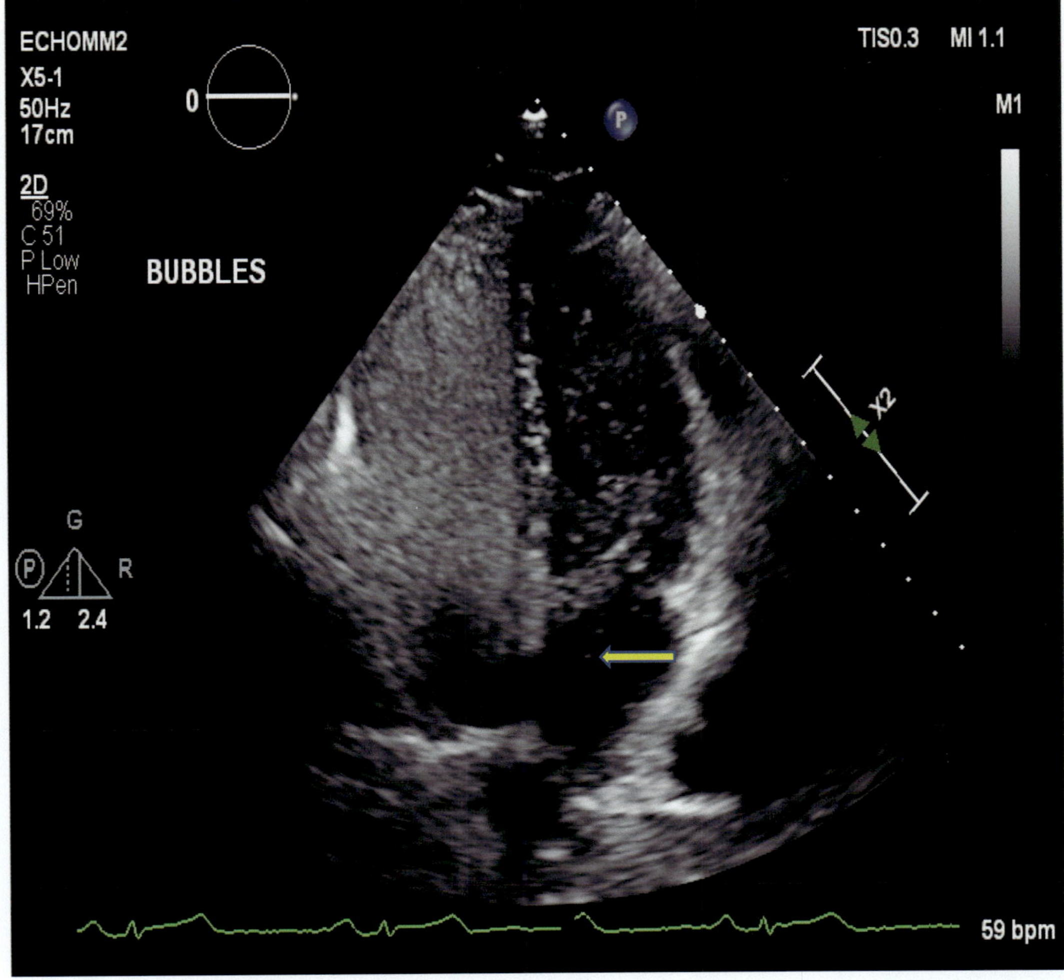

Fig. 47 Agitated saline ("bubble") injection showing the right side filled with saline bubbles some of which appear in the left side as well (yellow arrow), findings consistent with right to left shunt

compression should be performed. A hand should be placed on the right side of the epigastrium of the patient to depress the abdominal wall, with release immediately after opacification of the right atrium. If the patient is anesthetized and/or ventilated a Valsalva maneuver can be undertaken by applying and then releasing positive airway pressure.

In recent years microbubble contrast agents have been developed which can traverse the pulmonary vasculature and opacify the left ventricle, providing significantly improved LV endocardial border definition in patients with technically suboptimal echocardiograms. Suboptimal images limit the interpretation in approximately 30–40% of echocardiographic studies, thereby impairing the assessment of segmental and global LV systolic function. Contrast opacification of the LV cavity enhances border detection, decreasing the variability in the interpretation of regional wall motion abnormalities, LV volumes, and ejection fraction (Fig. 48). It is an accurate method for evaluating LV function in situations where obtaining a study is technically difficult, such as in the intensive care unit. Contrast agents may also be useful to assess LV pathology such as thrombus, noncompaction and apical hypertrophy.

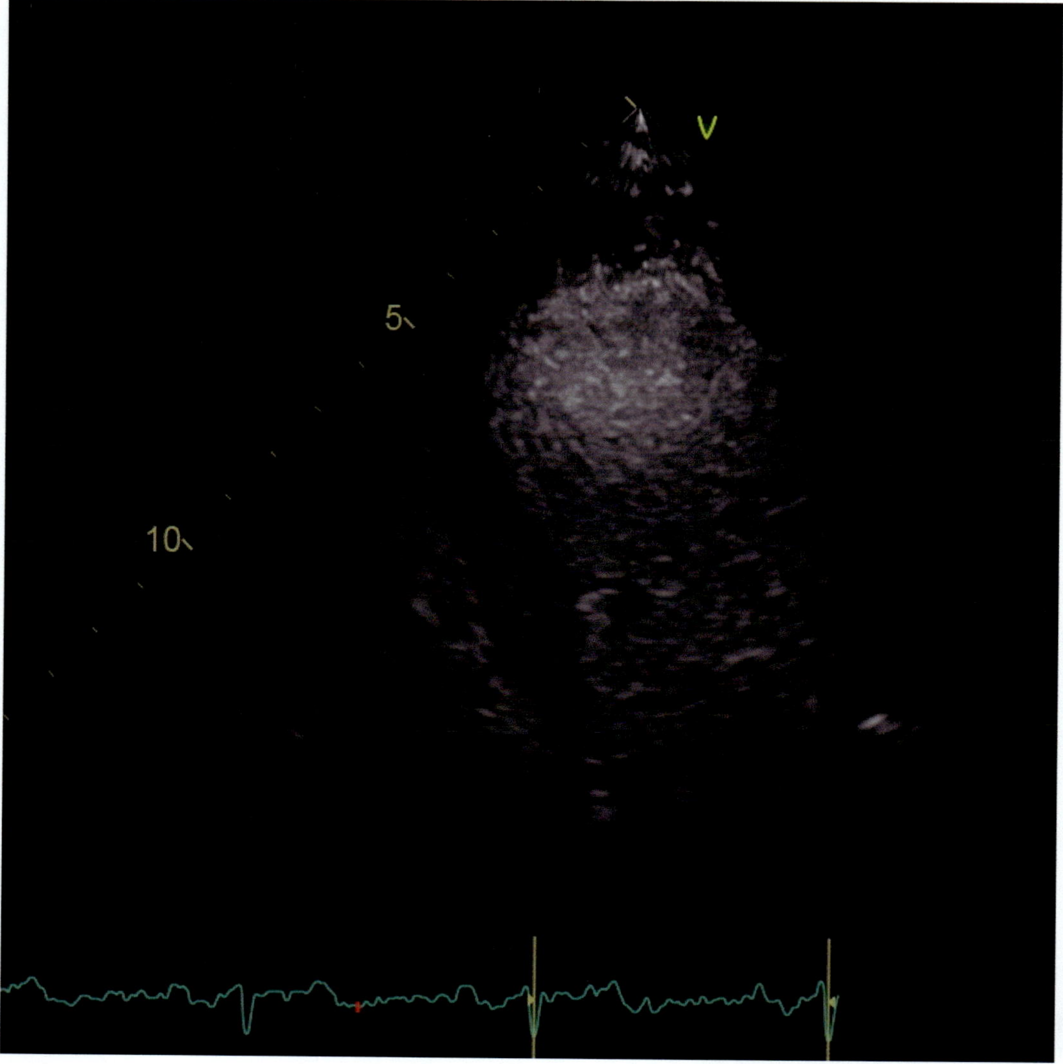

Fig. 48 Contrast injection showing complete opacification of the LV cavity. Note the well delineated endocardial borders

To ensure optimal use of contrast agents, a very low mechanical index (generally 0.3) should be used to avoid destruction of the bubbles by the ultrasound beam. Fist adequate apical 4 chamber view imaging should be performed using standard settings and only then should the mechanical index be reduced. Gain settings should be adjusted to reduce background noise. The contrast should be injected shortly after preparation in a bolus. The contrast will initially fill the right sided chambers and gradually will opacify the left side as well. Only then should imaging be performed from the apical 4, 2 and 3 chamber views. Our algorithms for the use of "contrast echo" in patients with chest pain and/or shortness of breath are presented in the chapter "Patient-Centered Care Cardiac Electrosonography" in Figs. 3 and 4.

References

Lancellotti P, Pibarot P, Chambers J, La Canna G, Pepi M, Dulgheru R, Dweck M, Delgado V, Garbi M, Vannan MA, Montaigne D, Badano L, Maurovich-Horvat P, Pontone G, Vahanian A, Donal E, Cosyns B. Scientific Document Committee of the European Association of Cardiovascular Imaging. Multi-modality imaging assessment of native valvular regurgitation: an EACVI and ESC council of valvular heart disease position paper. Eur Heart J Cardiovasc Imaging 2022;18:e171–232.

Lang RM, Badano LP, Mor-Avi V, Afilalo J, Armstrong A, Ernande L, Flachskampf FA, Foster E, Goldstein SA, Kuznetsova T, Lancellotti L, Muraru D, Picard MH, Rietzschel ER, Rudski L, Spencer KT, Tsang W, Voigt J-U. Recommendations for cardiac chamber quantification by echocardiography in adults: an update from the American Society of Echocardiography and the European Association of Cardiovascular Imaging. J Am Soc Echocardiogr. 2015;28:1–39.

Sorrell VL, Lindner JR, Pellikka PA, Kirkpatrick JN, Muraru D. Recognized and unrecognized value of echocardiography in guideline and consensus documents regarding patients with chest pain. J Am Soc Echocardiogr. 2023;36:146–53.

Tutorial for Chest Sonography: Performance and Interpretation

Alexander Davidovich, Adam Rothman, Janet Shapiro, Yair Elitzur, David Leibowitz, and Eyal Herzog

Abstract

This chapter describes the fundamentals of utilizing chest sonography in the evaluation of respiratory symptoms. It reviews pulmonary anatomy, ultrasound probe positioning, and common ultrasound findings. Unlike sonography of other organs, including cardiac sonography, sonography of the lungs produces mainly artifactual findings due to air interfering with the ultrasound waves. When pathology impairs air-filled alveoli or if fluid accumulates around the lung, the ultrasound can produce more clearly discernable structures. We describe the principal patterns of lung ultrasound starting with normal findings of *lung sliding* and *A-lines*, and abnormal findings including pulmonary edema with diffuse *B-lines*, pneumonia with *lung hepatization* and dynamic air-bronchograms, pleural effusions, and pneumothorax with its characteristic *lung point*. Finally, we present an important algorithm to guide the standardized incorporation of chest sonography into the bedside clinical evaluation of patients with respiratory symptoms.

Keywords

Ultrasound · Chest sonography · Pleura · A-lines · B-lines · Lung sliding · Pneumothorax · Pneumonia · Pulmonary edema

1 Overview of Chest Sonography

1.1 Basic Principles

Thoracic ultrasonography developed late compared to ultrasound usage for other organ systems, as ultrasound waves cannot be transmitted well through air-filled structures. Air is in fact a near total reflector of ultrasound, and so with normal healthy lungs, the pleural line will serve as a border and generator of reflecting signs. Within the lung itself, specific abnormal ultrasound findings are related to the ratio of air to fluid, as anything displacing air in the alveolar space (fluid, blood, or pus), or any process causing interstitial thickening, will lead to appreciable changes. Because many abnormal lung processes, including pulmonary edema,

A. Davidovich (✉) · J. Shapiro
Mount Sinai Morningside, Institute for Critical Care Medicine, Icahn School of Medicine at Mount Sinai, New York, NY, USA
e-mail: alexander.davidovich@mountsinai.org

A. Rothman
Mount Sinai West, Institute for Critical Care Medicine, Icahn School of Medicine at Mount Sinai, New York, NY, USA

Y. Elitzur · D. Leibowitz · E. Herzog
The Heart Institute, Department of Cardiology, Hadassah Medical Center, Hebrew University of Jerusalem, Jerusalem, Israel

E. Herzog et al. (eds.), *Cardiac Electrosonography*,
https://doi.org/10.1007/978-3-031-38469-1_4

pneumothorax, pleural effusion, and atelectasis extend to the lung periphery, ultrasound can distinguish air from other substances that produce various types of artifacts visible on imaging. The clinical interpretation of these artifacts is described below.

1.2 Lung Surface Anatomy

Reviewing the basic lung anatomy is important to properly interpret the images acquired during thoracic ultrasonography. The right lung contains three lobes, the right upper (RUL), right middle (RML), and right lower (RLL) lobes while the left lung contains two true lobes, the left upper (LUL) and left lower (LLL) lobes, and a vestigial third lobe called the lingula akin to the RML, which is not readily visualized on ultrasound (Figs. 1 and 2).

1.3 Lung and Pleural Examination

Thoracic ultrasonography can be performed using a linear or phased array transducer. The phased array probe is preferable as it may be

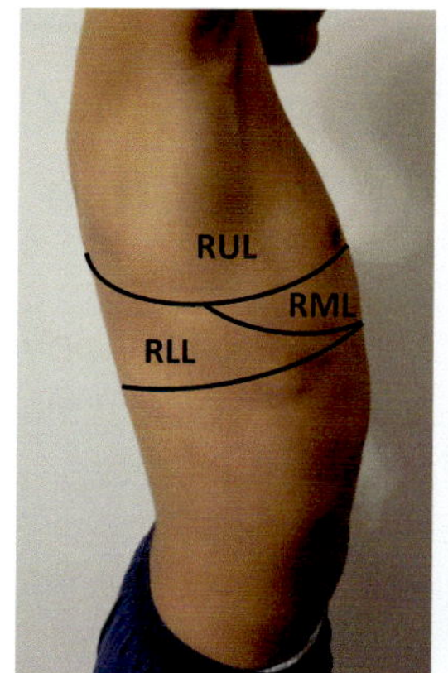

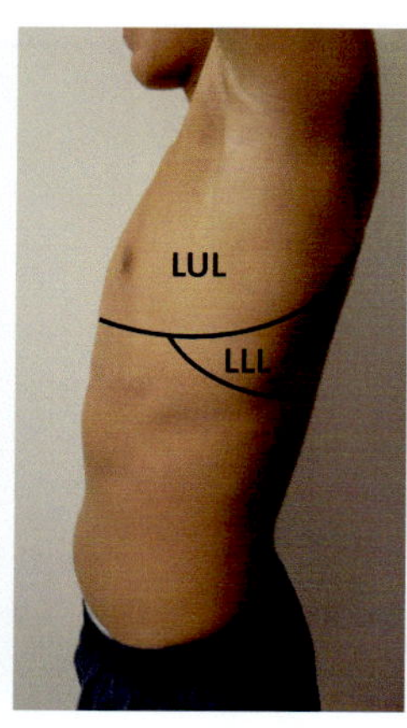

Fig. 2 Lateral views of chest with markings delineating lobe locations, right lateral and left lateral, respectively

used for cardiac imaging as well and can therefore be utilized for both exams. In addition, it has a smaller footprint, enabling it to fit between rib interspaces and provide superior imaging. A high frequency, linear transducer, designed for vascular access at superficial depths, can be utilized for detailed assessment of the pleural line. The probes should always be held with the probe marker facing cephalad (Fig. 3).

While there is no best way to perform thoracic ultrasonography, it is generally recommended to obtain two anterior lung views along the midclavicular line at least one to two rib spaces apart,

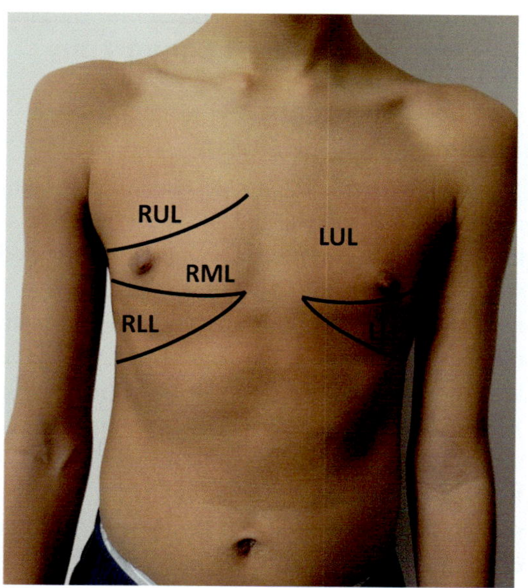

Fig. 1 Anterior view of chest with markings delineating lobe locations

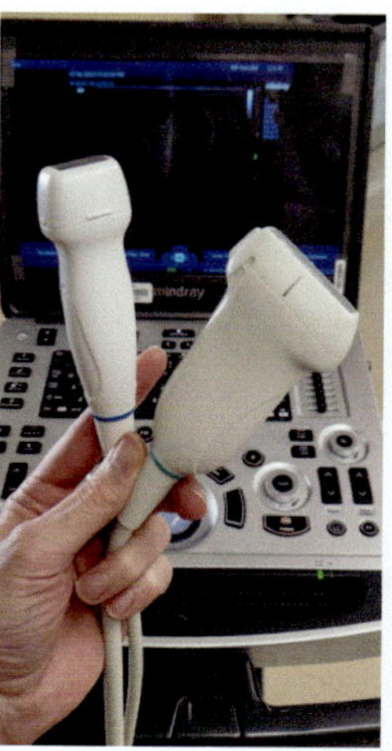
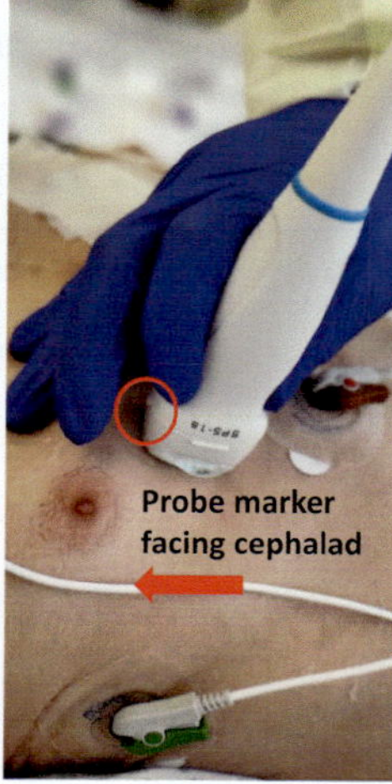

Fig. 3 Linear and phased array transducers; phased array probe facing cephalad, respectively

and then to obtain an additional one or two views along the mid-axillary and posterior axillary lines (Figs. 4 and 5). Assessment of the posterior chest should include the posterior and/or lateral alveolar and/or pleural syndrome (PLAPS) point, which is found at the intersection of the posterior axillary line and a rib space between the 10th and 12th ribs (Fig. 5). The PLAPS point is best for identifying pleural effusions and consolidations. The presence of a PLAPS pathology can aid in diagnosing conditions such as pneumonia (Lichtenstein and Mezière 2008). This comprehensive examination is then repeated in the same fashion on the opposite hemithorax. Representative locations of these points are referenced on a sample chest radiograph (Fig. 6).

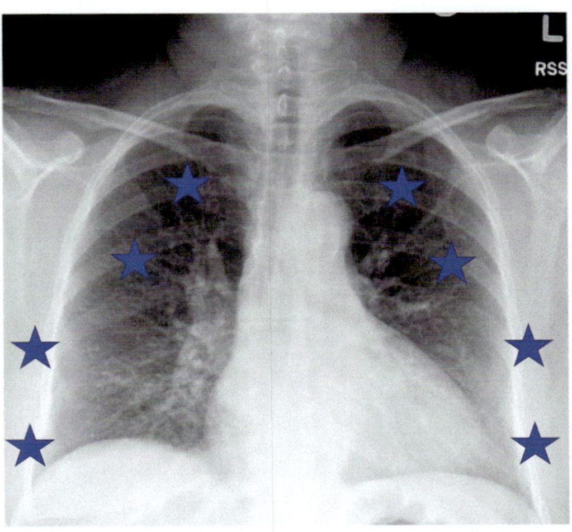

Fig. 6 Radiographic representation of the recommended ultrasound viewpoints

1.4 Probe Positioning

Proper positioning of the ultrasound probe with the probe marker facing cephalad and between two rib spaces is important to confirm correct probe placement. This will produce a standard lung ultrasound view, involving a pleural line at the top with a series of sequential A-lines (i.e., pleural reflections) in between an upper and lower rib each producing an anechoic shadowing extending beneath, known as a *batwing sign*, as it may resemble a bat flying out of the screen (Figs. 7 and 8).

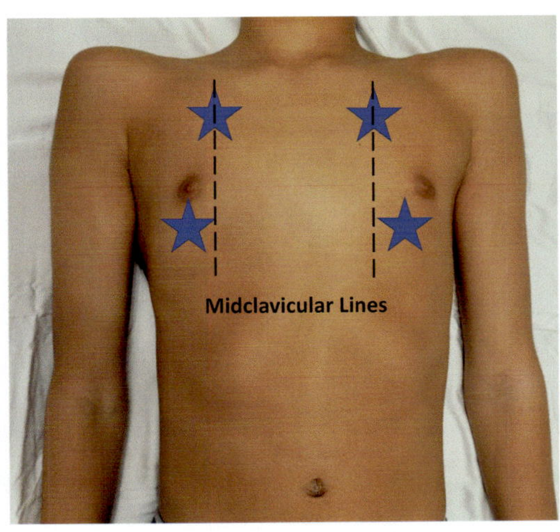

Fig. 4 Locations of recommended anterior chest views

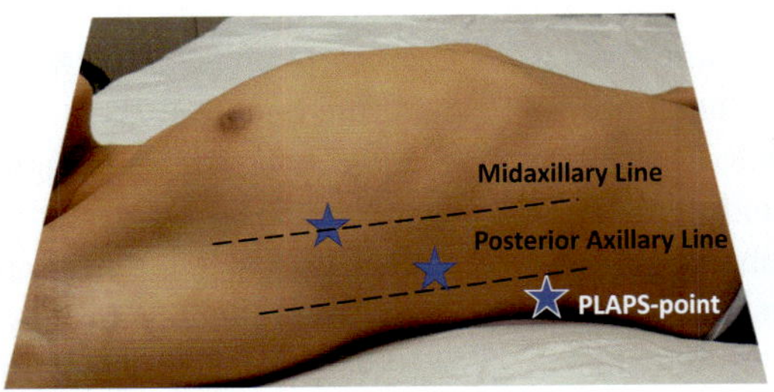

Fig. 5 Locations of recommended lateral chest views

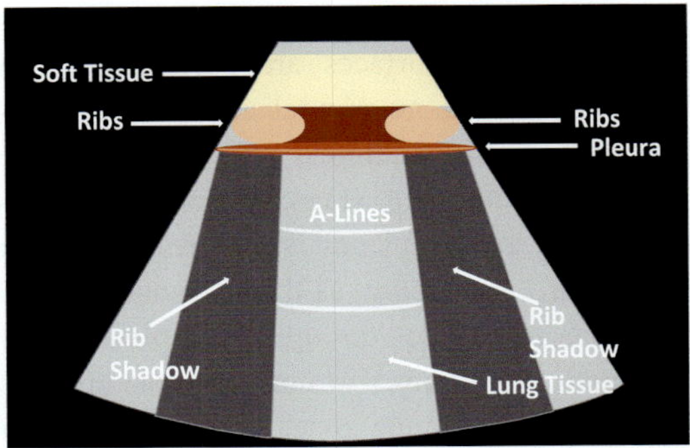

Fig. 7 Picture representation of standard lung ultrasound view

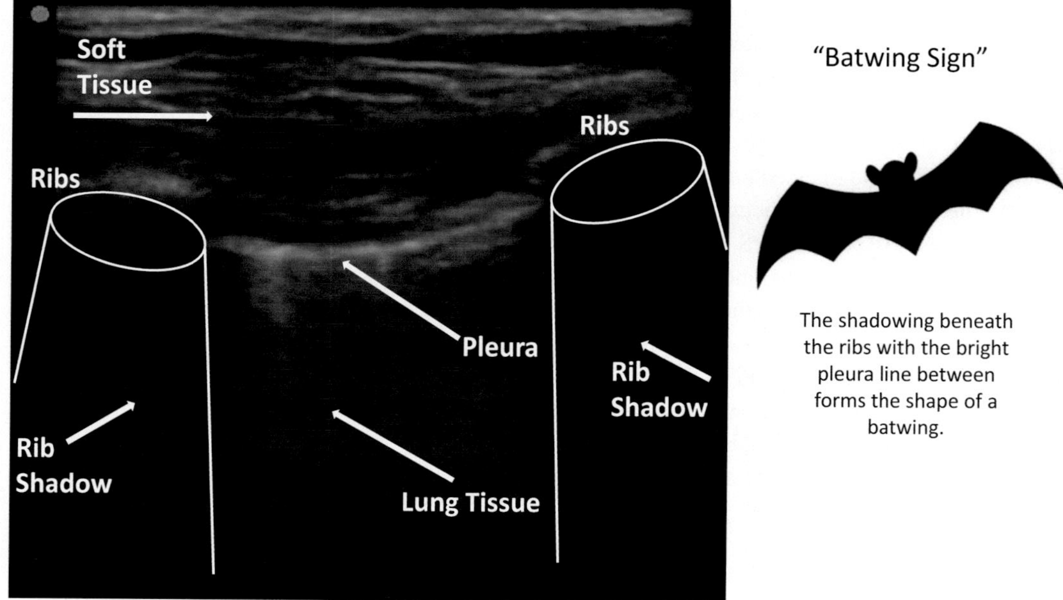

Fig. 8 Ultrasound image with labeled landmarks for standard lung ultrasound view; batwing sign described

2　Normal and Abnormal Lung and Pleural Signs

2.1　Lung Sliding

During the respiratory cycle, as the lungs expand, the visceral pleura surface will slide relative to the parietal pleura and chest wall. This creates a shimmering of the hyperechoic pleural line when visualized on ultrasound and is especially evident when utilizing a high-frequency transducer. This finding, called *lung sliding*, strongly suggests that the pleural surfaces are adjacent to one another (meaning no pleural effusion or pneumothorax in the examined area) and that the patient is ventilating (Figs. 9 and 10). Conversely, air in the pleural space will cause an absence of lung sliding, as the ultrasound waves will not propagate through the pleural air. Additional conditions that may cause an absence of lung sliding include apnea or hypoventilation (contralateral bronchial intubation, bronchial occlusion), prior pleurodesis, large bullae, or large dense lung consolidation. A finding called

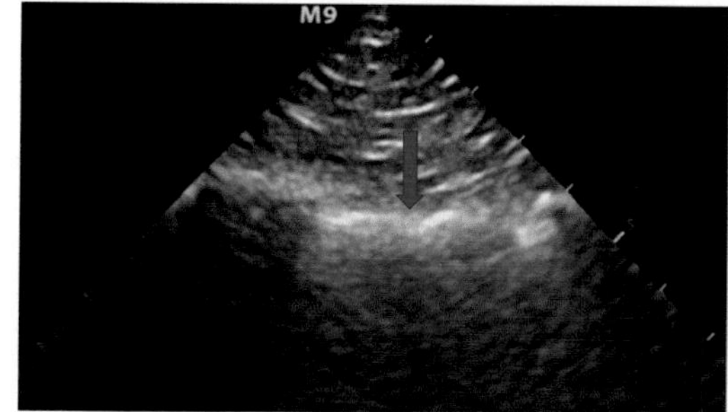

Fig. 9 Lung ultrasound view, the blue arrow points to the pleural line

lung pulse occurs when cardiac movement leads to a pulsating appearance of the pleural line. The *curtain sign* is seen at each bilateral PLAPS-point in normal aerated lungs indicating an air-filled lung extending down over the diaphragm and sub-diaphragmatic organs momentarily obliterating them from view during the inspiratory phase of respiration and returning to view during exhalation (i.e., liver/kidney on the right and spleen/kidney on the left) (Fig. 11) (Lichtenstein and Mezière 2008).

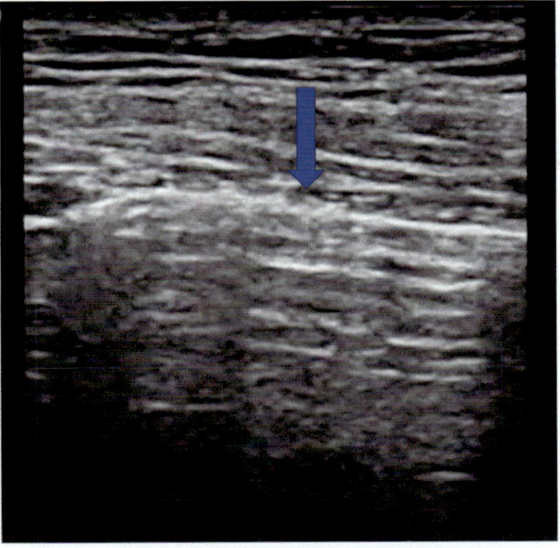

Fig. 10 Magnified image of pleural line, which under normal circumstances during the respiratory cycle, will have a shimmering appearance. This appearance is also occasionally described as "ants marching on a log"

2.2 A-lines

A-lines are hyperechoic horizontal lines that represent reverberation artifacts of the pleural line. A-lines will be equidistant from each other and the pleural line and are present whether there is air in the lung parenchyma or pleural space (Fig. 12). The presence of A-lines and lung sliding at a specific site signifies that that area of the lung is aerated normally.

2.3 B-lines

B-lines are vertical projections that start at the pleura and extend the entirety of the depth to the edge of the screen. They will move along with lung sliding and obliterate A-lines. B-lines represent either thickening of the interlobular septa and/or alveolar filling processes. 1–2 B-lines in a single view may be a normal finding, whereas the presence of 3 or more B-lines is abnormal (Fig. 13). B-lines in a single view may be reflective of a local infiltrative process (such as a focal pneumonia), whereas a generalized B-line pattern may indicate an interstitial syndrome, with a differential diagnosis consisting of pulmonary edema, multifocal pneumonia, acute respiratory distress syndrome, or interstitial lung disease (Fig. 14).

2.4 Alveolar Consolidation

As normally aerated alveoli are replaced with fluid and inflammation or become atelectatic, ultrasound waves can reveal echogenic tissue deep to the pleura. This solidification of the lung is described as *lung hepatization*, as the texture and appearance of the consolidation on ultrasound resembles that of the liver (Fig. 15). Within these consolidations, pinpoint hyperechoic opacities signify sonographic air

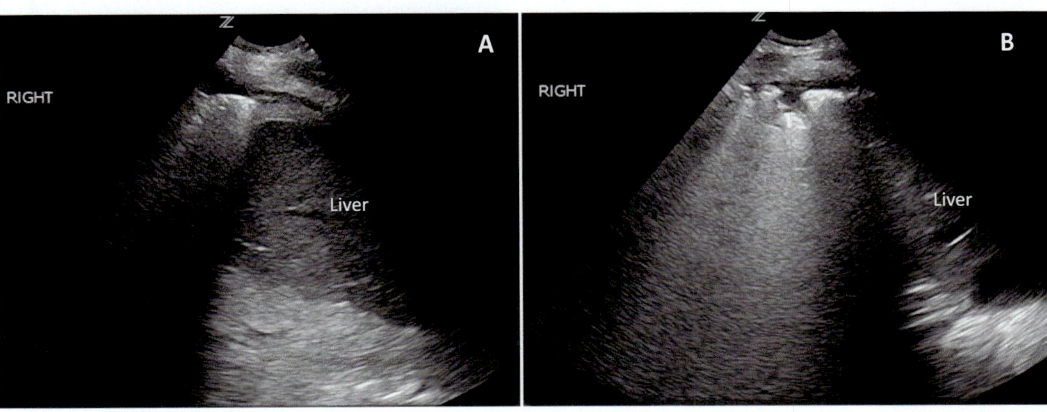

Fig. 11 Example of the *curtain sign* with image A captured during exhalation and image B captured during inhalation with air-filled lung extending down over the diaphragm and momentarily obliterating the liver from view

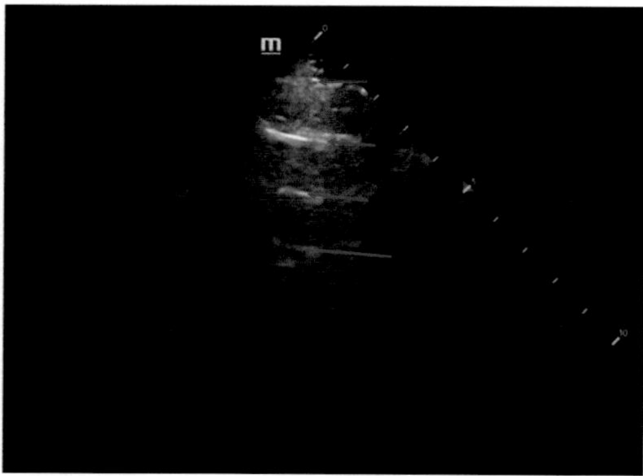

Fig. 12 The pleural line is denoted by the red arrow. In this lung view, there are three distinct A-lines, highlighted by the blue arrows, which are parallel to the pleural line and equidistant from each other

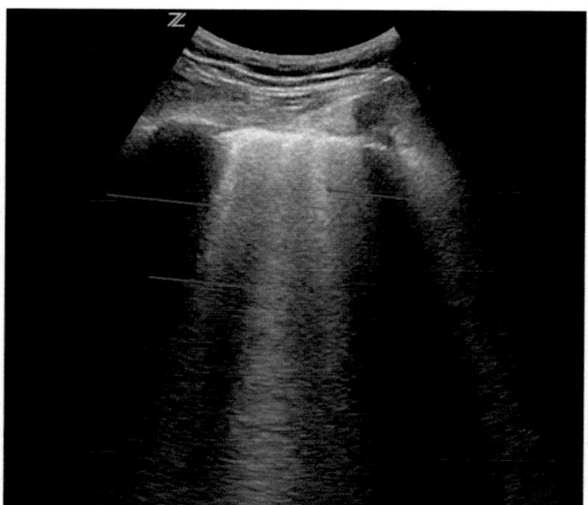

Fig. 13 The blue arrows indicate the three B-lines seen in this lung space, which start at the pleural line and descend the entirety of the depth of the image

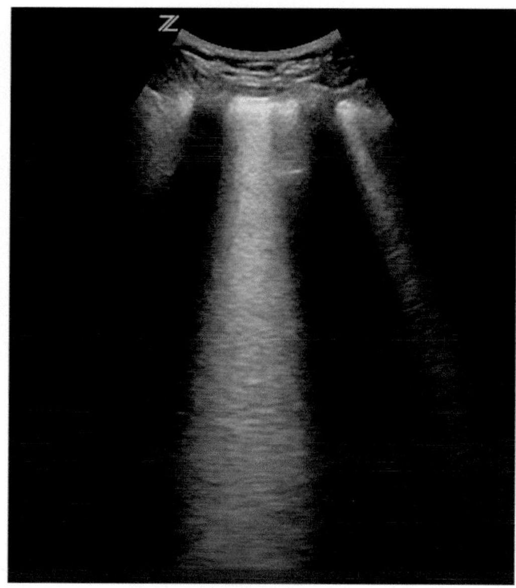

Fig. 14 Confluent B-lines that completely obliterate the A-line pattern

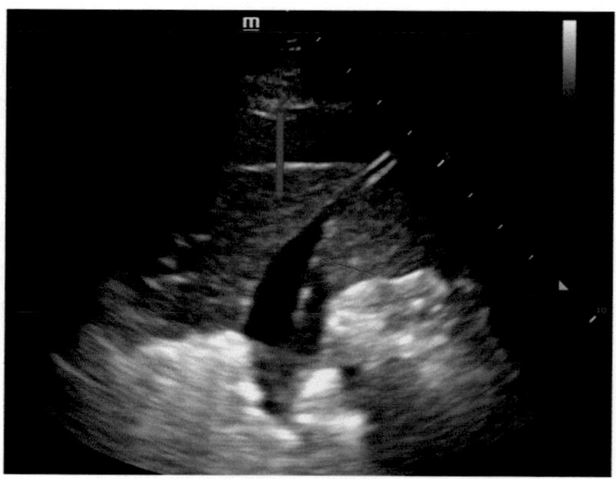

Fig. 15 Consolidated lung, or "lung hepatization," highlighted by the blue arrow. The red arrow denotes the curvilinear diaphragm, separating the thoracic cavity from the intraabdominal cavity. Note the similar appearance of the consolidated lung and the spleen below

bronchograms and indicate that air remains in the bronchioles. These air bronchograms can then be used to differentiate pneumonia from atelectasis. The presence of mobile or dynamic air bronchograms has a high specificity for the diagnosis of pneumonia, as air is still moving in and out of the bronchioles. In contrast, static air bronchograms are indicative of atelectasis (Lichtenstein et al. 2019, 2004).

2.5 Pleural Effusion

Ultrasound can easily detect pleural effusions and is significantly better at differentiating fluid from lung consolidation as compared to chest X-ray

(Mayo et al. 2019). When seen on ultrasound, a pleural effusion is an anechoic space with anatomic boundaries consisting of the chest wall, diaphragm, and lung, and with associated dynamic changes seen with the atelectatic lung and diaphragm. Simple, anechoic fluid suggests an uncomplicated pleural effusion. In contrast, septated and/or loculated fluid denotes a complicated pleural effusion. Depending on the size of the effusion, a *flapping lung* or *jellyfish sign*, which refers to the oscillating movement of an area of collapsed or atelectatic lung within the effusion, may be present (Fig. 16). Complex pleural effusions can occasionally contain strands of echogenic matter floating within it; this finding is called the *plankton sign*. When blood fills the pleural cavity, as occurs with a hemothorax, there may be a layering of echogenic material in a gravity-dependent fashion, with increasing echogenicity with increased depth. This finding is known as the *hematocrit sign*.

3 Clinical Applications

3.1 Detection of Lung Alveolar-Interstitial Syndrome (AIS)

Alveolar-interstitial syndrome refers to radiographic findings related to conditions with diffuse involvement of the interstitium and impairment of the alveolocapillary exchange

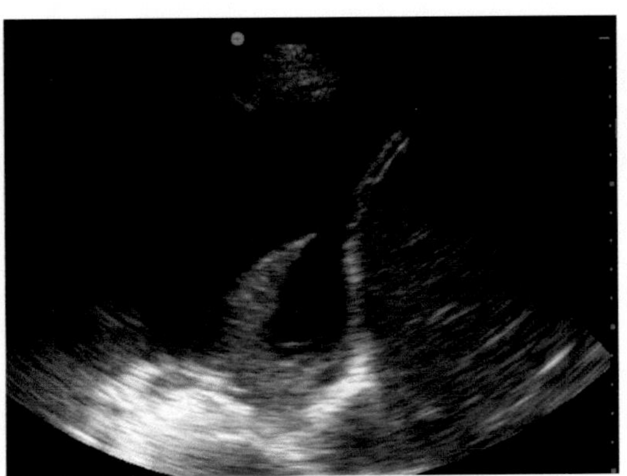

Fig. 16 A simple pleural effusion with *flapping lung* also known as *jellyfish sign*

capacity. Chronic conditions include pulmonary fibrosis and acute conditions include acute respiratory distress syndrome (ARDS). Lung ultrasound provides an easy bedside modality to detect AIS. The presence of diffuse B-lines corresponds to sonographic evidence of sub-pleural thickened interlobular septa. These B-lines produce characteristic confluent vertical echo beams that extend the entire depth of the image and do not decrease in intensity (Mayo et al. 2019).

3.2 Detection of Pneumothorax

The presence of lung sliding at the site of probe application rules out pneumothorax at that specific site, as this signifies that there is no air separating the visceral and parietal pleura. The presence of B-lines excludes pneumothorax as well, as these are visualized deep to the visceral pleura and would not be visualized in the presence of intrapleural air. While lung sliding rules out pneumothorax, the absence of it only suggests the possibility of it. *Lung point*, however, is pathognomonic of a pneumothorax and represents the intersection of the partially deflated lung and the air-filled pneumothorax space (Chan 2003). At this location, the partially collapsed lung moves in and out of the ultrasound view during the respiratory cycle, whereas the adjacent pneumothorax space is immobile (Fig. 17). The location of a lung point is helpful in determining the extent of a pneumothorax and determining the optimal location for chest tube placement.

3.3 Detection of Pulmonary Edema/Vascular Congestion

Cardiogenic pulmonary edema is most clearly characterized by an extensive B-line pattern on thoracic ultrasonography. Because B-lines are non-specific and indicate that there is something other than air within that specific area of the lung (fluid, infection, inflammation, etc.), additional clues must be relied upon to differentiate

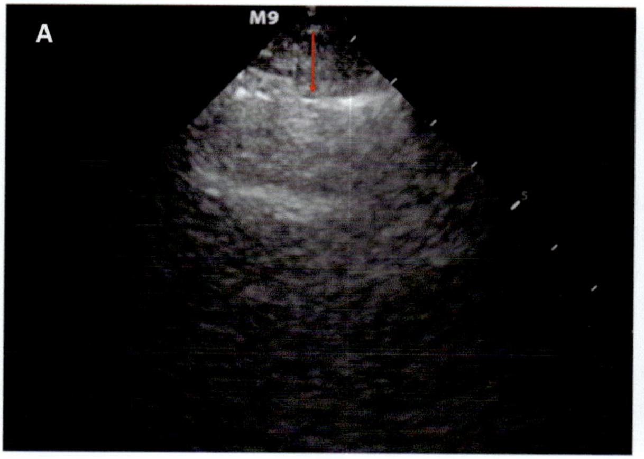 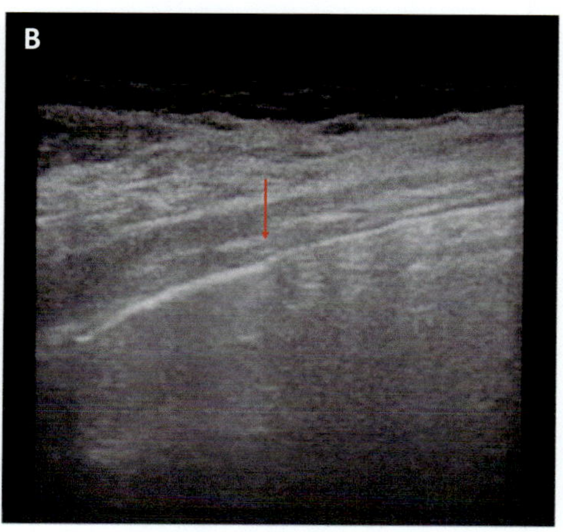

Fig. 17 The red arrows mark the border of the pneumothorax in both images. Image A: to the left (cephalad) of this point, there is an absence of lung sliding, while to the right (caudad) of this point, there is lung sliding, with shimmering and thickening of the pleural line; Image B: to the right (caudad) of this point, there is an absence of lung sliding, while to the left (cephalad), lung sliding is present with shimmering and thickening of the pleural line

pulmonary edema and/or vascular congestion from other pulmonary pathologies. In most circumstances, pulmonary edema will be bilateral and often gravity-dependent, so there will be B-lines seen in bilateral lung fields and with a potential worsening in the lower lung fields in patients with vascular congestion (Mayo et al. 2019; Kataoka and Takada 2000). This finding will often help differentiate this diagnosis from a multifocal pneumonia or acute respiratory distress syndrome (ARDS), where there would likely be asymmetry and areas of lung sparing (with normal A-line pattern). In addition, the pleural line may also help to differentiate pulmonary edema from an inflammatory or infectious process. For infectious or inflammatory processes, the pleural line will often be thickened (> 2 mm) and coarse or irregular in appearance, in contrast to vascular congestion or pulmonary edema, where the pleural line will have a thinner, smoother appearance. The classic ultrasound pattern then for patients with significant pulmonary edema and vascular congestion will be an extensive, bilateral B-line lung pattern and a smooth pleural line (+/− pleural effusions).

4 Summary

To outline the common approach of utilizing chest sonography clinically, we have adapted the frequently cited "Blue Protocol" (Lichtenstein et al. 2009) (Fig. 18). Additionally, the common lung ultrasound patterns and their clinical interpretation have been condensed in a table for reference (Table 1). In summary, chest sonography is invaluable in the evaluation of cardiopulmonary symptoms and, with practice, can quickly aid in the diagnosis of many conditions at the bedside.

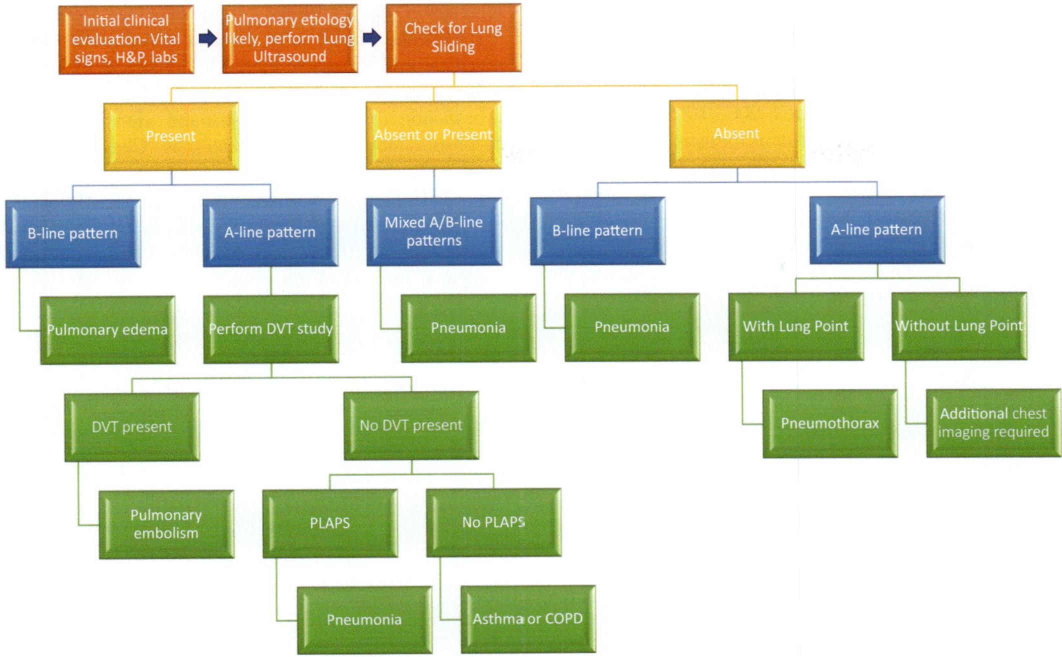

Fig. 18 This algorithm demonstrates how to incorporate lung ultrasound findings to guide the diagnosis of pulmonary symptoms

Table 1 This chart outlines common lung ultrasound patterns and their clinical interpretation

Lung ultrasound pattern	Clinical Interpretation
Lung sliding with A-line pattern	Normal lung aeration
Absent lung sliding with A-lines ± lung point	Pneumothorax
Moderate B-lines (4–5 visible)	Interlobular septal pathology
Diffuse B-lines (7–8 visible)	Alveolar-interstitial syndrome
Lung hepatization + dynamic air bronchograms	Pneumonia
Lung hepatization ± static air bronchograms	Atelectasis
Anechoic fluid collection without septations	Simple pleural effusion
Echogenic fluid collection with septations	Complicated pleural effusion

References

Chan SS. Emergency bedside ultrasound to detect pneumothorax. Acad Emerg Med. 2003;10(1):91–4.

Kataoka H, Takada S. The role of thoracic ultrasonography for evaluation of patients with decompensated chronic heart failure. J Am Coll Cardiol. 2000;35 (6):1638–46.

Lichtenstein DA, Mezière GA. Relevance of lung ultrasound in the diagnosis of acute respiratory failure: the BLUE protocol. Chest. 2008;134(1):117–25.

Lichtenstein DA, Lascols N, Mezière G, Gepner A. Ultrasound diagnosis of alveolar consolidation in the critically ill. Intensive Care Med. 2004;30(2):276–81.

Lichtenstein D, Mezière G, Seitz J. The dynamic air bronchogram. A lung ultrasound sign of alveolar consolidation ruling out atelectasis. Chest. 2009;135 (6):1421–1425.

Mayo PH, Copetti R, Feller-Kopman D, Mathis G, Maury E, Mongodi S, Mojoli F, Volpicelli G, Zanobetti M. Thoracic ultrasonography: a narrative review. Intensive Care Med. 2019;45(9):1200–11.

Clinical Cases in Cardiac Electrosonography

Clinical Cases of Electrosonography in Patients with Acute Chest Pain

Jonathan Koslowsky, Yair Elitzur,
David Leibowitz, Ronny Alcalai,
and Eyal Herzog

Abstract

Acute chest pain is one of the most frequent complaints in emergency facilities. The differential diagnosis of chest pain is wide and can vary from a benign complaint to a life-threatening illness. Although it is very common, it poses upon the treating physician a diagnostic challenge as the correlation between the quality and characteristics of the chest pain and a specific diagnosis is low, and the overlap is high. Electrocardiogram (ECG) and trans-thoracic echocardiography (TTE) are two of the most important tests in the early workup stages of the acute chest pain patient and can help diagnose correctly the etiology of the chest pain and rule out alternative diagnoses. The combined use of ECG and TTE in the workup process is termed **Electrosonography**, and in this chapter we present the use of electrosonography in the evaluation of acute chest pain patients. The chapter first presents an algorithm demonstrating the workflow for evaluating an acute chest pain patient. The algorithm lays out the recommended steps for evaluating the patient including the timing of when ECG and TTE should be done and the next step in the workup. The second part of the chapter includes 16 acute chest pain patients who presented at an emergency facility. Each case includes 4 pages in a learning-friendly format with the information gathering gradually allowing the reader to test his knowledge in ECG and TTE, leading to electrosonography, the combined information obtained from the ECG and TTE. The case number of each scenario is imbedded in the algorithm near the specific diagnosis. The cases in this chapter can be studied independently or as part of the algorithm, as an example for each diagnosis. Learning the algorithm and the different chest pain cases can aid the physician with the challenging yet critical process of evaluating and treating acute chest patients in an emergency setting.

Keywords

ECG · Chest pain · Coronary artery disease · Echocardiography · Pericarditis · Myocardial infarction · Aortic dissection · Pulmonary embolism · Aortic stenosis

J. Koslowsky (✉) · Y. Elitzur · D. Leibowitz ·
R. Alcalai · E. Herzog
Department of Cardiology, The Heart Institute,
Hadassah Medical Center, Hebrew University
of Jerusalem, Jerusalem, Israel

© The Author(s), under exclusive license to Springer Nature Switzerland AG 2023
E. Herzog et al. (eds.), *Cardiac Electrosonography*,
https://doi.org/10.1007/978-3-031-38469-1_5

1 Introduction

Acute chest pain is one of the most frequent complaints in an emergency department setting and may be a sign of a life-threatening illness. However, accurately diagnosing the etiology of the acute chest pain in an emergency setting is challenging and therefore other tests are required to achieve the correct diagnosis and implement the appropriate treatment.

Two of the most important tests in the early workup stages of the acute chest pain patient, are electrocardiogram (ECG) and trans-thoracic echocardiography (TTE). ECG and TTE, if done and interpreted properly, can help diagnose correctly the etiology of the chest pain and rule out alternative diagnoses. The combined use of ECG and TTE in the workup process is termed **Electrosonography**, and in this chapter we present the use of electrosonography in the evaluation of acute chest pain patients.

We first introduce an algorithm (Fig. 1) laying out the pathway for the use of electrosonography in patients with acute chest pain. This algorithm will aid the physician with decision making based on the primary evaluation upon presentation and the ECG and TTE findings. The algorithm defines the time each test should be done and the next step in the workup process. We include the ECG test code answers as well (Fig. 2) for easy preparation for the test.

We then demonstrate the use of the algorithm by presenting 16 cases of patients who presented with acute chest pain. Each case has a similar layout and contains 4 pages allowing the reader to test his or her knowledge of ECG and TTE interpretation:

- Page 1 includes the presenting complaint and additional clinical information as well as an ECG performed on arrival
- Page 2 includes the authors' interpretation of the ECG and a short discussion regarding the findings and the next recommended step. The ECG test answers are included for aiding students in preparation for the test
- Page 3 includes transthoracic echocardiography images with a legend of the views seen

- Page 4 includes the authors' interpretation of the echocardiography with a discussion of the combined electrosonography findings.

The algorithm lays out the workup process for chest pain patients. Initial evaluation includes a thorough and detailed history and physical examination including vital signs. If the chest pain is clearly not of cardiac origin, alternative diagnoses should be pursued.

If the chest pain appears to be of cardiovascular origin the initial evaluation should start with a 12-lead ECG. The ECG findings divide the patients into two groups:

- ECG findings suggestive of acute coronary syndrome (ACS)
- ECG findings non diagnostic of ACS

In addition to ECG, transthoracic echocardiography (TTE) plays a critical role in the evaluation of patients with chest pain. Nonetheless, the recommended timing for completing the TTE differs between patients based on their presumed diagnosis.

If the ECG findings are suggestive of ACS the patients are further divided into two groups:

- Patients with ST elevation on ECG who are diagnosed as ST elevation myocardial infarction (STEMI)
- Patients with ECG findings suggestive of ACS but without ST elevation who are diagnosed as Non ST elevation acute coronary syndrome (Non STE ACS)

It is well accepted that STEMI patients who present with acute chest pain and ST elevation on ECG, should undergo revascularization therapy. In a capable facility the best option for revascularization is usually percutaneous coronary intervention (PCI) in the cardiac catheterization laboratory. In these patients proceeding to immediate PCI is of great significance, therefore TTE should not be performed before the PCI as it can delay revascularization.

In contrast to STEMI patients, patients who are diagnosed with non-STE ACS should be treated medically as per current guidelines and TTE should be performed as soon as possible. TTE can assess for regional wall motion abnormalities supporting the diagnosis of ACS, evaluate for structural heart disease (such as valvular

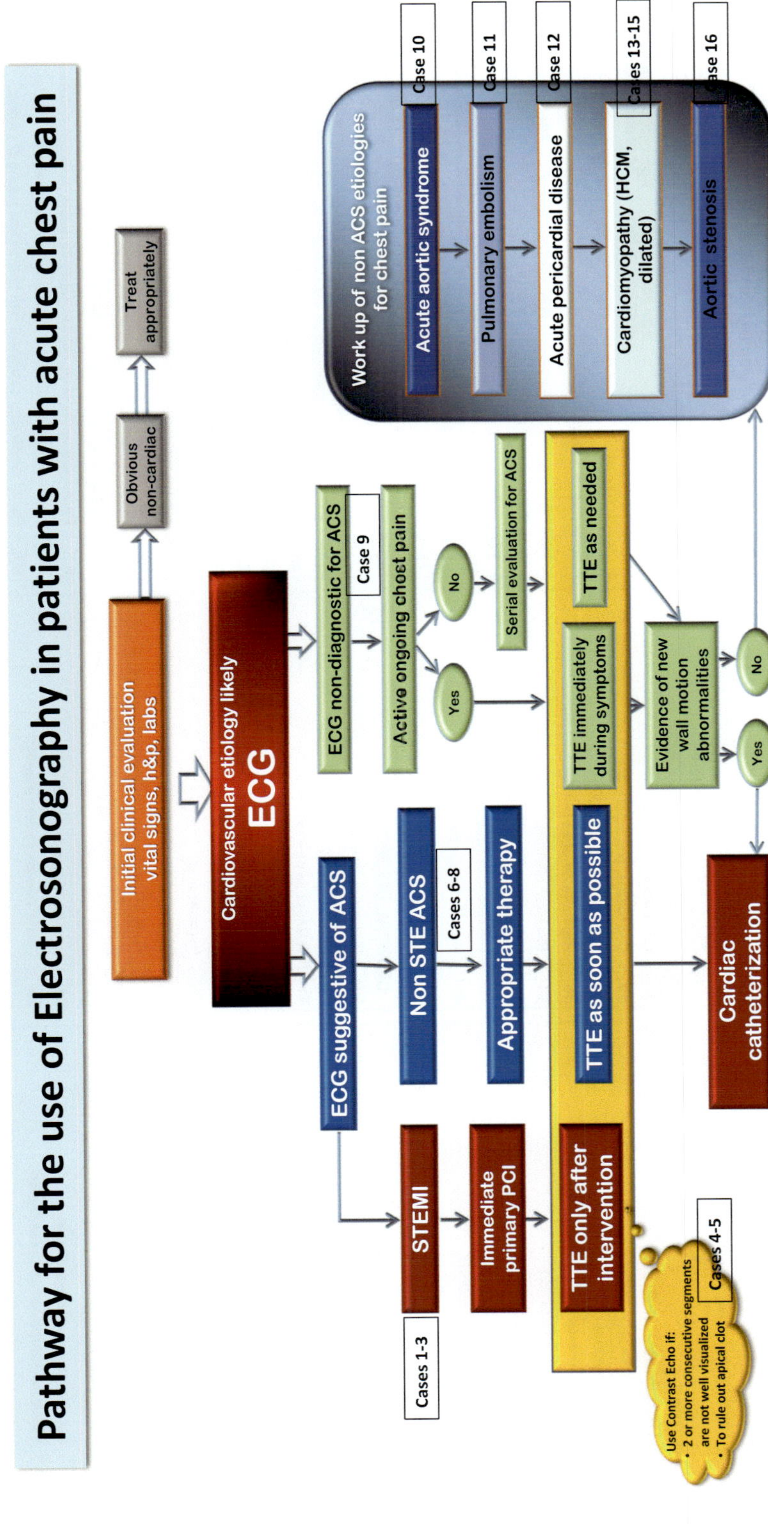

Fig. 1 Pathway for the use of electrosonography in patients with acute chest pain

GENERAL FEATURES & P WAVE ABNORMALITIES

General Features

1 ☐ Normal ECG
2 ☐ Normal variant
3 ☐ Incorrect electrode placement
4 ☐ Artifact

P Wave Abnormalities

5 ☐ Right atrial abnormality/enlargement
6 ☐ Left atrial abnormality/enlargement

RHYTHMS

Atrial Rhythms

7 ☐ Sinus rhythm
8 ☐ Sinus arrhythmia
9 ☐ Sinus bradycardia (<60)
10 ☐ Sinus tachycardia (>100)
11 ☐ Sinus pause or arrest
12 ☐ Sinoatrial exit block
13 ☐ Atrial premature complexes
14 ☐ Atrial tachycardia
15 ☐ Atrial tachycardia, multifocal
16 ☐ Supraventricular tachycardia
17 ☐ Atrial flutter
18 ☐ Atrial fibrillation

AV Junctional Rhythms

19 ☐ AV junctional premature complexes
20 ☐ AV junctional escape complexes
21 ☐ AV junctional rhythm/tachycardia

Ventricular Rhythms

22 ☐ Ventricular premature complex(es)
23 ☐ Ventricular parasystole
24 ☐ Ventricular tachycardia (3 or more consecutive complexes)
25 ☐ Accelerated idioventricular rhythm
26 ☐ Ventricular escape complexes or rhythm
27 ☐ Ventricular fibrillation

ATRIOVENTRICULAR CONDUCTION

28 ☐ AV block, 1°
29 ☐ AV block, 2° - Mobitz type I (Wenckebach)
30 ☐ AV block, 2° - Mobitz type II
31 ☐ AV block, 2:1
32 ☐ AV block, 3°
33 ☐ Wolff-Parkinson-White pattern
34 ☐ AV dissociation

VOLTAGE OR AXIS/HYPERTROPHY

Abnormal QRS Voltage or Axis

35 ☐ Low voltage, limb leads
36 ☐ Low voltage, precordial leads
37 ☐ Left axis deviation (> -30°)
38 ☐ Right axis deviation (> +100°)
39 ☐ Electrical alternans

Ventricular Hypertrophy

40 ☐ Left ventricular hypertrophy
41 ☐ Right ventricular hypertrophy
42 ☐ Combined ventricular hypertrophy

CLINICAL DISORDERS

43 ☐ Brugada syndrome
44 ☐ Digitalis toxicity
45 ☐ Torsades de pointes
46 ☐ Hyperkalemia
47 ☐ Hypokalemia
48 ☐ Hypercalcemia
49 ☐ Hypocalcemia
50 ☐ Dextrocardia, mirror image
51 ☐ Acute cor pulmonale including pulmonary embolus
52 ☐ Pericardial effusion
53 ☐ Acute pericarditis
54 ☐ Hypertrophic cardiomyopathy
55 ☐ Central nervous system disorder
56 ☐ Hypothermia

INTRAVENTRICULAR CONDUCTION

57 ☐ RBBB, complete
58 ☐ RBBB, incomplete
59 ☐ Left anterior fascicular block
60 ☐ Left posterior fascicular block
61 ☐ LBBB, complete
62 ☐ LBBB, incomplete
63 ☐ Aberrant conduction (including rate-related)
64 ☐ Intraventricular conduction disturbance, nonspecific type

MYOCARDIAL INFARCTION

	Age recent, or probably acute	Age indeterminate, or probably old
Anterolateral	65 ☐	66 ☐
Anterior or anteroseptal	67 ☐	68 ☐
Lateral	69 ☐	70 ☐
Inferior	71 ☐	72 ☐
Posterior	73 ☐	74 ☐

ST, T, U WAVE ABNORMALITIES

75 ☐ Normal variant, early repolarization
76 ☐ Normal variant, juvenile T waves
77 ☐ Nonspecific ST and/or T wave abnormalities
78 ☐ ST and/or T wave abnormalities suggesting myocardial ischemia
79 ☐ ST and/or T wave abnormalities suggesting myocardial injury
80 ☐ ST and/or T wave abnormalities suggesting electrolyte disturbances
81 ☐ ST and/or T wave abnormalities secondary to hypertrophy
82 ☐ Prolonged Q-T interval
83 ☐ Prominent U waves

PACEMAKER FUNCTION

84 ☐ Atrial or coronary sinus pacing
85 ☐ Ventricular demand pacemaker (VVI), normally functioning
86 ☐ Dual-chamber pacemaker (DDD), normally functioning
87 ☐ Pacemaker malfunction, not constantly capturing (atrium or ventricle)
88 ☐ Pacemaker malfunction, not constantly sensing (atrium or ventricle)
89 ☐ Paced morphology consistent with biventricular pacing or cardiac resynchronization therapy

Fig. 2 Codes for ECG reading

abnormalities) and rule out alternative diagnoses. If regional wall motion abnormalities are found on the TTE, supporting the diagnosis of ACS, the patients are usually referred for cardiac catheterization and revascularization as needed. Patients who present with symptoms and signs suggestive of ACS and the ECG is not diagnostic for ACS, divide as well into two groups based on the clinical scenario. If the patient has ongoing chest pain, a TTE should be performed immediately, ideally during the pain. If the chest pain symptoms resolved, we recommend serial evaluation for ACS and TTE as needed. In both scenarios, a finding of regional wall motion abnormality on TTE supports the diagnosis of ACS, and the patient should be referred for cardiac catheterization.

For patients without regional motion abnormality, in whom a diagnosis of ACS is unlikely, other cardiac etiologies should be considered. We recommend performing a thorough work up ruling out the following conditions in this order, based on the urgency and the risk they pose to the patient:

– Acute aortic syndrome
– Acute pulmonary embolism
– Acute pericardial disease
– Cardiomyopathy (dilated, hypertrophic)
– Aortic stenosis.

In this chapter we present 16 different scenarios of patients presenting with acute chest pain. In each case we discuss the electrosonography which is the combined findings of the ECG and TTE. We demonstrate how electrosonography leads to the likely diagnosis and the next recommended step. The case number of each scenario is imbedded in the algorithm near the specific diagnosis. The cases in this chapter can be studied independently or as part of the algorithm, as an example of each diagnosis.

In conclusion, acute chest pain is a very common complaint in emergency facilities. The differential diagnosis of acute chest pain is wide and can vary from a benign complaint to a life-threatening illness. Although it is very common, it poses a serious diagnostic challenge. We hope this chapter will lay out a clear and easy-to-use algorithm for the evaluation of acute chest pain, using two of the most important tools we have—ECG and echocardiography, guiding the physician through the challenging yet critical process.

2 Case 1

Clinical History

A 48-year old male with a history of heavy smoking and exertional chest pain in the past few months, presented with 3 hours of severe mid sternal chest pain.

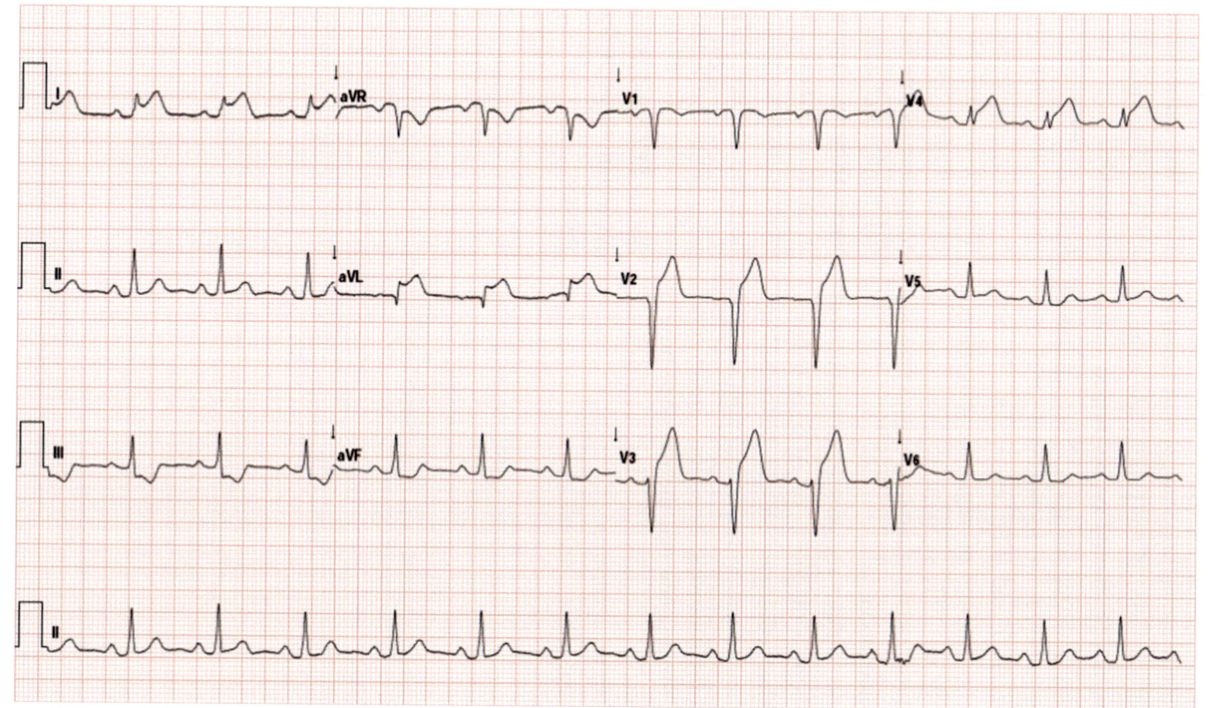

ECG Interpretation

Rhythm: Sinus
Rate: 82 bpm
Intervals: PR = 160 ms, QRS = 100 ms, QT = 340 ms, QTC Baz = 382 ms– normal intervals.
Axis: Normal.

Abnormalities on the ECG

- ST elevation in I, aVL, V1, V2, V3, V4
- ST depression in III, aVF, aVR
- Poor R wave progression in V1, V2, V3.

ECG Test Answers
7, 65, 67, 78, 79.

ECG Synthesis

This ECG shows sinus rhythm at 82 bpm, normal intervals and axis.

Abnormalities include ST elevation in the anterior septum, anterior and lateral leads with poor R wave progression in leads V1, V2 and V3. In addition, there are ST depressions in the inferior leads. The finding of ST depression in the inferior leads in the presence of ST elevation in the anterior leads is most probably due to reciprocal changes and not a sign of inferior ischemia.

A patient with ST elevation on ECG in a setting of acute substernal chest pain requires immediate revascularization, usually by percutaneous cardiac angioplasty.

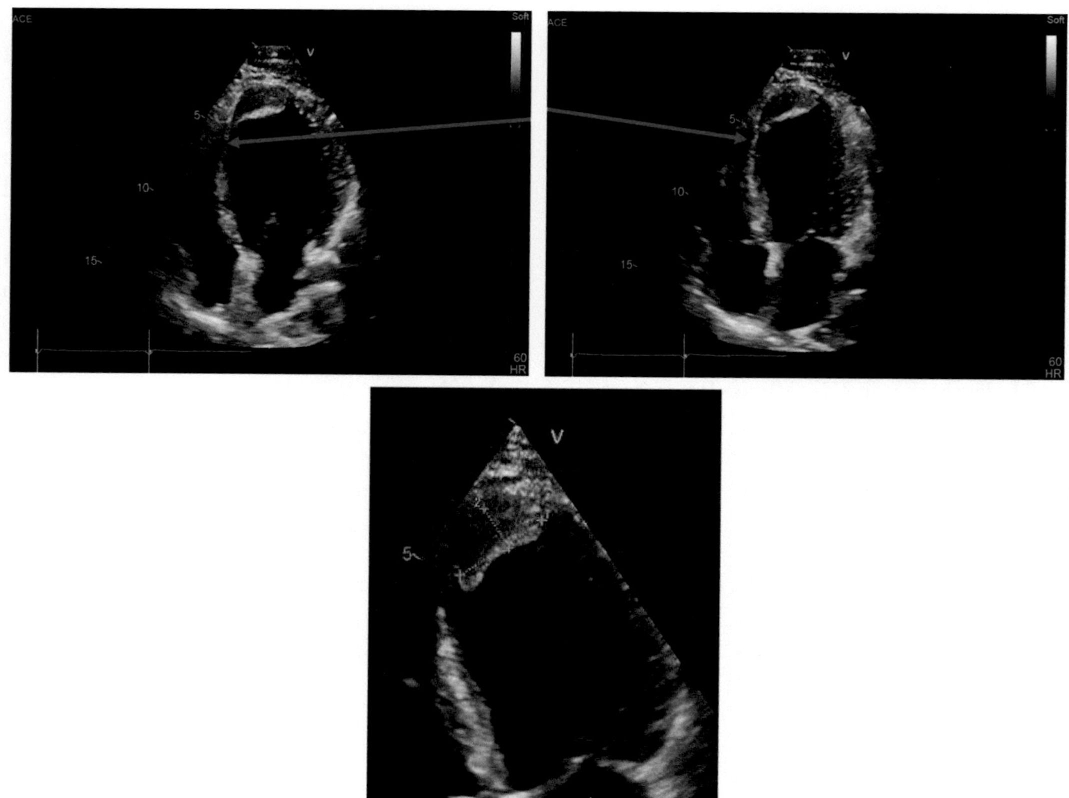

Top images: Apical 4-chamber views with mitral valve opened in diastole (left) and closed in systole (right). The blue arrows show part of the area of akinesis. Bottom image: Apical 4-chamber image with focus on the apex demonstrating a hyperechogenic finding

Echo Interpretation

The left ventricle is normal size

The left ventricular systolic function is severely decreased with estimated LVEF = 30%.

A large, regional wall motion abnormality is seen with akinesis of the mid septum and the apex. A large (14 mm × 30 mm) hyperechoic finding is seen in the apex

Echo Synthesis

The finding of akinesis of the mid inferior septum, the apex and the apical anterior wall is consistent with severe ischemia in the LAD (left anterior descending) territory. The hyperechoic finding is most consistent with mural thrombus. This is a common complication of a large akinetic segmental wall motion abnormality in particular in the apical region after an anterior wall myocardial infarction.

Cardiac Electrosonography Synthesis

The patient presented with classic substernal chest pain with ECG changes demonstrating ST elevation in the antero-lateral leads with inferior reciprocal changes, corresponding with an acute antero-lateral myocardial infarction mandating immediate revascularization therapy. In this setting, completing an echo should not delay the immediate treatment and is not required before the coronary angiography.

The patient was taken to the cardiac catheterization laboratory, and the LAD artery was found to be occluded. PCI (percutaneous coronary intervention) of the LAD was done with improvement in symptoms and ECG findings. Echo that was done post PCI demonstrated akinesis in the LAD region (blue arrows) and an hyperechogenic finding in the apical region (blue measurement) consistent with a mural thrombus.

3 Case 2

Clinical History

A 65-year-old male with a prior history of smoking, hypertension and hypercholesterolemia presented with 2 hours of severe chest pain

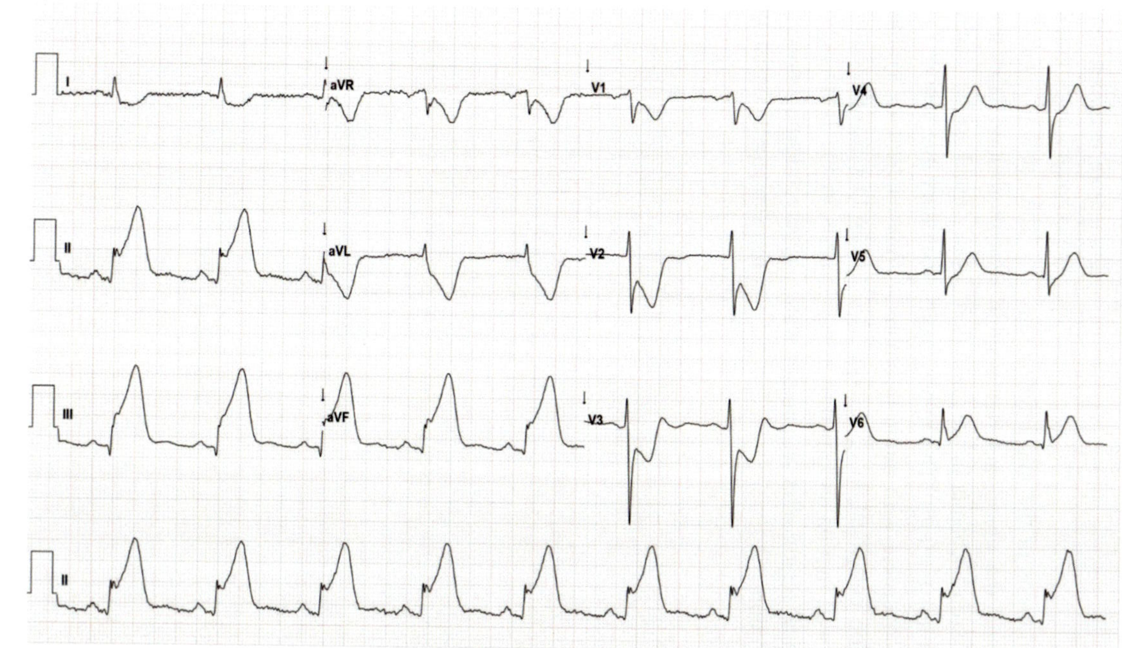

Additional Clinical History

While being treated in the emergency department, the patient developed ventricular fibrillation treated with emergent defibrillation

ECG Interpretation

Rhythm: Sinus
Rate: 60 bpm
Intervals: PR = 195 ms, QRS = 111 ms, QT = 427 ms, QTC Baz = 428 ms– normal intervals.
Axis: Normal.

Abnormalities on the ECG

- ST elevation in II, III, aVF, V6.
- ST depression in I, aVL, aVR, V1. V2, V3.

ECG Test Answers
7, 71, 73, 78, 79.

ECG Synthesis
This ECG shows sinus rhythm at 60 bpm with normal intervals and axis.

Abnormalities seen in this ECG are ST elevation in the inferior leads and ST depression in the posterior and the high lateral leads.

The finding of ST depression in leads V1-V3 in the presence of ST elevation in the inferior leads most likely are due to posterior wall involvement and occasionally (less likely) due to additional anterior wall injury.

A patient with ST elevation on ECG in a setting of acute substernal chest pain requires immediate revascularization, usually by percutaneous cardiac angioplasty.

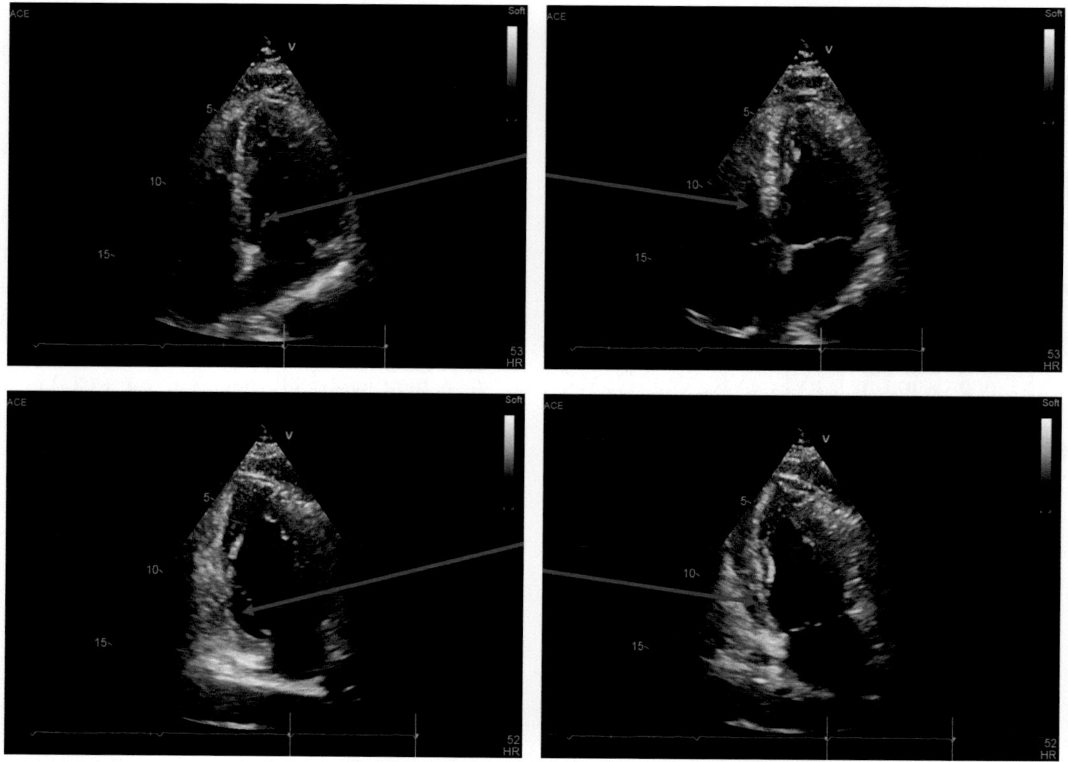

Top images: Apical 4-chamber views with mitral valve opened in diastole (left) and closed in systole (right) Bottom images: Apical 2-chamber views with mitral valve opened in diastole (left) and closed in systole (right)

Echo Interpretation

The left ventricle is normal size.

The left ventricular systolic function is mildly reduced with estimated LVEF of 40–45%.

Regional wall motion abnormalities are seen with akinesis of the inferior and the inferior-septal walls (blue arrows).

Echo Synthesis

The findings of very specific regional wall motion abnormalities in a distribution of a specific coronary artery usually support a diagnosis of involvement of that coronary artery. In this case, as seen in the 2-chamber view, involvement of the inferior wall suggests involvement of either the RCA artery or the circumflex (LCx) artery. Wall motion abnormalities in the 4-chamber view can help distinguish between RCA and LCx, as the RCA causes wall motion abnormalities in the inferior septum while the LCx affects the anterior lateral wall. In this case, the wall motion abnormalities are seen in the inferior septum, hence the coronary artery involved is most likely the RCA.

Cardiac Electrosonography Synthesis

The patient presented with classic substernal chest pain with ECG changes including ST elevation in the inferior leads and ST depression in the posterior leads, corresponding with an acute inferior and posterior myocardial infarction and mandating immediate revascularization therapy. In this setting, completing an echo should not delay the immediate treatment and is not required before the coronary angiography.

The patient was taken to the cardiac catheterization laboratory and a coronary angiogram demonstrated an occluded right coronary artery which was treated with PCI (percutaneous coronary intervention) with immediate improvement in patient's symptoms and ECG findings. Echocardiography that was performed post PCI demonstrated regional wall motion akinesis involving the RCA territory.

4   Case 3

Clinical History

A 67 years old male with past medical history of heavy smoking, hypertension, and hypercholesterolemia presented with 3 hours of severe substernal chest pain

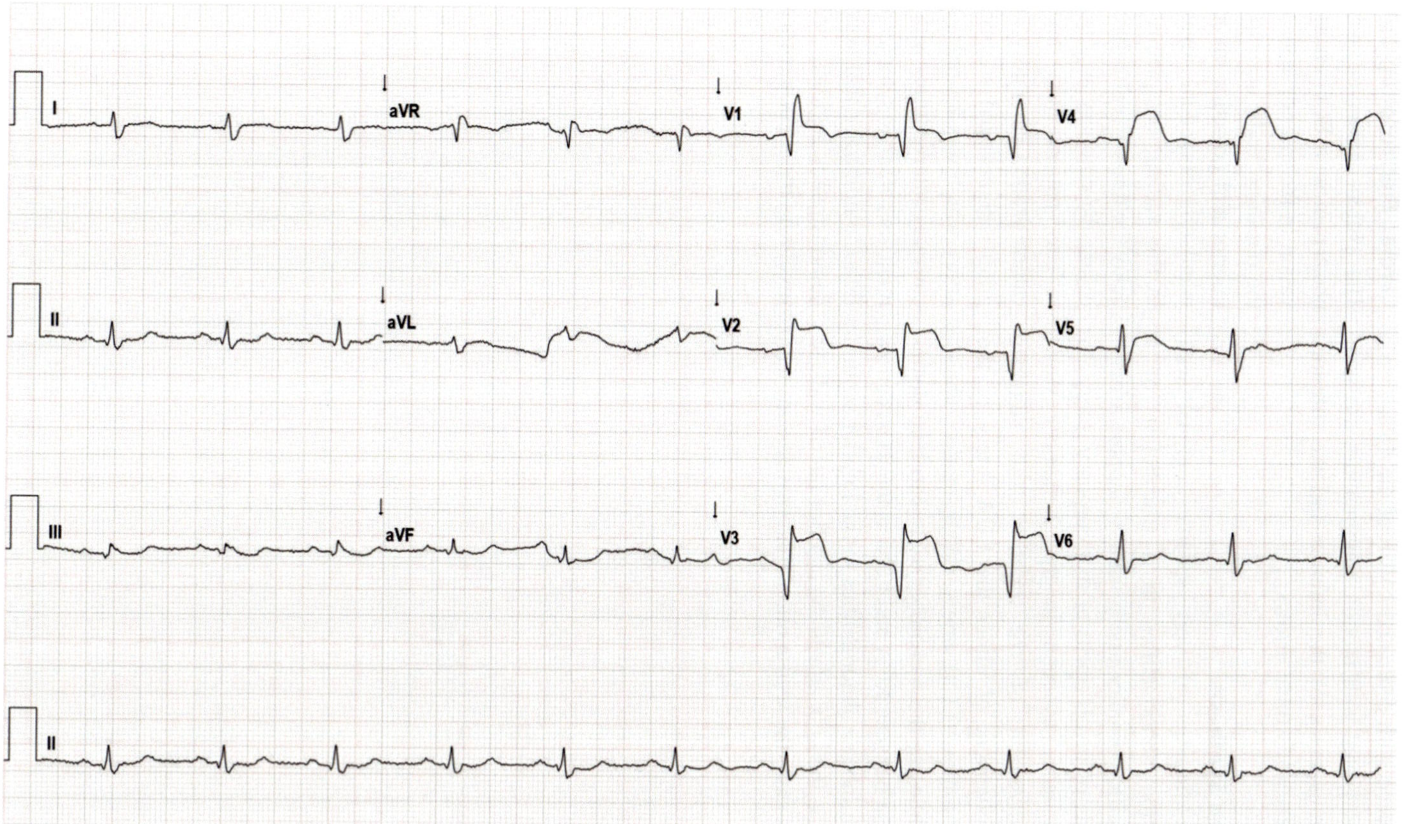

ECG Interpretation

Rhythm: Sinus
Rate: 72 bpm
Intervals: PR = 180 ms, QRS = 135 ms, QT = 385 ms, QTC Baz = 410 ms
Axis: Normal.

Abnormalities on the ECG

- RBBB, complete
- ST elevation in V1, V2, V3, V4, V5
- ST depression in II, III, aVF
- Q waves in V1, V2, V3, V4, q waves in II, III, aVF

ECG Test Answers

7, 57, 65, 67, 68, 72, 78, 79.

ECG Synthesis

This ECG shows sinus rhythm at 72 bpm, complete RBBB and normal axis.

Abnormalities seen in this ECG are Q waves in V1-V4 with ST elevation in the anterior and antero-septal leads. There are very small q waves and mild ST depression in the inferior leads, in the setting of a complete RBBB. In the setting of compete RBBB, usually the first 0.04 ms of the QRS complex can be appropriately interpreted, while the ST-T changes are more difficult to interpret if they are dis-concordant (opposite direction) to the R wave. In this case the Q waves in leads V1-V4 suggest infarct of undetermined duration of the anterior septum and the anterior walls. The finding of a RBBB, if new, in the setting of acute anterior wall infarction is an ominous prognostic sign.

The concordant ST elevation in V1-V4 seen here in the setting of RBBB, suggest acute myocardial injury in the same coronary artery distribution. The small q wave seen in the inferior leads may suggest involvement of the inferior wall (likely due to a large LAD that supplies the apical inferior wall).

Q waves in the anterior leads can develop in acute MI cases and, in some studies, has been correlated with worse prognosis compared to patients who did not develop Q waves.

A patient with ST elevation on ECG in a setting of acute substernal chest pain requires immediate revascularization, usually by cardiac angioplasty.

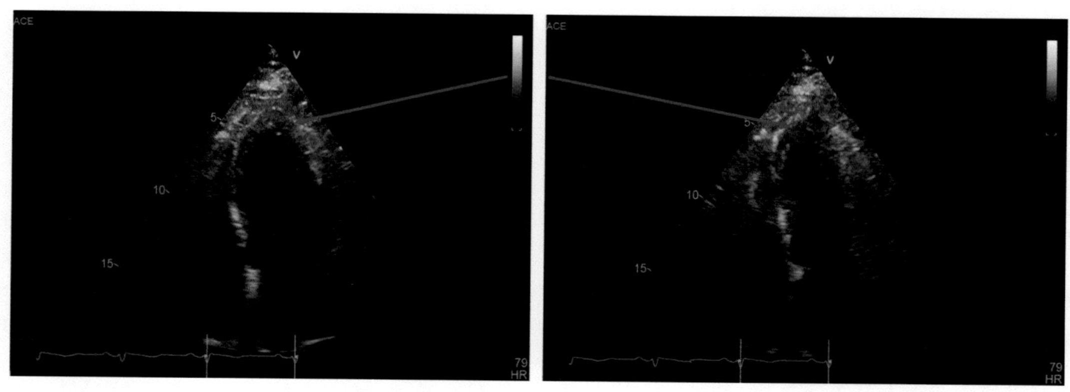

Apical 4-chamber views with mitral valve opened in diastole (left) and closed in systole (right)

Echo Interpretation

The left ventricle is normal size.

The left ventricular systolic function is mildly decreased with estimated LVEF = 45% Regional wall motion abnormality demonstrates akinesis of the apex.

Echo Synthesis

The finding of akinesis of the apex without involvement of the base and mid-septum is consistent with ischemia or injury in the mid to distal LAD territory.

Cardiac Electrosonography Synthesis

The patient presented with classic substernal chest pain with ECG changes including ST elevation in the antero-septal leads in the setting of RBBB, consistent with an acute myocardial injury that mandates immediate revascularization therapy. In this setting, completing an echocardiogram should not delay immediate treatment and is not recommended before the coronary angiography.

The patient was taken to the cardiac catheterization laboratory, and the mid portion of the LAD (left anterior descending) artery was found to be occluded. PCI (percutaneous coronary intervention) to the LAD was done with improvement in the patient's symptoms and the ECG findings.

Echocardiography that was performed after the PCI demonstrated akinesis in the apex which correlates with the LAD territory.

Of note, the findings on echocardiography were less impressive compared to the ECG findings, which occurs occasionally in a setting of ST elevation myocardial infarction. This can be explained by rich collateral arteries supplying a prior infarcted territory.

5 Case 4

A 60 years old male with history of anxiety and depression, presented to the ED with new onset severe sub-sternal chest pain, which awoke him from sleep early in the morning. Upon arrival to the ED, the pain subsided.

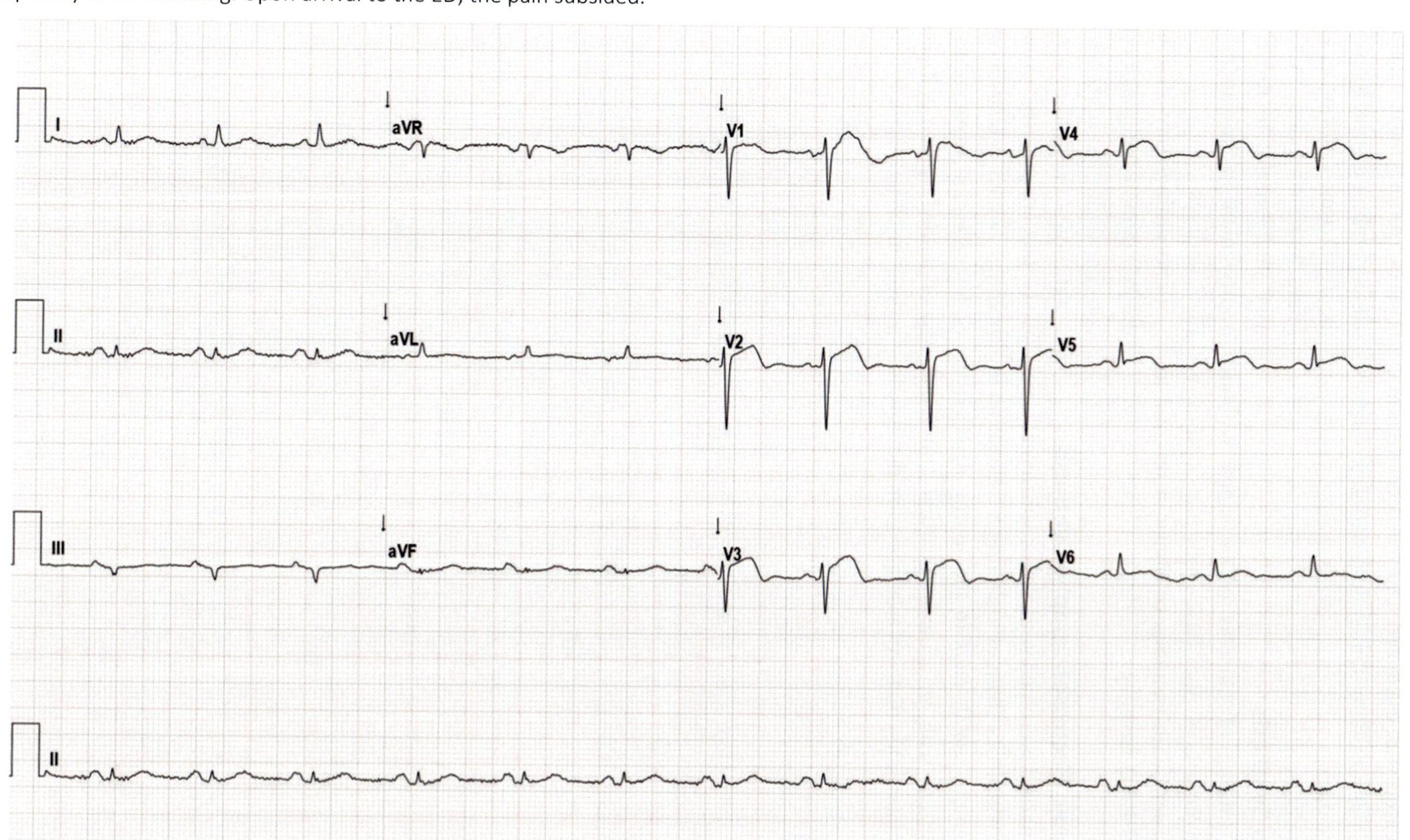

ECG Interpretation

Rhythm: Sinus
Rate: 80 bpm
Intervals: PR = 145 ms, QRS = 86 ms, QT = 375 ms, RR = 750 ms, QTC Baz = 410 ms
Axis: Normal

Abnormalities on the ECG

- ST elevation in V1-V5
- Bi-phasic T wave in V1-V4
- Poor R wave progression in V1-V4
- Low voltage limb leads.

ECG Test Answers

7, 35, 67, 78, 79.

ECG Synthesis

This ECG shows sinus rhythm at 80 bpm, normal intervals and axis.

Abnormalities include ST elevation in the anterior and the anterior-septal leads with poor R wave progression in V1-V4 and noticeable biphasic T waves in V1-V4.

This patient with high suspicion for a severe LAD coronary stenosis, as other patients with ST elevation on ECG in a setting of acute substernal chest pain should be taken to the cardiac catheterization laboratory for angiography of the coronary arteries and revascularization.

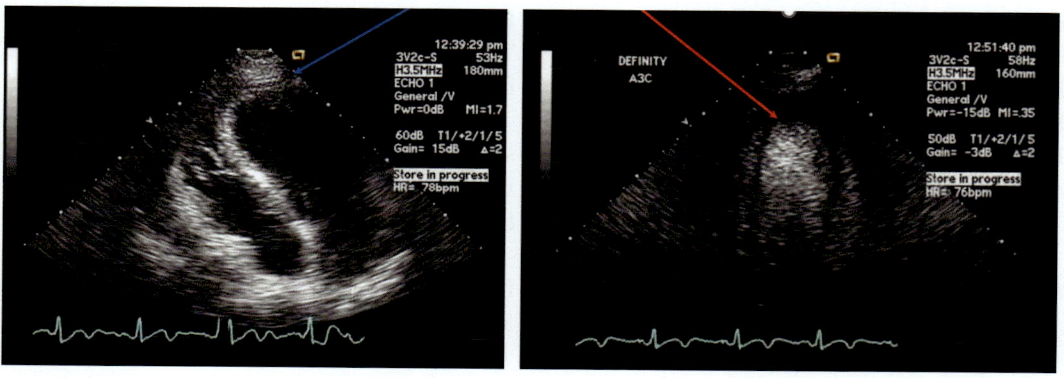

Unenhanced 4 chambers apical imaging (left) and the same view with imaging enhancing agent (right)

Echo Interpretation

The left ventricle is normal size.

The left ventricular systolic function is moderately decreased, estimated LVEF—35 to 40%.

Regional wall motion abnormalities include akinesis of the mid inferior-septal wall and the apical segments. Unenhanced echocardiography 4 chambers apical views raised the suspicion for apical thrombus (blue arrow).

Using an imaging enhancing agent (contrast echocardiography)—no signs of filling defect in the apical region (red arrow).

Echo Synthesis

The finding of akinesis of the mid inferior-septal wall and the apex is consistent with ischemia of the LAD.

Echo contrast can be used to better delineate the endocardial borders and to visualize filling defects such as a thrombus. In this case a finding in the apical region seen on unenhanced echocardiography raised the suspicion for an apical thrombus which was ruled out by repeating the echo using imaging enhancing agent.

Cardiac Electrosonography Synthesis

The patient presented with classic substernal chest pain with ECG changes including ST elevation in the anterior and anterior-septal leads with clear biphasic T waves in V2-V3, consistent with severe stenosis of the proximal LAD. This situation mandates immediate revascularization therapy. In this setting, completing an echo should not delay the immediate treatment and is not required before the coronary angiography.

The patient was taken to the cardiac catheterization laboratory, and the proximal portion of the LAD (left anterior descending) artery was found to be occluded. PCI (percutaneous coronary intervention) to the LAD was done with improvement in symptoms and ECG findings.

Echo was done post PCI demonstrating akinesis of the mid inferior-septal wall and the apical segments with a suspected apical thrombus, a common complication post anterior myocardial infarction. Repeating the echocardiography with use of an imaging enhancing agent ruled out this possibility.

6 Case 5

Clinical History

A 68 years old female presented to the emergency department with complaints of three days of severe substernal chest pain

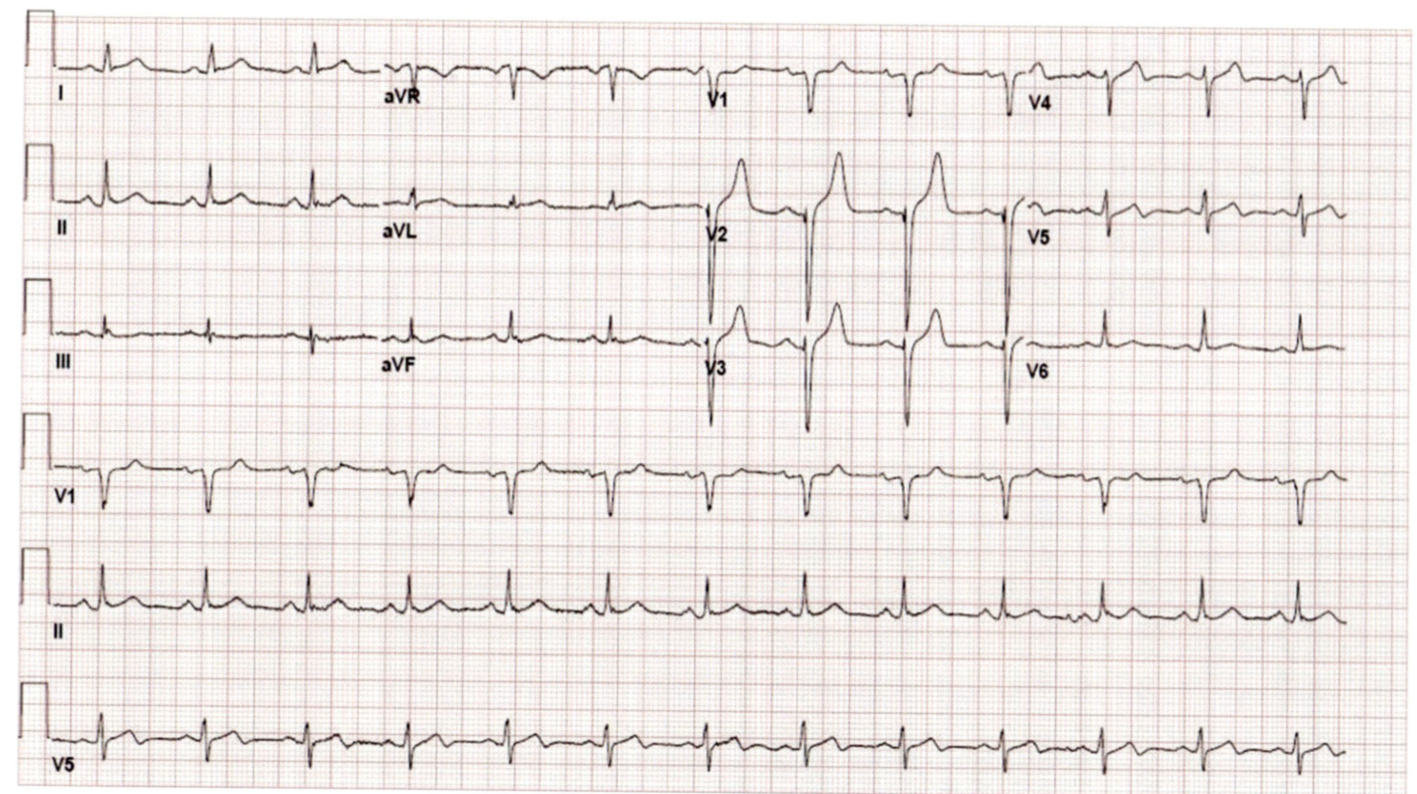

ECG Interpretation

Rhythm: Sinus
Rate: 76 bpm
Intervals: PR = 160 ms, QRS = 110 ms, QT = 350 ms, RR = 780 ms, QTC Baz = 396 ms
Axis: Normal.

Abnormalities on the ECG

- The T wave in lead V2 seems somewhat tall and peaked; however, is not very tall when compared to the depth of the QRS complex in the same lead.
- There is an upright T wave in lead V1 which is greater than the T wave in V6.

ECG Test Answers
7, 77.

ECG Synthesis

The findings on this ECG are not specific and further imaging is required. Of note, an upright T wave in lead V1, especially when new or greater than the T wave in V6, is associated with a higher chance of significant coronary artery disease.

The presentation of a patient with risk factors and typical chest pain accompanied with non-specific changes in the ECG, requires a thorough workup including an echocardiography early in the workup process, as echocardiography can aid in confirming an ischemic etiology of the patient's complaints and rule out alternative diagnosis.

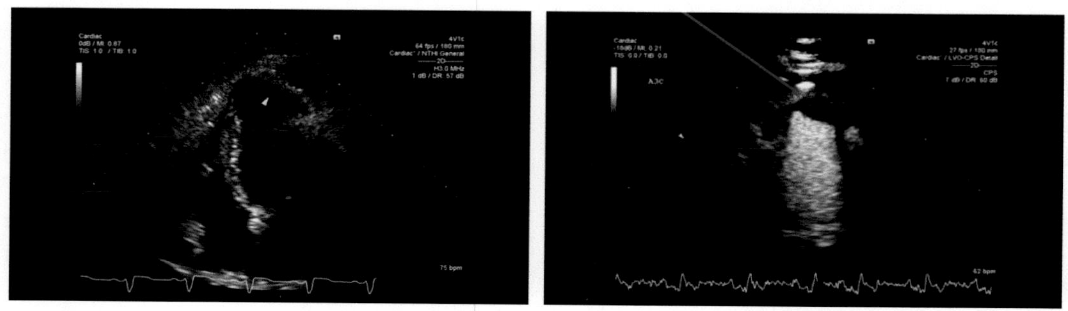

Unenhanced 4 chambers apical imaging (left) and view with imaging enhancing agent (right)

Echo Interpretation

The left ventricle is mildly dilated.

The left ventricular systolic function is moderately decreased, estimated LVEF—35 to 40%.

Regional wall motion abnormalities include akinesis of all apical segments as well as the mid inferior-septal wall. Unenhanced echocardiography (left image)—can not exclude apical thrombus (yellow arrow-head).

Using imaging enhancing agent (contrast echocardiography)—clear sign of filling defect in the apical region (blue arrow), caused by an apical thrombus.

Echo Synthesis

The finding of akinesis of the mid inferior-septal wall and all the apical segments is consistent with ischemia of the LAD territory. Akinetic areas are a predisposing factor for developing a mural thrombus.

Imaging enhancing agents (contrast echo) are used to better visualize the endocardial borders and to identify filling defects such as a thrombus. In this case, contrast echocardiography confirmed the presence of an apical mural thrombus.

Cardiac Electrosonography Synthesis

The patient presented with classic substernal chest pain with nonspecific ECG changes including peaked T waves in V1-V3. In this setting, echocardiography plays a critical role in the workup of the patient and should be done as early as possible. The echocardiogram demonstrated LV dysfunction with regional wall motion abnormalities including akinesis of the mid inferior-septal wall and all apical segments. Although there was no clear sign of an apical thrombus in the unenhanced echocardiogram, the echocardiogram was repeated using an imaging enhancing agent which confirmed the presence of an apical clot.

Due to the clear findings on echo suggesting ischemia of the LAD (left anterior descending) artery, the patient was taken to the cardiac catheterization laboratory, and the LAD artery was found to be occluded. PCI (percutaneous coronary intervention) to the LAD was done with improvement in the patient's symptoms. The patient was treated with anticoagulation therapy in addition to antiplatelet treatment.

7 Case 6

Clinical History

A 60 years old female with past medical history of hypertension and diabetes, presented with 2 days of exertional substernal chest pain

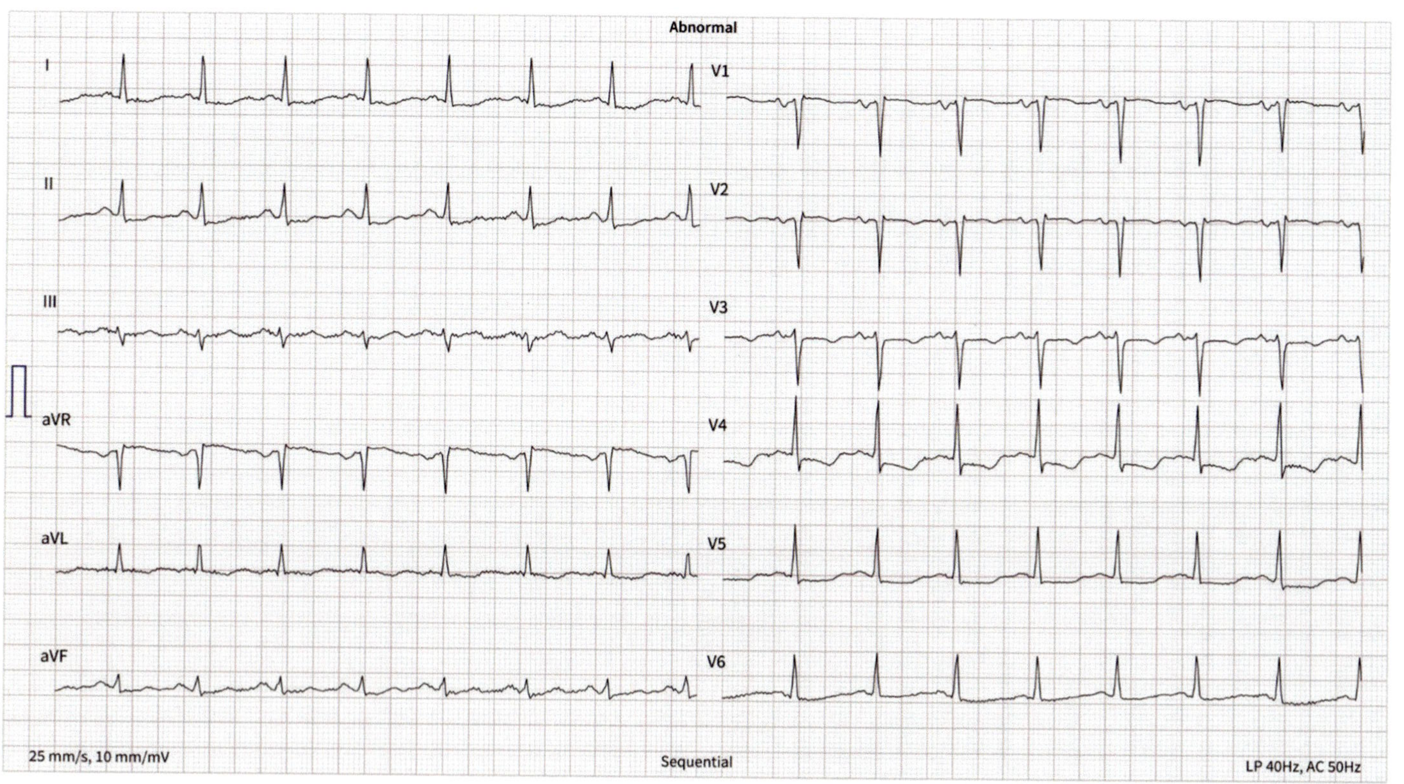

ECG Interpretation

Rhythm: Sinus
Rate: 95 bpm
Intervals: PR = 145 ms, QRS = 86 ms, QT = 375 ms, QTC Baz = 410 ms
Axis: Normal

Abnormalities on the ECG

- Poor R wave progression in leads V1-V3 (R wave less than 3 mm in lead V3)
- Horizontal ST depression in leads II, III, AVF, V3-V6. This ST depression of 2-3 mm is best seen in leads V4-V6
- ST elevation is seen in lead AVR (1.5 mm) and in lead V1 (0.5 mm)

ECG test Answers

7, 67, 78, 79.

ECG Synthesis

This ECG shows sinus rhythm at 95 bpm with markedly abnormal ST-T changes.

The combination of ST elevation in the odd leads (AVR & V1), with horizontal ST depression in most of the other ECG leads, is suggestive of marked ischemia. The differential diagnosis of such marked ST-T abnormalities includes:

1. Significant coronary artery disease such as: severe left-main disease, severe three-vessel coronary disease or its equivalent, and proximal LAD disease.
2. Severe valvular disease such as severe fixed aortic-valve disease
3. Dynamic hypertrophic cardiomyopathy
4. Hemodynamic instability resulting in severe global ischemia.

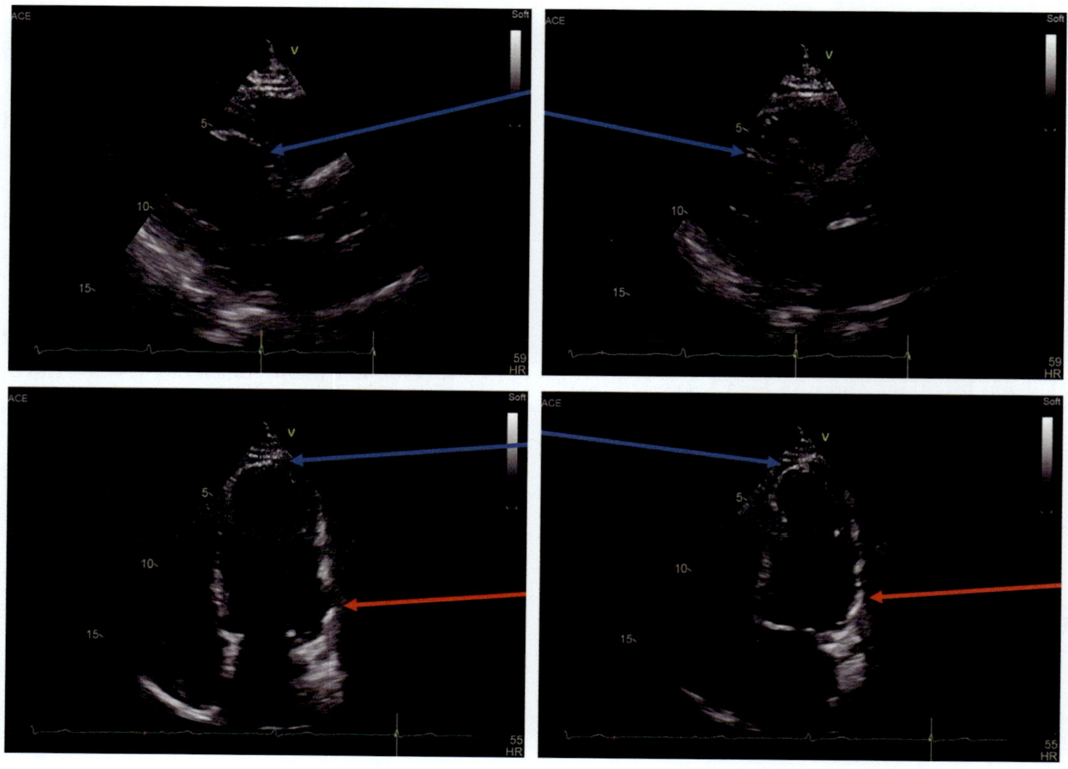

Top images: Para-sternal long axis view with mitral valve opened in diastole (left) and closed in systole (right) Bottom images: Apical 4-chamber view with mitral valve opened in diastole (left) and closed in systole (right)

Echo Interpretation

The left ventricle is normal size

The left ventricular systolic function is moderately decreased with estimated LVEF = 35–40%.

The blue arrows demonstrate an akinetic apex (4 chamber view) and an akinetic mid anterior-septum (parasternal long axis view). The red arrows in the 4 chambers view demonstrate an akinetic basal anterior-lateral wall.

Echo Synthesis

This imaging demonstrates multiple wall motion abnormalities including the territory of the mid left-anterior-descending artery territory (blue arrows) and left circumflex artery (red arrows).

Cardiac Electrosonography Synthesis

The patient presented with symptoms of substernal chest pain accompanied with alarming ECG changes of ST elevation in leads aVR and V1 with diffuse ST depression in almost all other leads. This combination is suggestive of global ischemia usually caused by marked coronary artery disease including involvement of the left-main coronary artery or its equivalent. Nonetheless, there is a differential diagnosis for these findings and echocardiography has a critical role in diagnosis and treatment.

The echo in this case demonstrated ischemia of multiple regions as noted above.

The patient was taken to the cardiac catheterization laboratory and was found to have severe triple-vessel-disease. After discussing the case with the local 'heart team' of the hospital, bypass surgery was recommended and performed.

8 Case 7

Clinical History

A 64 years old male presented to the emergency department with complaints of one week history of continued severe substernal chest pain. On presentation to the emergency department, he suffered a cardiac arrest and was successfully resuscitated

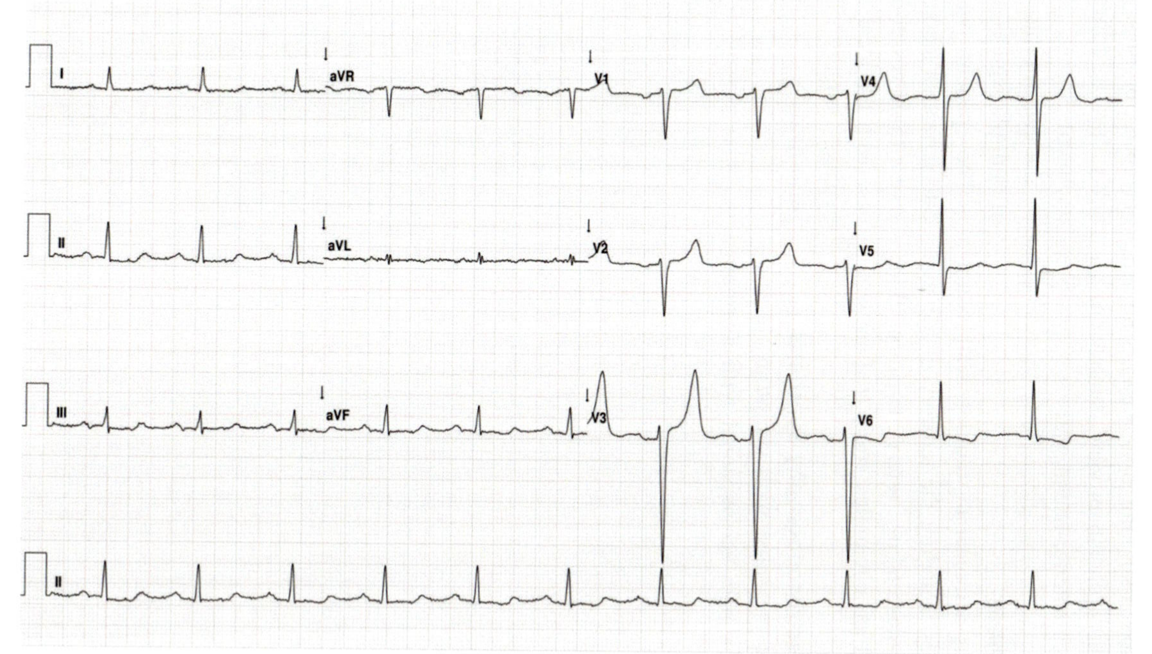

ECG Interpretation

Rhythm: Sinus
Rate: 80 bpm
Intervals: PR = 175 ms, QRS = 86 ms, QT = 375 ms, RR = 750 ms, QTC Baz = 410 ms
Axis: Normal.

Abnormalities on the ECG

- Peaked T waves in V3 and positive T wave in V1.
- Poor R wave progression in V1-V3.
- Horizontal ST depression in II, III, aVF and V5.

ECG Test Answers
7, 78.

ECG Synthesis
This ECG shows sinus rhythm at 80 bpm, normal intervals and axis.

Abnormalities include peaked T waves in V3, positive T wave in V1 which is larger than the T wave in V6, poor R wave progression in V1-V4 and horizontal ST depression in the inferior leads and in V5.

Hyperacute T waves can be an early sign of acute myocardial ischemia and can appear prior to ST changes (depression or elevation). Besides a sign of early ischemia, the finding of hyperacute T waves has a wide differential diagnosis. Hyperacute T waves may be a normal variant, they can be a finding secondary to other cardiac pathologies such as left ventricular hypertrophy (LVH) or left bundle branch block (LBBB) and they can be secondary to electrolyte abnormalities such as hyperkalemia.

In the setting of acute substernal chest pain, accompanied with other ischemic changes (ST depression in the inferior leads) and especially if the patient went into cardiac arrest the possibility of acute ischemia should be considered the probable cause.

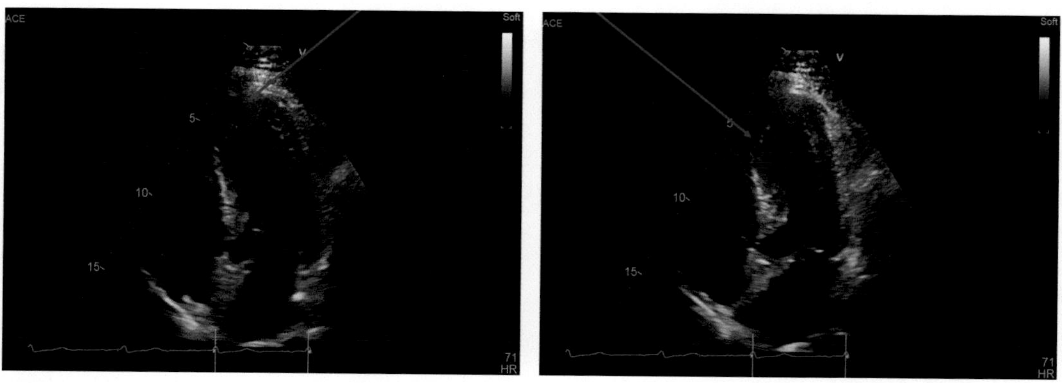

Apical 4-chambers views. Diastole with mitral valve open (left) and systole with mitral valve closed (right)

Echo Interpretation

The left ventricle is normal size.

The left ventricular systolic function is moderately decreased, estimated LVEF—35 to 40%.

Regional wall motion abnormalities including akinesis of the mid inferior-septal and apical walls (blue arrow).

Echo Synthesis

The finding of akinesis of the mid inferior-septal and apical walls is consistent with ischemia of the LAD.

Cardiac Electrosonography Synthesis

The patient presented with classic substernal chest pain accompanied with ST-T changes on ECG changes including ST depression in the inferior leads and peaked T wave in the anterior leads. This case warrants a thorough workup and echocardiography is critical in evaluating the patient, and thus should be done early in the process. The echocardiography findings confirm the likely diagnosis of acute coronary ischemia and based on the regional involvement support the involvement of the left anterior descending (LAD) coronary artery.

The combination of typical angina, ischemic ECG changes and involvement of a discrete coronary artery on echocardiography, mandate a coronary angiogram and usually revascularization therapy.

The patient was taken to the cardiac catheterization laboratory, and the mid portion of the LAD artery was found to be occluded. PCI (percutaneous coronary intervention) to the LAD was performed with improvement in symptoms and ECG findings.

9 Case 8

Clinical History

72 years old male with history of hyperlipidemia presented with 8 hours of substernal chest pain

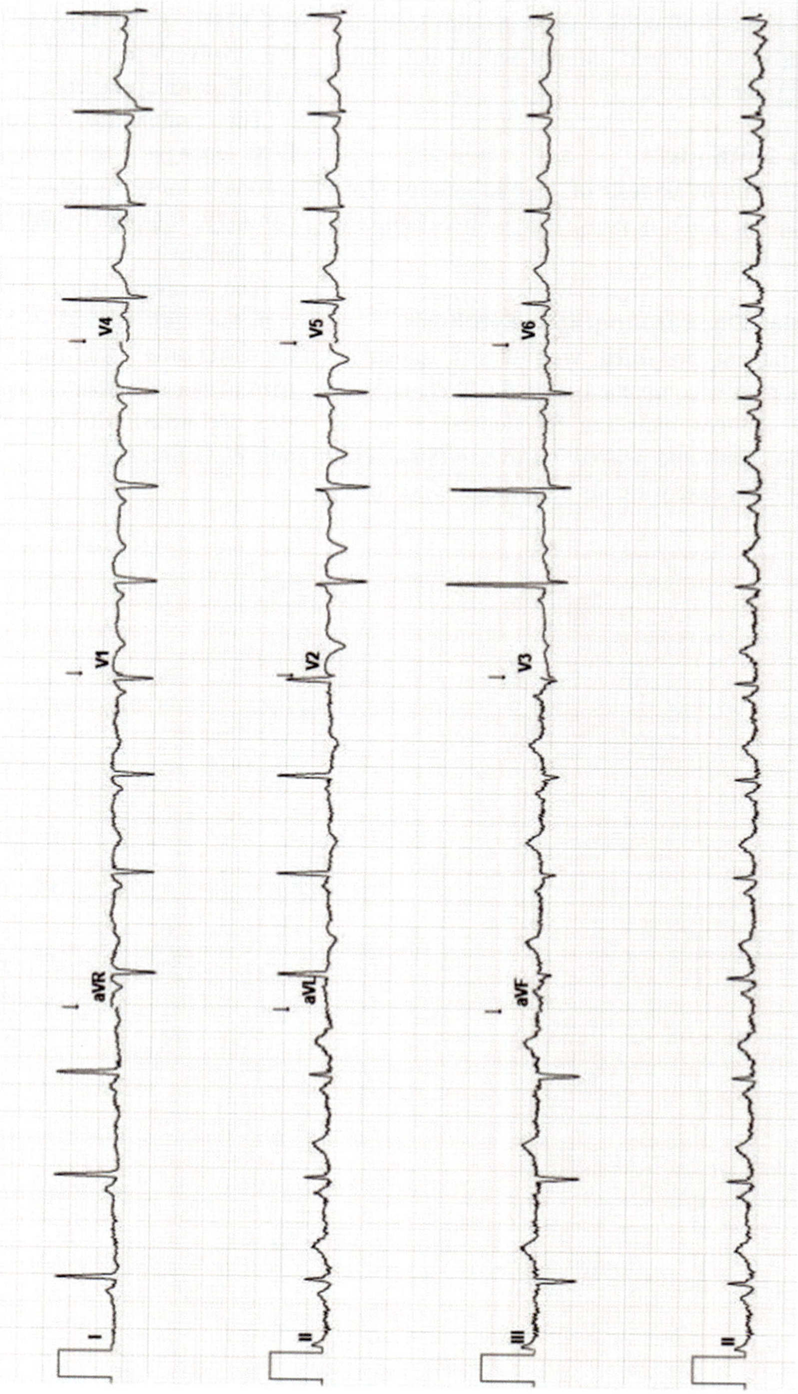

ECG Interpretation

Rhythm: Sinus
Rate: 85 bpm
Intervals: PR = 145 ms, QRS = 86 ms, QT = 375 ms, RR = 750 ms, QTC Baz = 410 ms
Axis: Normal.

Abnormalities on the ECG

T wave inversion in aVL, V1, V2 Biphasic T wave in I, V3.

ECG test Answers

7, 78.

ECG Synthesis

This ECG shows sinus rhythm at 85 bpm, normal intervals and axis.

Abnormalities include T wave inversion in I, aVL & V1-V3. T wave changes usually correspond with myocardial ischemia. T wave inversion in V1-V3 can be a sign of anterior-septal ischemia usually corresponding with a narrowing or blockage of the left anterior descending (LAD) coronary artery. The differential diagnosis includes apical hypertrophic cardiomyopathy and involvement of the right ventricle (RV) as may be seen in pulmonary embolism or other pulmonary disorders involving primarily the RV.

In this case, the echocardiography plays a critical role in further understanding the cause of the patient's complaints and ECG findings and should be done early in the workup process.

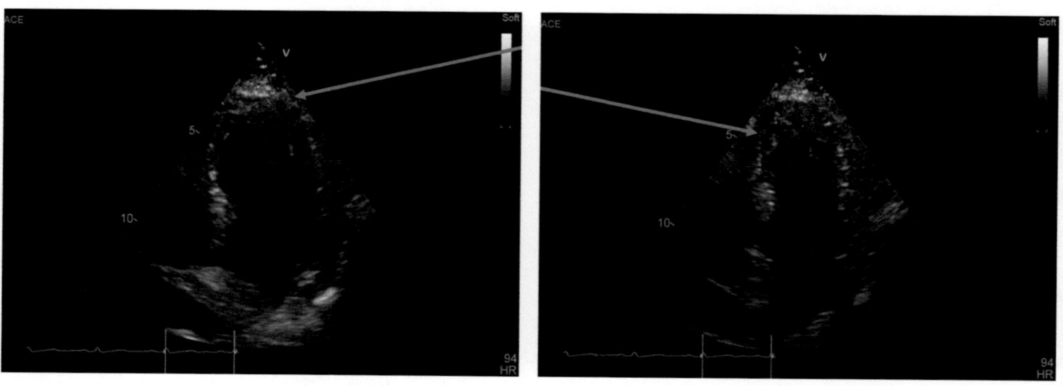

Apical 4-chamber views. Diastole with mitral valve open (left) and systole with mitral valve closed (right)

Echo Interpretation

The left ventricle is normal size

The left ventricular systolic function is moderately decreased, estimated LVEF—35 to 40%.

Regional wall motion abnormality with akinesis of the mid anterior-septum and the apex (blue arrows).

Echo Synthesis

The findings of regional wall motion abnormality support ischemia of a single coronary artery, and in this case the akinesis of the antero-septal and apex correspond with involvement of the LAD. The right ventricle looks normal in size, reducing the likelihood for the diagnosis of an acute pulmonary disorder including PE.

Cardiac Electrosonography Synthesis

The patient presented with classic substernal chest pain with ECG changes including T wave inversion in the antero-septal and lateral leads. The differential diagnosis includes myocardial ischemia, an acute pulmonary disorder and hypertrophic cardiomyopathy. In this case the role of an early echocardiography is of much importance and can guide the diagnostic and treatment plan. The findings of the ehco support the diagnosis of myocardial ischemia involving the LAD.

These ECG and echocardiography findings in the setting of acute chest pain, necessitate coronary investigation.

The patient was taken to the cardiac catheterization laboratory and a coronary angiogram demonstrated severe narrowing of the proximal portion of the LAD coronary artery which was treated with PCI (percutaneous coronary intervention) and immediate improvement in the patient's symptoms and ECG findings were noticed.

10   Case 9

Clinical History

60 years old male with hypertension, presented with exertional substernal chest pain radiating down the left arm that started 3 days ago

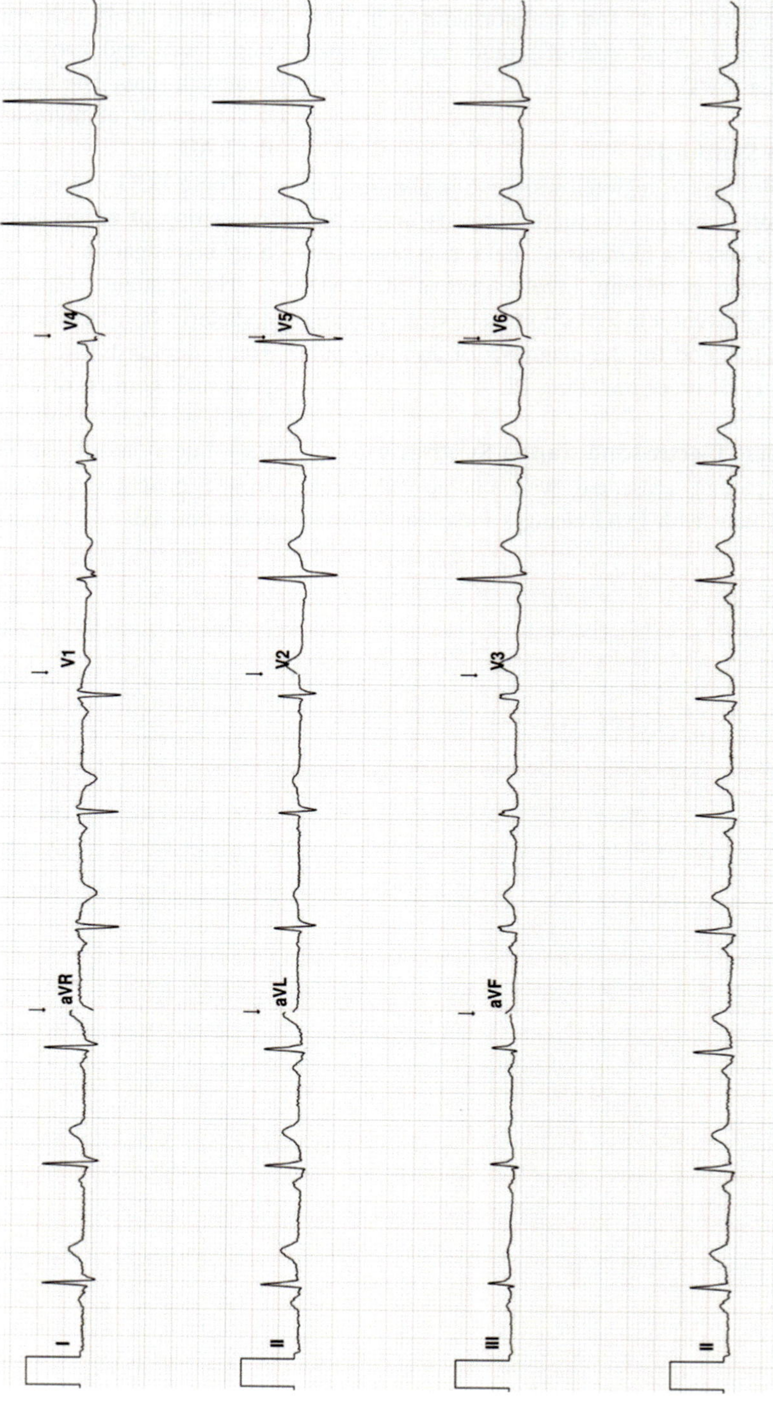

ECG Interpretation

Rhythm: Sinus
Rate: 70 bpm
Intervals: PR = 158 ms, QRS = 90 ms, QT = 370 ms, RR = 870 ms, QTC Baz = 390 ms
Axis: Normal.

Abnormalities on the ECG

-Normal ECG

ECG Test Answers
1, 7.

ECG Synthesis
This ECG shows normal sinus rhythm at 70 bpm with no pathologies.

The presentation of a 60-year-old male with new onset typical substernal chest pain and no ECG abnormalities requires a thorough investigation starting with the patient's past medical history, an in-depth understanding of the patient's complaints and a systemic physical examination. Additional tests can include a wide array of blood tests, different imaging tests and a stress test.

One of the most important tests, that should be done early in the work up process, is a cardiac echocardiogram. The echocardiogram can help establish the diagnosis of an acute coronary syndrome, as well as rule out numerous other pathologies involving the cardiac and respiratory systems.

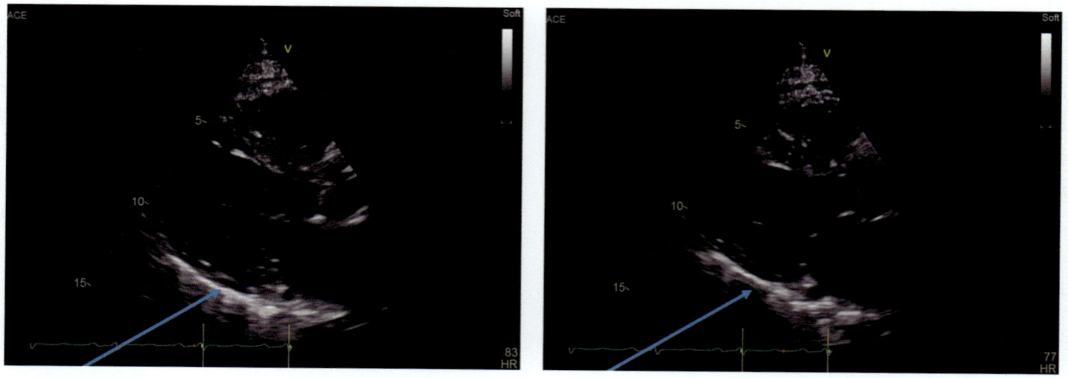

Para-sternal long axis views. Diastole with mitral valve open (left) and systole with mitral valve closed (right)

Echo Interpretation

The left ventricle is normal size.

The left ventricular systolic function is mildly decreased, estimated LVEF—45%.

Regional wall motion abnormality with akinesis of the basal-inferolateral wall (blue arrows).

Echo Synthesis

This imaging demonstrates wall motion abnormalities in the territory supplied by a single coronary artery. This area is usually supplied by the left circumflex (LCx) artery. In addition, this echo can help rule out many other potential differential diagnosis, such as involvement of the proximal ascending aorta, disease in one of the heart valves or involvement of right ventricle (as seen in acute pulmonary disorders such as pulmonary embolism).

Cardiac Electrosonography Synthesis

This 60 year old patient presented with typical chest pain and with no abnormalities in the ECG. Thorough investigation of the patient's complaints, completing a systemic physical examination and completing additional tests is necessary for diagnosis of the chest pain. As part of that, echocardiography plays a critical role in supporting the diagnosis an acute coronary syndrome and ruling out many other diagnostic possibilities.

The echo showed regional wall motion abnormality consistent with myocardial ischemia caused by a single coronary vessel. These findings necessitate coronary imaging, usually completed by angiography in the cardiac catheterization laboratory.

Occasionally, even severe disease in a coronary artery doesn't present on the ECG ("silent ECG"), and is more common in the left circumflex artery.

The patient was taken to the cardiac catheterization laboratory and a coronary angiogram demonstrated severe narrowing of the left circumflex coronary artery which was treated with PCI (percutaneous coronary intervention).

11 Case 10

Clinical History

Clinical History
A 62 years old male with a history of high blood pressure presented to the ED with three hours of stabbing chest pain radiating to the upper back

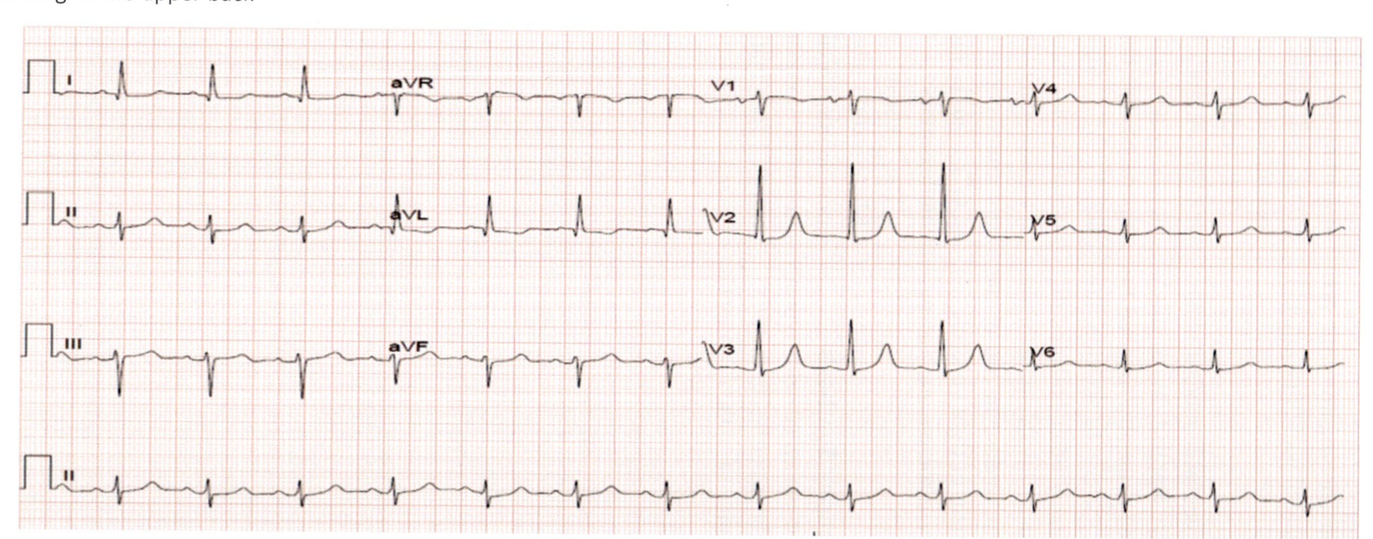

Additional Clinical History
The patient states he had a brief episode of right arm weakness and blurred vision which spontaneously resolved

Additional information
Patients BP was 161/103 in both arms, cardiac enzymes were elevated

ECG Interpretation

Rhythm: Sinus
Rate: 84 bpm
Intervals: PR = 168 ms QRS = 92 ms QTC 444 ms
Axis: − 27.

Abnormalities on the ECG

− Borderline left axis deviation
− Tall R waves in V2-3
− Mild ST depressions in 1,L.

ECG Test Answers
7, 74, 78, 79.

ECG Synthesis
In general in the precordial leads the transition zone where R waves become larger than s waves should occur at leads V3-4. In this patient, the R wave in V2 is significantly larger than the s wave of the same lead. The differential diagnosis of "early transition" with a normal QRS interval includes: incorrect lead placement, counter clockwise rotation of the heart, posterior wall infarction, and right ventricular hypertrophy (RVH).

The mild ST depressions in 1,L, the clinical story of chest pain and the lack of other ECG changes associated with RVH such as right axis deviation or p pulmonale make posterior wall myocardial infarction the most likely diagnosis in this patient. An emergent echo was performed to confirm the diagnosis prior to referral for cardiac catheterization.

A

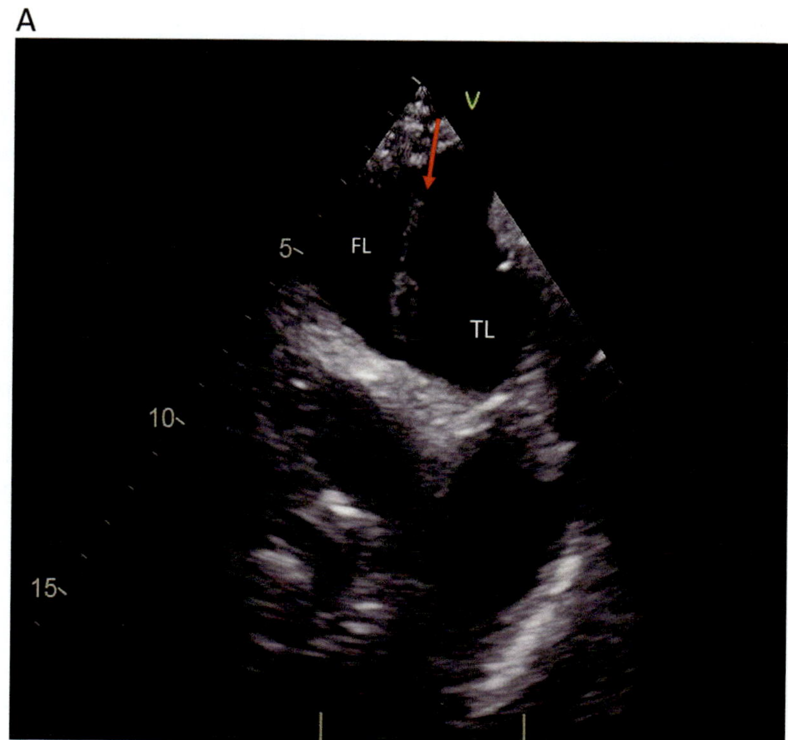

B

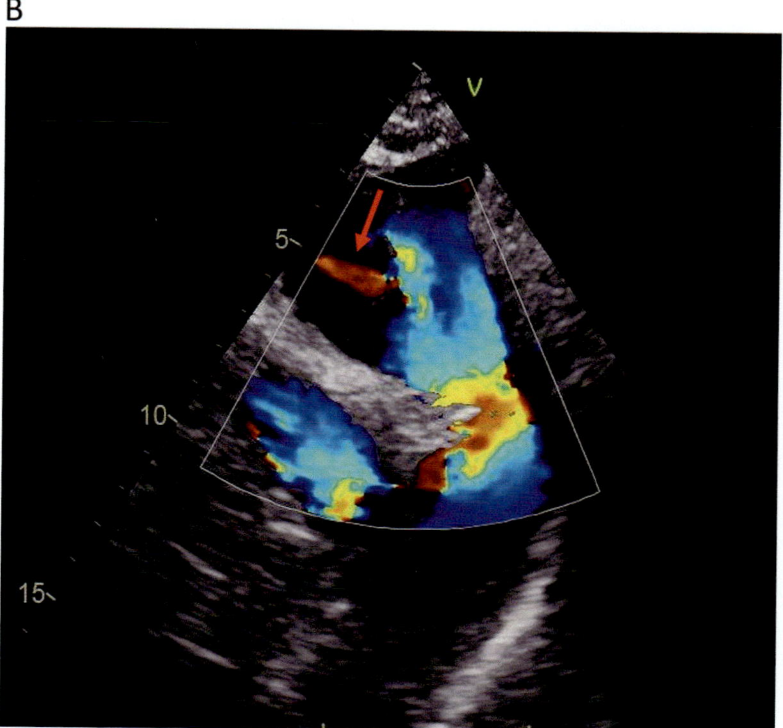

Echocardiographic suprasternal views: (A) showing a thin membrane dissecting across the mid aortic arch (red arrow) ((B) the same image with color Doppler imaging

Echo Interpretation

Suprasternal views (A) showing a thin membrane dissecting across the mid aortic arch (red arrow) dividing the aortic arch into a true lumen (TL) and false lumen (FL). Image (B) shows the same image with color Doppler imaging. The presence of color (in blue on the right side of the image confirms that this is the true lumen. A small connection between the true and false lumens (red arrow) is noted with red flow on color Doppler.

Echo Synthesis

The echo findings are consistent with an aortic dissection involving the aortic arch.

Cardiac Electrosonography Synthesis

The patient presented with chest pain and ECG changes consistent with an acute myocardial infarction. The findings on electrosonography were discordant with initial ECG suggesting a posterior wall infarction and echocardiography demonstrating an aortic dissection. This case vividly illustrates the utility of echocardiography in the setting of acute chest pain as the diagnosis of dissection would have been missed without it and the patient would have undergone a potentially life-endangering coronary angiogram. An important clue to the diagnosis was the patient's complaint of transient visual disturbance and arm weakness. Neurologic or peripheral vascular complaints in the setting of acute chest pain should always raise the clinical suspicion of acute aortic dissection compromising systemic perfusion.

12 Case 11

Clinical History

56 years old male, active smoker, presented with 3 days of worsening shortness of breath, right sided chest pain, dry cough and 3 hours of hemoptysis

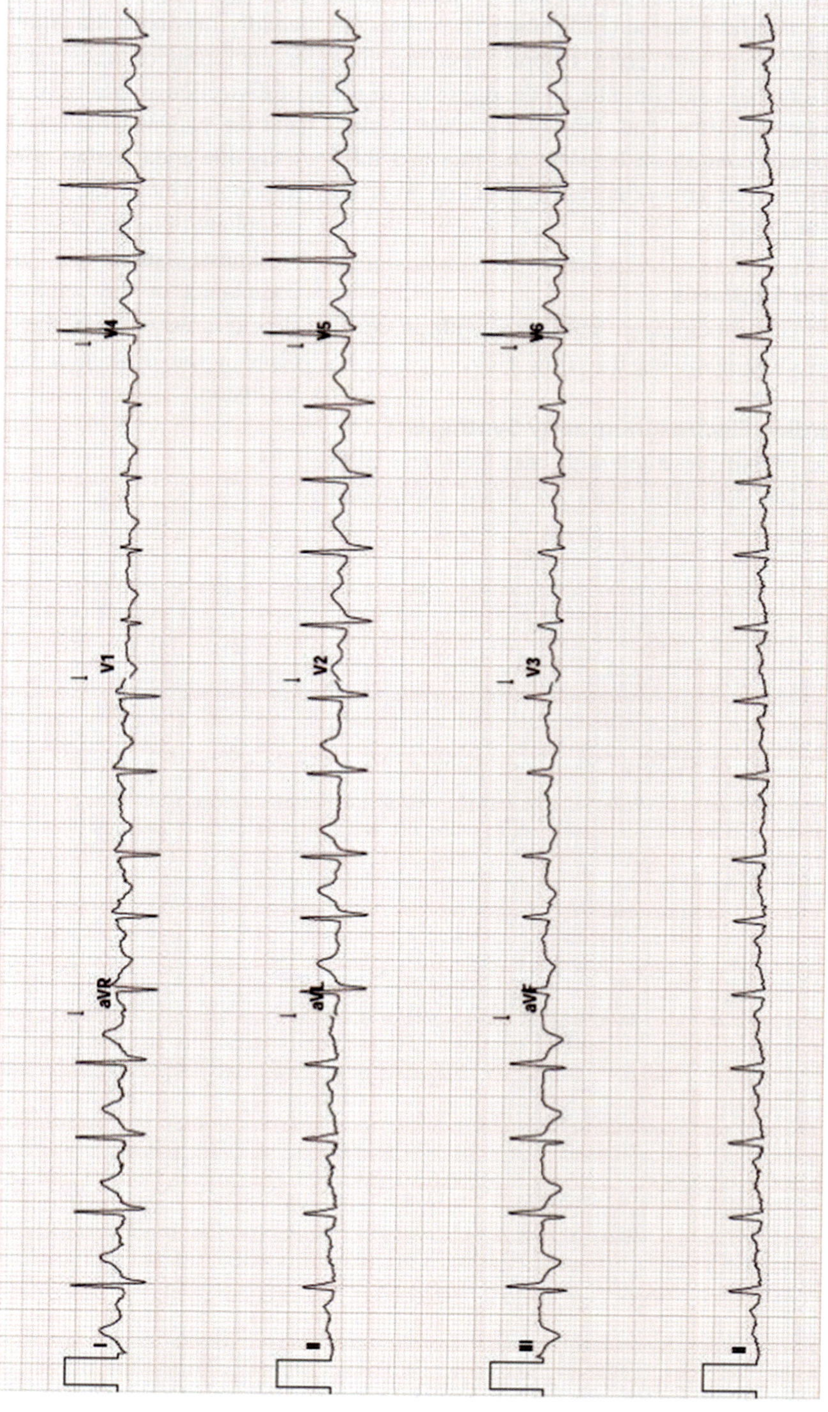

ECG Interpretation

Rhythm: Sinus
Rate: 110 bpm
Intervals: PR = 175 ms, QRS = 97 ms, QT = 325 ms, RR = 540 ms, QTC Baz = 440 ms – normal intervals.
Axis: Normal.

Abnormalities on the ECG

- Sinus tachycardia (110 bpm)
- Incomplete right bundle branch block (iRBBB)
- Large S wave in lead I and Q wave & T wave inversion in lead III (S1Q3T3)
- T wave inversion in V1, V3
- Dominant R wave in V2
- ST elevation in AVR.

ECG Test Answers

10, 41, 51, 58, 77.

ECG Synthesis

This ECG shows sinus tachycardia at 110 bpm accompanied with incomplete-RBBB pattern and T wave inversion in the right precordial leads (V1-V3). These findings are compatible with right ventricle strain pattern and are associated with elevated pulmonary pressure.

The differential diagnosis for elevated pulmonary pressure is wide and includes left-heart disease (heart failure, mitral or aortic valvular disease), chronic or acute lung disease, systemic diseases and primary pulmonary hypertension. Nonetheless, the setting of *acutely* elevated pulmonary pressure the likelihood for a pulmonary emboli (PE) is very high, specifically in this case with a classic clinical presentation with high suspicion for PE and sinus tachycardia, which is the most common pathology seen on ECG in PE patients.

Although the finding of S1Q3T3 on ECG (as this patients has) is considered a 'classic' finding in PE patients, it appears only in a minority of patients and is neither specific nor sensitive for the diagnosis of PE.

The workup of patients who are suspected to have PE include blood tests and imaging modalities. Echocardiography plays a critical role in the workup. It can aid in getting to a clear diagnosis, rule out alternative diagnoses and is part of the assessment of the PE severity, and should therefore be completed early in the workup process.

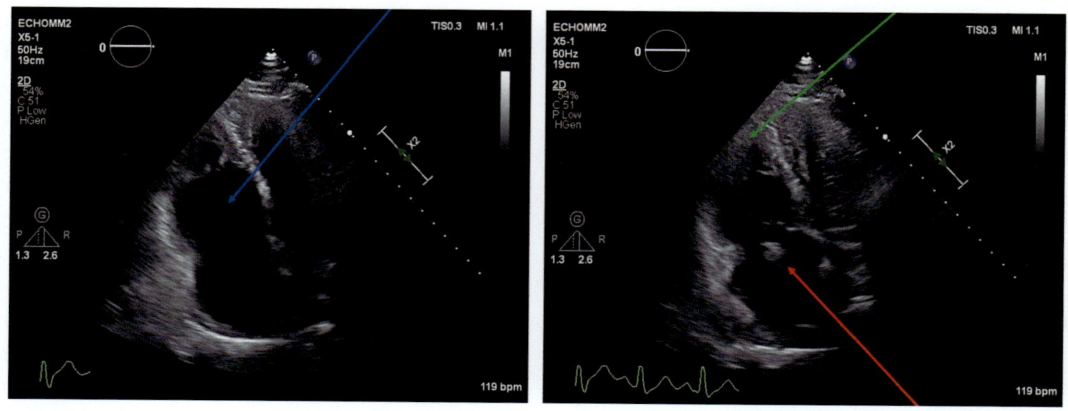

Apical 4-chambers views. Diastole with tricuspid valve open (left) and systole with tricuspid valve closed (right)

Echo Interpretation

Severely enlarged right ventricle (blue arrow) with RV:LV ratio >> 1. Severely reduced function of right ventricle.

Distinct regional RV dysfunction with akinesis of the base and mid portions of the RV free wall and sparing of the RV apex (green arrow).

Large echogenic finding in the right atrium (RA) near the tricuspid valve (red arrow).

Echo Synthesis

These findings on echocardiography demonstrate significant RV enlargement and severe *regional* dysfunction with akinesis of the RV free wall and preserved apical contraction (occasionally the RV apex is hypercontractile). These findings are known as McConell's sign, which is considered a specific, although not a sensitive, sign of acute PE. In addition, the echo demonstrated a large echogenic finding in the RA which is very suggestive of a thrombus. This thrombus, which is most probably a clot that embolized from a thrombus located in a distinct location in the body (for instance—deep vein thrombosis), is called 'clot in transit'. This situation may be life threatening as the clot can embolize further to the pulmonary vasculature at any moment and cause a more severe PE and hemodynamic collapse.

Cardiac Electrosonography Synthesis

The case is a classic presentation of an acute PE. The patient presented with shortness of breath and chest pain and has classic ECG findings of an acute PE, including sinus tachycardia and signs of right ventricle strain pattern which are associated with elevated pulmonary pressure. These ECG findings should immediately raise the suspicion of PE and as part of the early work up echocardiography should be done. Echocardiography can help confirm the diagnosis of PE and help in assessing the severity of the PE and guide the immediate treatment recommended.

Due to the hemodynamic status of the patient and the findings on ECG and echocardiography, the patient was brought up to discussion with the hospital PERT (Pulmonary Embolus Response Team) and surgery with embolectomy was recommended.

13 Case 12

Clinical History

A 37 years old woman with a history of smoking presented to the emergency department with 2 days of intermittent chest pain which worsened with inspiration and lying down.

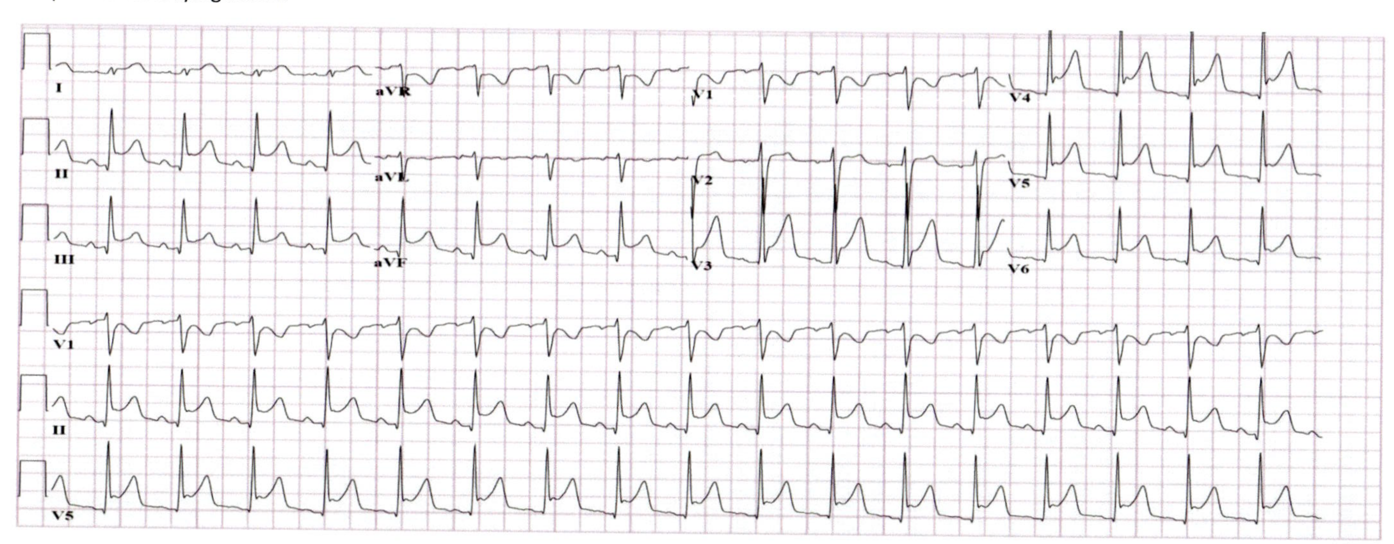

Additional Clinical History

The patient reported a recent upper respiratory infection. Exam revealed a fever of 37.8 C and a harsh bi phasic systolic murmur

Additional information

Labs were significant for elevated c-reactive protein while troponin was negative. CXR revealed an enlarged cardiac silhouette

ECG Interpretation

Rhythm: Sinus
Rate: 92 bpm
Intervals: PR 192 ms, QRS 80 ms, QTc 398 ms
Axis: Normal.

Abnormalities on the ECG

- ST elevations in 1, 2, 3, AVF and V2-V6
- ST depression in leads AVR and V1
- PR depressions in 2, 3, F, V2-V6
- PR elevation in AVR.

ECG Test Answers
7, 53, 77.

ECG Synthesis

The ECG in this patient is notable for diffuse ST segment elevations which do not conform anatomically to a specific distribution of a coronary artery. The differential diagnosis includes early repolarization and acute peri and/or myocarditis. Depressions of the PR segment are a relatively insensitive but highly specific ECG finding in acute pericarditis. There is PR segment elevation in leads AVR and V1 which is highly specific of acute pericarditis. The negative troponin ruled out significant myocarditis. Given the clinical complaints, the lab findings and the ECG findings a diagnosis of acute pericarditis was highly suspected and urgent echocardiography performed.

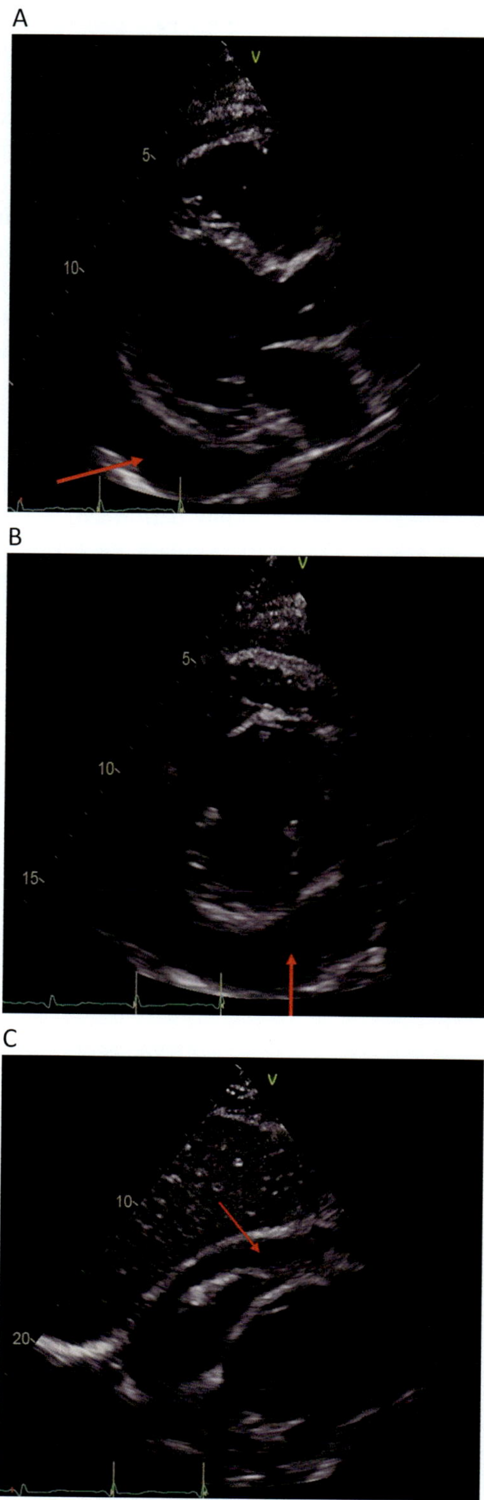

Parasternal long-axis (panel A), short-axis (panel B) and subcostal (panel C) views showing an echo-free space surrounding the heart

Echo Interpretation

Echo revealed normal left ventricular (LV) function with a an echo-free space surrounding the heart consistent with a pericardial effusion (arrows) without echocardiographic evidence of tamponade physiology.

Echo Synthesis

The echo findings of a pericardial effusion in the clinical setting described is very supportive of the diagnosis of acute pericarditis.

Cardiac Electrosonography Synthesis

In this patient with cardiovascular risk factors and chest pain, initial ECG was suggestive of acute pericarditis. Emergent echo revealed normal left ventricular function which definitively ruled out acute coronary occlusion in the setting of ST elevation as well as a significant pericardial effusion, confirming the diagnosis suspected by ECG. The patient received treatment with anti-inflammatory medication with resolution of her clinical complaints and ECG and echo findings.

14   Case 13

Clinical History

Clinical History

A 68 years old man with a history of hypertension and diabetes presented to the ED with 5 days of intermittent substernal chest pain

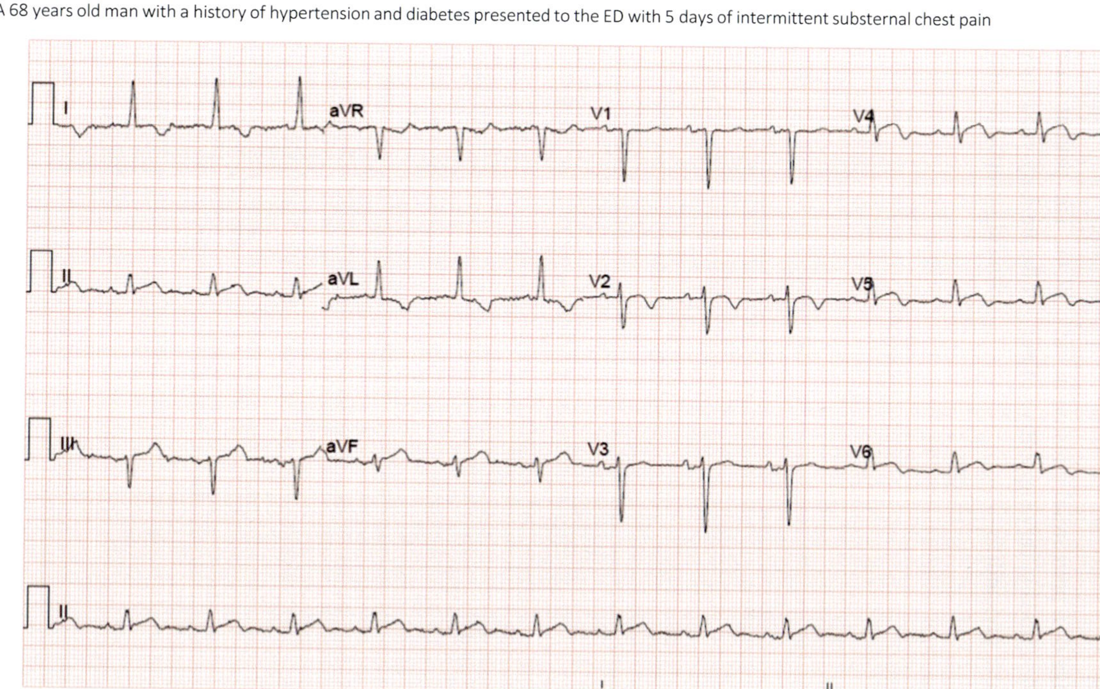

Additional Clinical History

The patient reports being told of an "abnormal" ECG performed in the past. Family history is positive for a "cardiac incident" in the patient's father at age 45

ECG Interpretation

Rhythm: Sinus
Rate: 76 bpm
Intervals: PR 179 ms QRS 101 ms QTc 433 ms
Axis: Normal.

Abnormalities on the ECG

- ST elevations in 2, V4-6
- T wave abnormalities
- Misplaced leads V2 and V3

ECG Test Answers
3, 7, 79

ECG Synthesis

The ECG in this patient is notable for profound ST segment and T wave abnormalities in the anterolateral wall consistent with myocardial injury. The presence of biphasic t waves in leads V4-V6 and inverted t waves in leads 1 and L suggests a chronic process possibly related to left ventricular hypertrophy although the voltage is not elevated. The clinical history of a known abnormal ECG supports this possibility. The small decrease in r wave in V3 compared to lead V2 and V4 suggests that leads V2 and V3 have been reversed. Given the patients clinical complaints of chest pain and ECG changes possibly consistent with anterior wall ischemia, emergent echocardiography was performed.

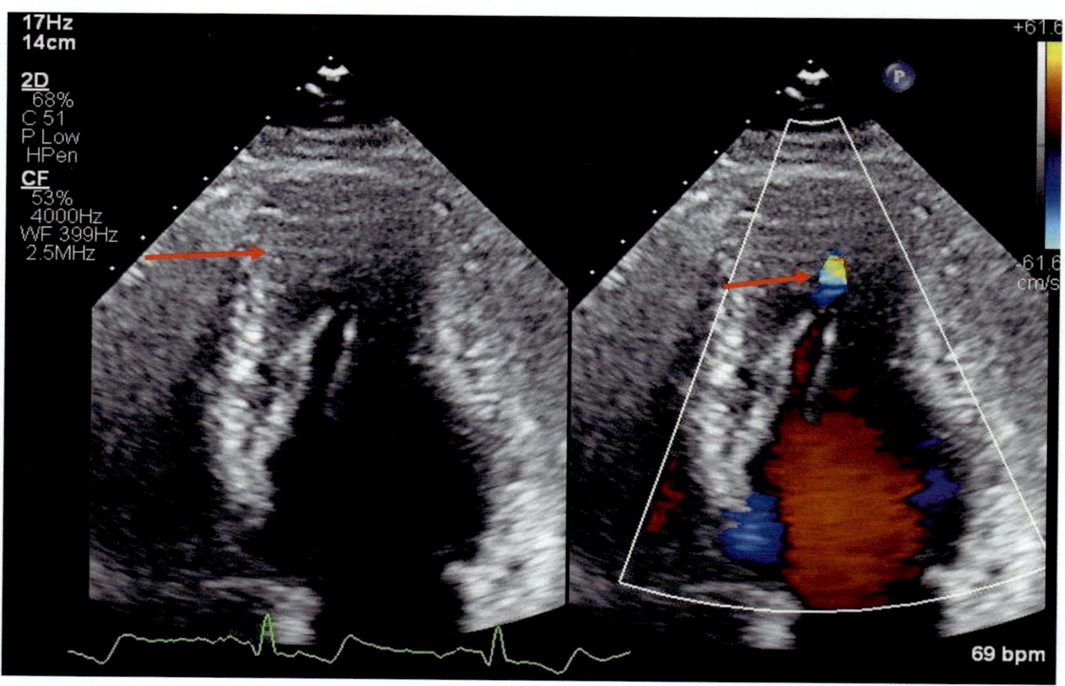

Apical 2D two chamber view (left image) showing prominent apical hypertrophy (arrow) and corresponding color Doppler image (right) showing acceleration of flow in the apex due to the localized hypertrophy (arrow)

Echo Interpretation

Echo revealed overall normal left ventricular function without evidence of regional wall motion abnormalities. There was very prominent hypertrophy of the apical segments with intraventricular acceleration of flow in the apex due to the localized hypertrophy.

Echo Synthesis

This echo is suggestive of significant apical left ventricular hypertrophy with a small intraventricular pressure gradient.

Cardiac Electrosonography Synthesis

In this patient with cardiovascular risk factors and chest pain, initial ECG was suggestive of myocardial pathology and raised the question of whether emergent angiography was indicated. Emergent echo revealed evidence of severe apical hypertrophy without evidence of acute ischemia and angiography was postponed. The localized hypertrophy explains the absence of elevated voltage on the ECG. The chest pain is probably due to apical ischemia due to the extensive hypertrophy and elevated end diastolic pressures.

15   Case 14

Clinical History

67 years old female with no significant past medical history presented to the ED with three hours of chest pain radiating to the left arm.

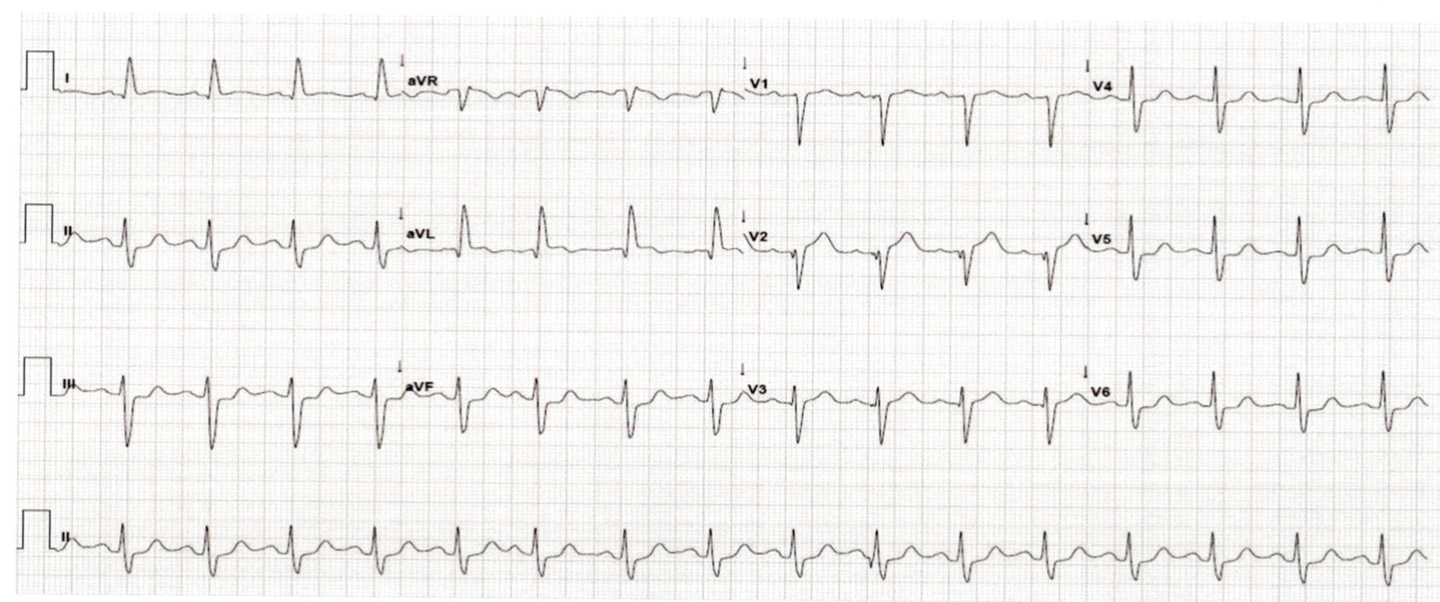

Additional Clinical History

The patient states she has felt weak and depressed since the death of her husband one week prior to admission

Additional information

Physical examination was normal. High sensitive troponin was mildly elevated

ECG Interpretation

Rhythm: Sinus
Rate: 100 bpm
Intervals: PR 180 ms, QRS 120 ms, QTC 400 ms
Axis: Normal.

Abnormalities on the ECG

- Interventricular conduction delay
- Poor R wave progression V1-V3
- Horizontal ST elevations in lead avL (1 mm) and lead I (0.5 mm) which are concordant to R wave in these leads
- Horizontal ST depressions in leads 2, 3, F, V4-V6.

ECG Test Answers

7, 64, 69, 78, 79

ECG Synthesis

This ECG demonstrates normal sinus rhythm with interventricular conduction delay. The poor R wave progression in V1-V3 has a wide differential diagnosis including: anteroseptal infarction, left ventricular hypertrophy, left bundle branch block, and incorrect lead position. The ST segment elevation in leads 1 and avL suggests acute myocardial injury in the high lateral territory. There are marked diffuse horizontal ST depressions in almost all other leads which may raise the possibility of more global myocardial current of injury.

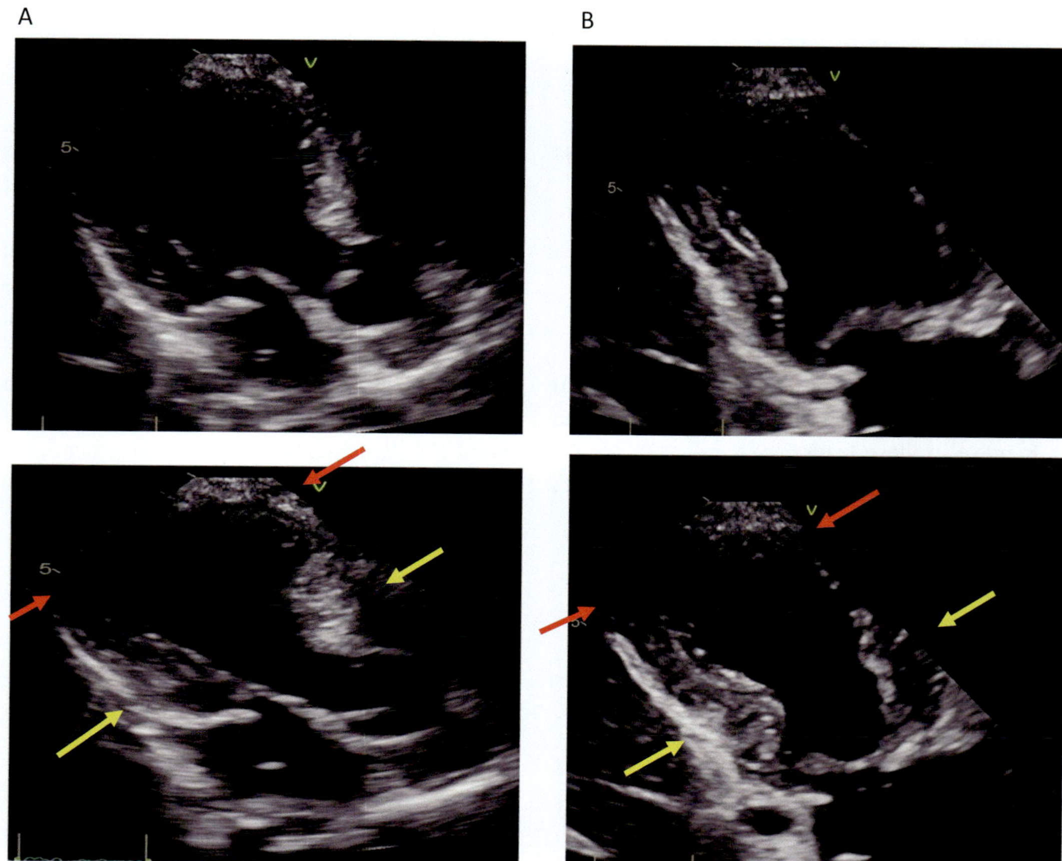

(A) Apical three chamber view in diastole (top) and systole (bottom) demonstrates akinesis and "ballooning" of the apical segments (red arrows) with thickening and hyperdynamic function of the basal segments (yellow arrows). (B) Apical two chamber view in diastole (top) and systole (bottom) demonstrates akinesis and "ballooning" of the apical segments (red arrows) with thickening and hyperdynamic function of the basal segments (yellow arrows)

Echo Interpretation

Apical three chamber (A) and apical two chamber (B) views demonstrate akinesis and "ballooning" of the apical segments (red arrows) with thickening and hyperdynamic function of the basal segments (yellow arrows).

Echo Synthesis

The echo findings are consistent with an extensive regional wall motion abnormalities involving all the apical segments with hyperdynamic function of the basilar segments.

Cardiac Electrosonography Synthesis

The patient presented with chest pain and ECG changes consistent with an acute myocardial infarction. The findings on electrosonography were potentially consistent with a high lateral wall myocardial infarction. However, the apical ballooning which included portions of the apical and anteroapical walls and the hyperdynamic function of the basilar segments raised the diagnosis of stress (or takotsubo) cardiomyopathy. This diagnosis was supported by the clinical history of recent death of a spouse. The patient underwent emergent cardiac catheterization that revealed normal coronary arteries which supported a diagnosis of stress cardiomyopathy.

16 Case 15

Clinical History

A 74 years old male with no significant past medical history presented to the ED with one week of chest and back pain and several hours of extreme weakness and diaphoresis.

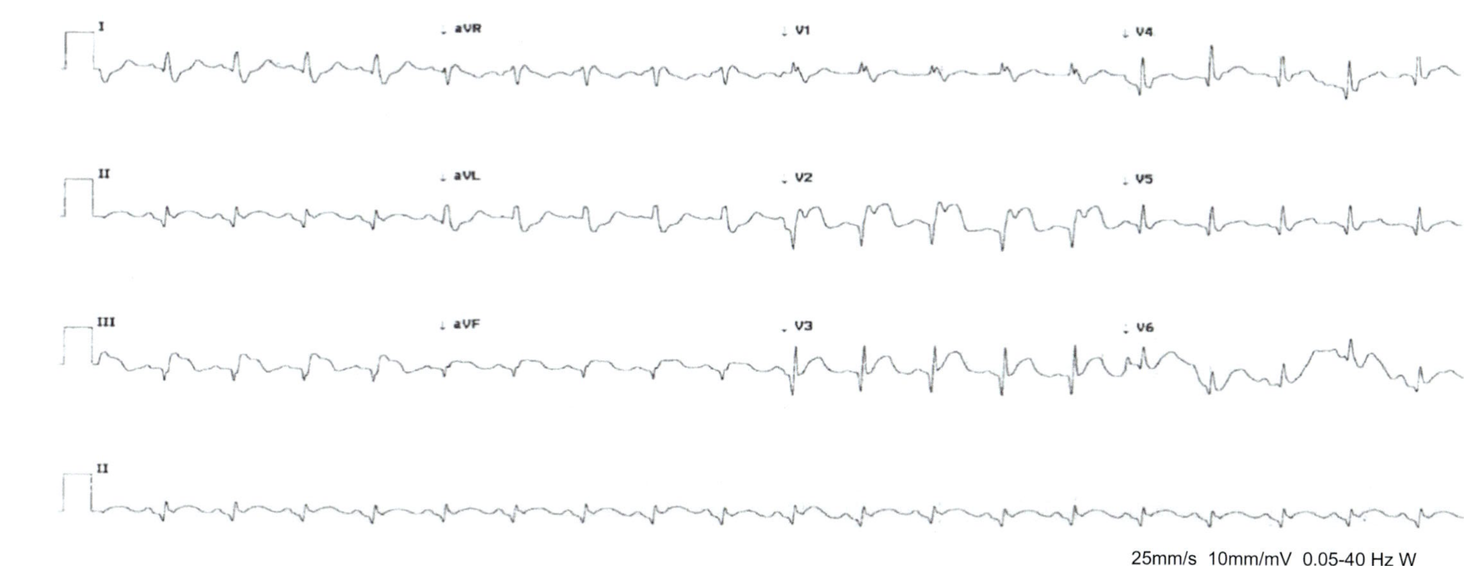

Additional Clinical History

Upon arrival – patient had severe dyspnea and diaphoresis with blood pressure of 82/53 mmHg.

Physical exam - JVP was elevated, lungs were clear. A soft 2\6 systolic murmur was heard at the left sternal border

Blood tests - CPK 392 u/L, TroT HS 15,092 ng/L, Creatinine 2.5 mg/dL

ECG Interpretation

Rate: 120 bpm
Rhythm: Sinus tachycardia
Intervals: PR 146 ms, QRS 150 ms, QTC 410 ms
Axis: Borderline left.

Abnormalities on the ECG

- Sinus tachycardia
- ST elevation and q waves in inferior leads (II, III and aVF) and V2 to V5.
- ST depression and inverted T waves in I, aVL.

ECG Test Answers

10, 68, 72.

ECG Synthesis

This patient has ECG signs of a recent extensive myocardial infarction. There are q waves and ST elevation in inferior as well as anterior leads. Q waves usually indicate that the MI is not acute, as known from the medical history in this case.

Involvement of both inferior and anterior territories is not common and raises the question of coronary anatomy and the identity of the infarcted artery. One possibility is a large, 'wrap around' LAD supplying both anterior and inferior walls. Other possibilities are previous coronary occlusion with a new subacute occlusion or coronary artery anomalies.

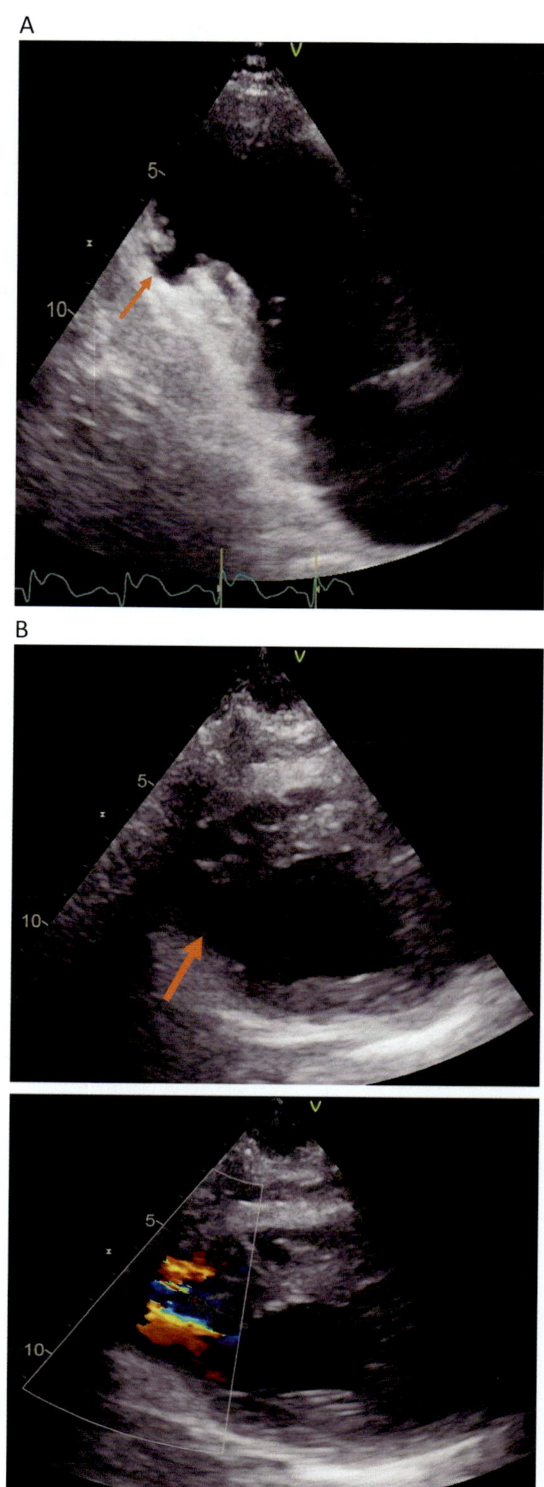

Panel A shows an apical 2 chamber view with a defect in the wall of the inferior apex (arrow). The parasternal short axis images in panel B confirm the finding of a defect in the wall of the left ventricle in the inferior apex with color

Echo Interpretation

Apical 2 chamber view shows a defect in the wall of the inferior apex (arrow). The parasternal short axis images of the apex confirm the finding of a defect in the wall of the left ventricle in the area of the inferior apex with color flow demonstrating a left to right shunt from the left to right ventricle.

Echo Synthesis

Possible explanations for cardiogenic shock in the setting of myocardial infarction include significant left and/or right ventricular dysfunction or a mechanical complication including free wall rupture, ventricular septal defect or papillary muscle rupture causing severe mitral regurgitation. The emergent echo revealed evidence of an inferior infarct with a ventricular septal defect in the inferior septum.

Cardiac Electrosonography Synthesis

The ECG findings in this patient were suggestive of a subacute inferoposterior infarct. The physical exam suggested hemodynamic impairment of the right side with elevated JVP and clear lungs leading to a low output state as reflected by the elevated creatinine. The emergency echo demonstrated a very large presumably acute ventricular septal defect associated with a recent acute inferoposterior wall MI seen on ECG. An intraaortic balloon pump was placed and the patient was referred to cardiothoracic surgery for emergent repair of the acute ventricular septal defect.

17 Case 16

Clinical History

82 years old female with 2 months of exertional substernal chest pain and shortness of breath, presented with worsening of her symptoms

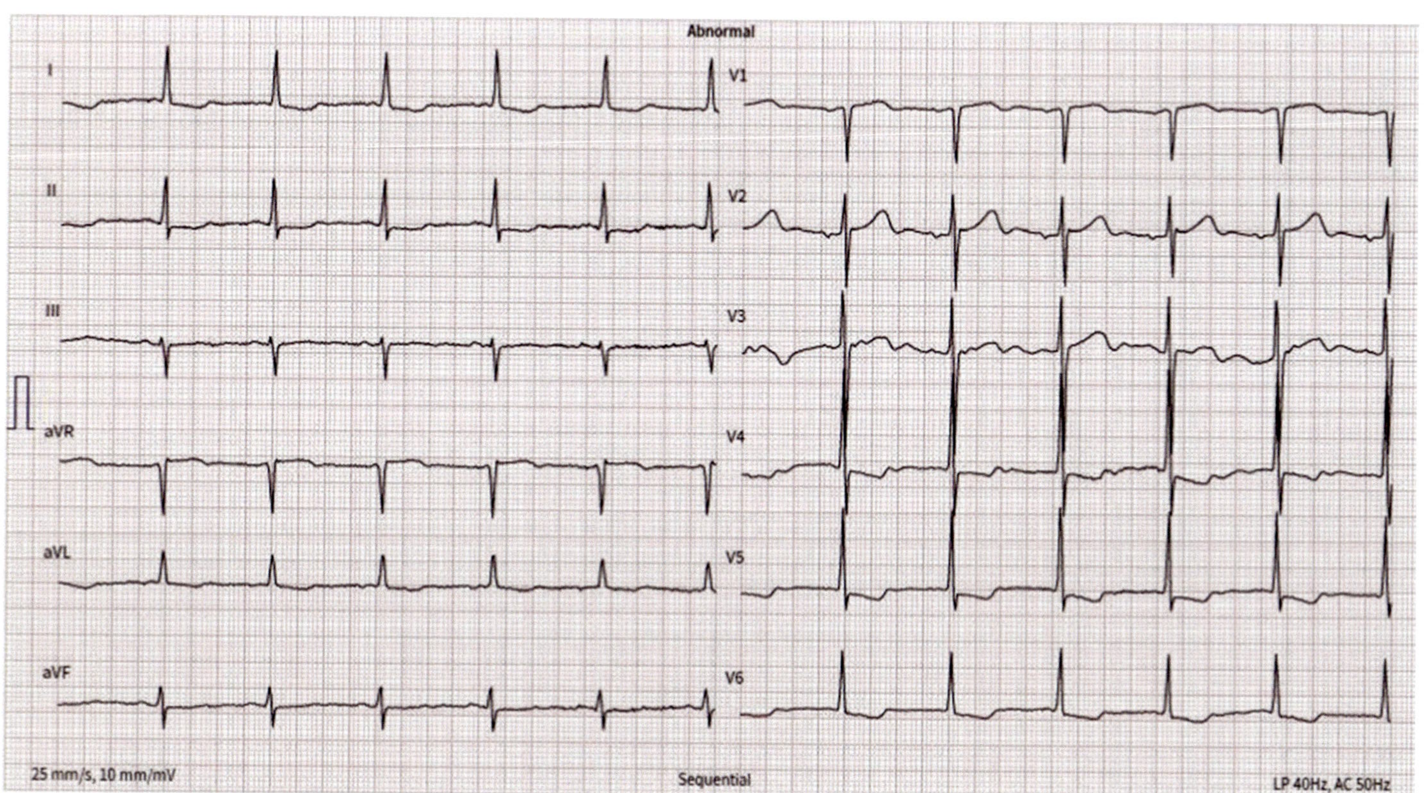

ECG Interpretation

Rhythm: Sinus
Rate: 72 bpm
Intervals: PR = 140 ms, QRS = 78 ms, QT = 420 ms, RR = 830 ms, QTC Baz = 440 ms – normal intervals.
Axis: Normal

Abnormalities on the ECG

- Left ventricular hypertrophy
- T wave inversion in I, aVL, V5, V6
- Downward-sloping ST depression in II, aVF, V4. V5. V6
- ST elevation in aVR.

ECG Test Answers

7, 40, 81

ECG Synthesis

This ECG shows sinus rhythm at 72 bpm, normal intervals and axis.

Abnormalities include left ventricular hypertrophy (based on 'Cornell criteria' – R wave in aVL + S wave in V3 > 20 mm in females) and ST-T changes in the lateral + inferior leads including down-sloping ST depression and T wave inversion.

The finding of LVH can be caused by several pathologies including long standing hypertension or outflow obstruction as seen in hypertrophic cardiomyopathy or significant aortic stenosis (AS).

The ST-T changes seen here in the lateral + inferior leads are nonspecific but are seen frequently in a setting of left ventricular hypertrophy (LVH). In that scenario these changes are termed 'left ventricular strain pattern'.

The most important next step in further investigating the patient's symptoms and ECG findings is completing an echocardiography which can confirm the ECG findings, assist defining the etiology and rule out other pathologies.

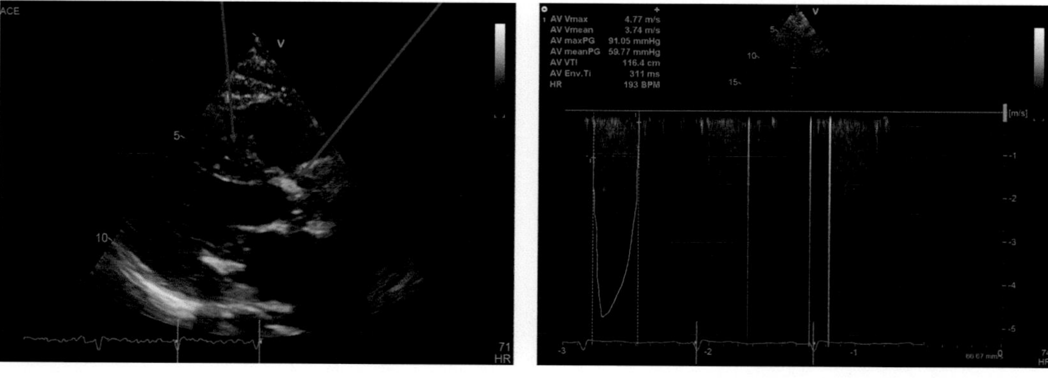

Left. Parasternal lang axis view showing the aortic valve (blue arrow) and the interventricular septum (red arrow) Right. Continuous-wave (CW) doppler echocardiography of the aortic valve

Echo Interpretation

Significant left ventricular hypertrophy Heavily calcified aortic valve.

Continuous wave (CW) doppler of the aortic valve measuring peak and mean velocities of 4.8 m/s and 3.7 m/s respectively; corresponding with 91 mmHg and 60 mmHg peak and mean gradients, respectively.

Echo Synthesis

These findings on echocardiography demonstrate significant LVH and a heavily calcified aortic valve with limited mobility and Doppler measurements of severe aortic stenosis (AS).

Cardiac Electrosonography Synthesis

This 82 year old female patient presented with a few months of exertional substernal chest pain, with a wide differential diagnosis. The ECG demonstrated LVH and ST-T changes which are most probably 'LV strain pattern'. The echo confirms the finding of LVH as well as severe aortic stenosis which is most probably the cause of the LVH and of the chest pain this patient is suffering from.

The patient was presented in the hospital 'heart team' and the best option for aortic-valve replacement was discussed. The patient was taken for transcatheter aortic valve replacement (TAVR) and her chest pain complaints resolved with marked reduction in her aortic gradients.

References

Abo Y, Yokoi H, et al. Electrocardiographic diagnosis of the coronary artery culprit site in ischemic heart disease. Circ J. 2003;67(9):775–80.

Allahwala UK, Nour D, et al. Prognostic implications of the rapid recruitment of coronary collaterals during ST elevation myocardial infarction (STEMI): a meta-analysis of over 14,000 patients. J Thromb Thrombolysis. 2021;51(4):1005–16.

Camaj A, Fuster V, et al. Left ventricular thrombus following acute myocardial infarction: JACC state-of-the-art review. J Am Coll Cardiol. 2022;79(10):1010–22.

Carrrel, et al. Acute aortic dissection. Lancet. 2023;401:773–88.

Cruz Rodriguez JB, Okajima K, Greenberg BH. Management of left ventricular thrombus: a narrative review. Ann Transl Med. 2021;9(6):520.

Hughes RK, et al. Apical ischemia is a universal feature of apical hypertrophic cardiomyopathy. Circ Cardiovasc Imaging. 2023;16: e014907.

Istolahti T, Lyytikäinen LP, et al. The prognostic significance of T-wave inversion according to ECG lead group during long-term follow-up in the general population. Ann Noninvasive Electrocardiol. 2021;26 (1):e12799.

Kazemi E, Mansoursamaei A, et al. The prognostic effect of ST-elevation in lead aVR on coronary artery disease, and outcome in acute coronary syndrome patients: a systematic review and meta-analysis. Eur J Med Res. 2022;27(1):302.

Kobo O, Marcusohn E, et al. Prognosis of patients with left circumflex artery acute myocardial infarction in relation to ST-segment on admission electrocardiogram. J Invasive Cardiol. 2021;33(1):E20–4.

Lazarou E, et al. Acute pericarditis: update. Curr Cardiol Rep. 2022;24(8):905–13.

Lindner JR. Contrast echocardiography: current status and future directions. Heart. 2021;107(1):18–24.

López-Candales A, Edelman K, Candales MD. Right ventricular apical contractility in acute pulmonary embolism: the McConnell sign revisited. Echocardiography. 2010;27(6):614–20.

Manno B, et al. Significance of the upright T wave in precordial lead VI in adults with coronary artery disease. J AM Coll Cardiol. 1983;1(5):1213–5.

Ogah OS, Oladapo OO, et al. Electrocardiographic left ventricular hypertrophy with strain pattern: prevalence, mechanisms and prognostic implications. Cardiovasc J Afr. 2008;19(1):39–45.

Rodriguez F, Mahaffey KW. Management of patients with NSTE-ACS: a comparison of the recent AHA/ACC and ESC guidelines. J Am Coll Cardiol. 2016;68 (3):313–21.

Ruiz-Mateos B, García-Borbolla R, et al. Identification of the culprit artery in inferior myocardial infarction through the 12-lead ECG. Coron Artery Dis. 2020;31 (1):20–6.

Shah AS, Chin CW, et al. Left ventricular hypertrophy with strain and aortic stenosis. Circulation. 2014;130 (18):1607–16.

Shahreyar M, et al. Post-myocardial infarction ventricular septal defect: a comprehensive review. Cardiovasc Revasc Med. 2020;21:1444–1449.

Singh, et al. Takotsubo syndrome: pathophysiology, emerging concepts and clinical implications. Circulation. 2022;145:1002–19.

Sovari AA, Assadi R, Lakshminarayanan B, Kocheril AG. Hyperacute T wave, the early sign of myocardial infarction. Am J Emerg Med. 2007;25 (7):859.e1-7.

Thomson D, Kourounis G, et al. ECG in suspected pulmonary embolism. Postgrad Med J. 2019;95 (1119):12–7.

Utsunomiya H, Hidaka T, et al. Value of resting echocardiographic findings and dobutamine stress echocardiography for diagnosing myocardial ischemia in patients with suspected angina pectoris. Echocardiography. 2015;32(6):993–1002.

Vaidya GN, Antoine S, et al. Reciprocal ST-segment changes in myocardial infarction: ischemia at distance versus mirror reflection of ST-elevation. Am J Med Sci. 2018;355(2):162–7.

Clinical Cases of Electrosonography in Patients with Shortness of Breath

David Leibowitz, Donna Zwas, Eldad Rachamim, Yair Elitzur, and Eyal Herzog

Abstract

In this chapter the authors provide representative cases of patients presenting with shortness of breath. Using the algorithm presented in the chapter "Patient-Centered Care Cardiac Electrosonography", the use of cardiac electrosonography in the evaluation of these complex patients is demonstrated in a variety of clinical scenarios including congestive heart failure of differing etiologies and valvular disease. The use of the algorithm in patients with acute coronary syndrome is similar to the cases presented in the chapter "Clinical Cases of Electrosonography in Patients with Acute Chest Pain" and is not repeated here.

Keywords

ECG · Echocardiography · Shortness of breath

D. Leibowitz (✉) · D. Zwas · E. Rachamim ·
Y. Elitzur · E. Herzog
The Heart Institute, Department of Cardiology,
Hadassah Medical Center, Hebrew University
of Jerusalem, 12000 Jerusalem, Israel
e-mail: oleibo@hadassah.org.il

1 Introduction

Shortness of breath is one of the most frequent complaints in an emergency department setting and may be a sign of a life-threatening illness. However, accurately diagnosing the etiology of the shortness of breath is challenging and other tests are required to achieve the correct diagnosis and implement the appropriate treatment.

Two important tests in the early workup of the patient with dyspnea, are the electrocardiogram (ECG) and trans-thoracic echocardiography (TTE). ECG and TTE, if done and interpreted properly, can help diagnose correctly the etiology of the dyspnea. The combined use of ECG and TTE in the workup process is termed **Electrosonography**, and in this chapter we present the use of electrosonography in the evaluation of patients with shortness of breath.

We first introduce an algorithm (Fig. 1) laying out the pathway for the use of electrosonography in patients with shortness of breath. This algorithm will aid the physician with decision making based on the primary evaluation upon presentation and the ECG and TTE findings. The algorithm defines the time each test should be done and the next step in the workup process. We include the ECG test code answers as well (Fig. 2) for easy preparation for the board review test.

We then demonstrate the use of the algorithm by presenting 13 cases of patients who presented with shortness of breath. Each case has a similar

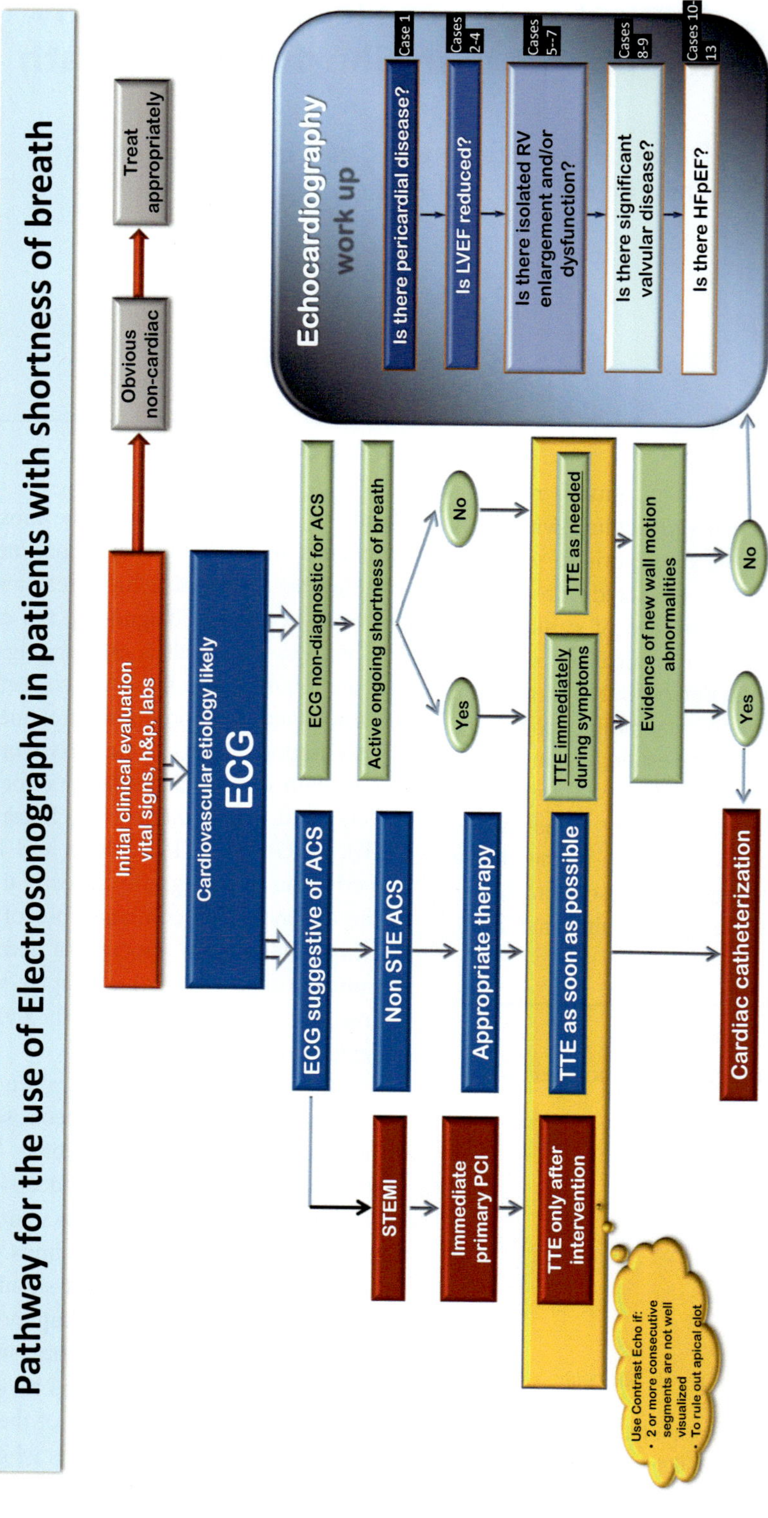

Fig. 1 Pathway for the use of electrosonography in patients with shortness of breath

GENERAL FEATURES & P WAVE ABNORMALITIES

General Features

1 ☐ Normal ECG
2 ☐ Normal variant
3 ☐ Incorrect electrode placement
4 ☐ Artifact

P Wave Abnormalities

5 ☐ Right atrial abnormality/enlargement
6 ☐ Left atrial abnormality/enlargement

RHYTHMS

Atrial Rhythms

7 ☐ Sinus rhythm
8 ☐ Sinus arrhythmia
9 ☐ Sinus bradycardia (<60)
10 ☐ Sinus tachycardia (>100)
11 ☐ Sinus pause or arrest
12 ☐ Sinoatrial exit block
13 ☐ Atrial premature complexes
14 ☐ Atrial tachycardia
15 ☐ Atrial tachycardia, multifocal
16 ☐ Supraventricular tachycardia
17 ☐ Atrial flutter
18 ☐ Atrial fibrillation

AV Junctional Rhythms

19 ☐ AV junctional premature complexes
20 ☐ AV junctional escape complexes
21 ☐ AV junctional rhythm/tachycardia

Ventricular Rhythms

22 ☐ Ventricular premature complex(es)
23 ☐ Ventricular parasystole
24 ☐ Ventricular tachycardia (3 or more consecutive complexes)
25 ☐ Accelerated idioventricular rhythm
26 ☐ Ventricular escape complexes or rhythm
27 ☐ Ventricular fibrillation

ATRIOVENTRICULAR CONDUCTION

28 ☐ AV block, 1°
29 ☐ AV block, 2° - Mobitz type I (Wenckebach)
30 ☐ AV block, 2° - Mobitz type II
31 ☐ AV block, 2:1
32 ☐ AV block, 3°
33 ☐ Wolff-Parkinson-White pattern
34 ☐ AV dissociation

VOLTAGE OR AXIS/HYPERTROPHY

Abnormal QRS Voltage or Axis

35 ☐ Low voltage, limb leads
36 ☐ Low voltage, precordial leads
37 ☐ Left axis deviation (> -30°)
38 ☐ Right axis deviation (> +100°)
39 ☐ Electrical alternans

Ventricular Hypertrophy

40 ☐ Left ventricular hypertrophy
41 ☐ Right ventricular hypertrophy
42 ☐ Combined ventricular hypertrophy

CLINICAL DISORDERS

43 ☐ Brugada syndrome
44 ☐ Digitalis toxicity
45 ☐ Torsades de pointes
46 ☐ Hyperkalemia
47 ☐ Hypokalemia
48 ☐ Hypercalcemia
49 ☐ Hypocalcemia
50 ☐ Dextrocardia, mirror image
51 ☐ Acute cor pulmonale including pulmonary embolus
52 ☐ Pericardial effusion
53 ☐ Acute pericarditis
54 ☐ Hypertrophic cardiomyopathy
55 ☐ Central nervous system disorder
56 ☐ Hypothermia

INTRAVENTRICULAR CONDUCTION

57 ☐ RBBB, complete
58 ☐ RBBB, incomplete
59 ☐ Left anterior fascicular block
60 ☐ Left posterior fascicular block
61 ☐ LBBB, complete
62 ☐ LBBB, incomplete
63 ☐ Aberrant conduction (including rate-related)
64 ☐ Intraventricular conduction disturbance, nonspecific type

MYOCARDIAL INFARCTION

	Age recent, or probably acute	Age indeterminate, or probably old
Anterolateral	65 ☐	66 ☐
Anterior or anteroseptal	67 ☐	68 ☐
Lateral	69 ☐	70 ☐
Inferior	71 ☐	72 ☐
Posterior	73 ☐	74 ☐

ST, T, U WAVE ABNORMALITIES

75 ☐ Normal variant, early repolarization
76 ☐ Normal variant, juvenile T waves
77 ☐ Nonspecific ST and/or T wave abnormalities
78 ☐ ST and/or T wave abnormalities suggesting myocardial ischemia
79 ☐ ST and/or T wave abnormalities suggesting myocardial injury
80 ☐ ST and/or T wave abnormalities suggesting electrolyte disturbances
81 ☐ ST and/or T wave abnormalities secondary to hypertrophy
82 ☐ Prolonged Q-T interval
83 ☐ Prominent U waves

PACEMAKER FUNCTION

84 ☐ Atrial or coronary sinus pacing
85 ☐ Ventricular demand pacemaker (VVI), normally functioning
86 ☐ Dual-chamber pacemaker (DDD), normally functioning
87 ☐ Pacemaker malfunction, not constantly capturing (atrium or ventricle)
88 ☐ Pacemaker malfunction, not constantly sensing (atrium or ventricle)
89 ☐ Paced morphology consistent with biventricular pacing or cardiac resynchronization therapy

Fig. 2 Codes for ECG reading

layout and contains 4 pages allowing the reader to test his or her knowledge of ECG and TTE interpretation:

Page 1 includes the presenting complaint and additional clinical information as well as an ECG performed on arrival.
Page 2 includes the authors' interpretation of the ECG and a short discussion regarding the findings and the next recommended step. The ECG test answers are included for aiding students in preparation for the test.
Page 3 includes transthoracic echocardiography images with a legend of the views seen.
Page 4 includes the authors' interpretation of the echocardiography with a discussion of the combined electrosonography findings.

2 Case 1

76 year old male, history of smoking with 2 weeks of hemoptysis, several days of worsening shortness of breath and chest pain.

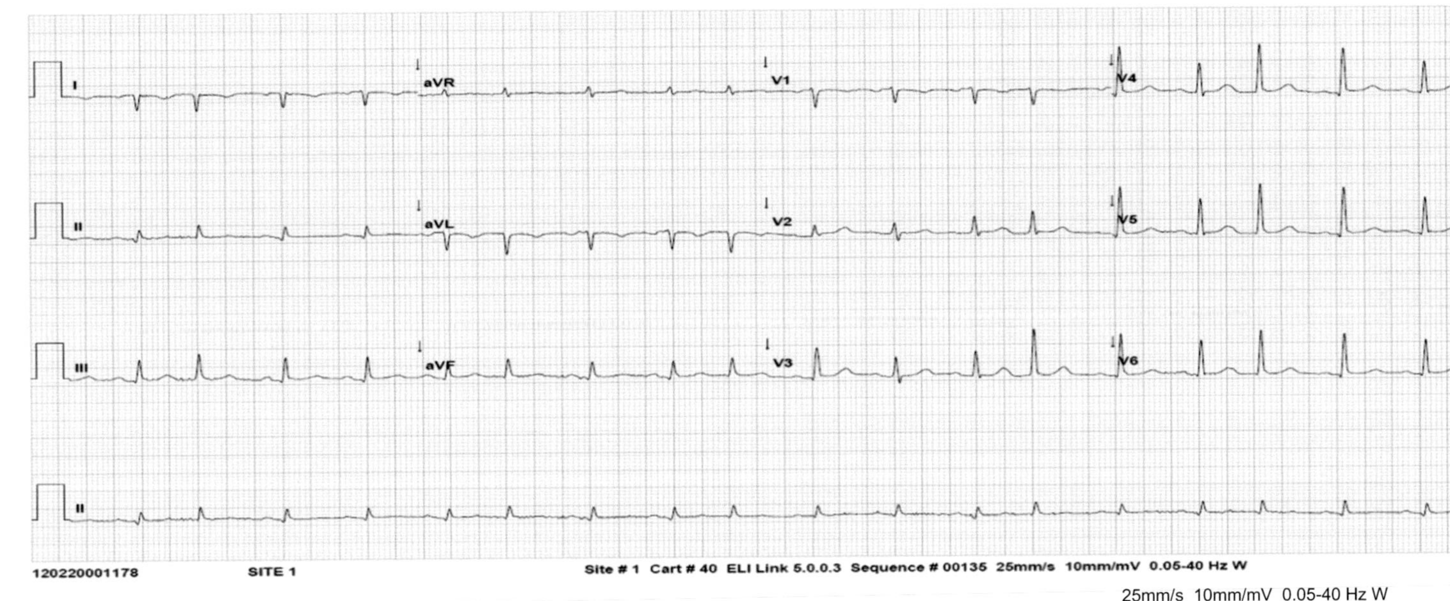

Additional Clinical History

One month of decreased appetite and weight loss. On physical examination jugular venous pressure was elevated. Heart sounds were decreased with no murmurs.

Additional information

CXR revealed a small pleural effusion, cardiomegaly and suspected mediastinal mass

ECG Interpretation

Rhythm: Sinus Tachycardia
Rate: 110 bpm
Intervals: PR = 140 ms, QRS = 70 ms, QTc = 385 ms
Axis: Right axis deviation

Abnormalities on the ECG

- Sinus tachycardia
- Right axis
- Atrial premature beats
- Borderline low voltage in limb leads
- Nonspecific ST-T abnormality
- Electrical alternans.

ECG Test Answers

8, 35, 38, 39, 52, 77.

ECG Synthesis

The ECG shows sinus tachycardia which is a sensitive but non specific sign of acute cardiovascular pathology. Borderline low voltage in limb leads suggests pericardial effusion, or an extra-cardiac cause such as COPD or morbid obesity. There are no signs of pericarditis, such as ST elevation, T wave inversion or PR depression. The finding of electrical alternans in the presence of low voltage ECG suggests a large pericardial effusion; possibly with a 'rocking heart' which may be a cause of the alternans. The presence of atrial premature beats is non specific but is consistent with the suspicion of pericardial disease. The right axis deviation is most likely a sign of underlying pulmonary disease in this elderly smoker.

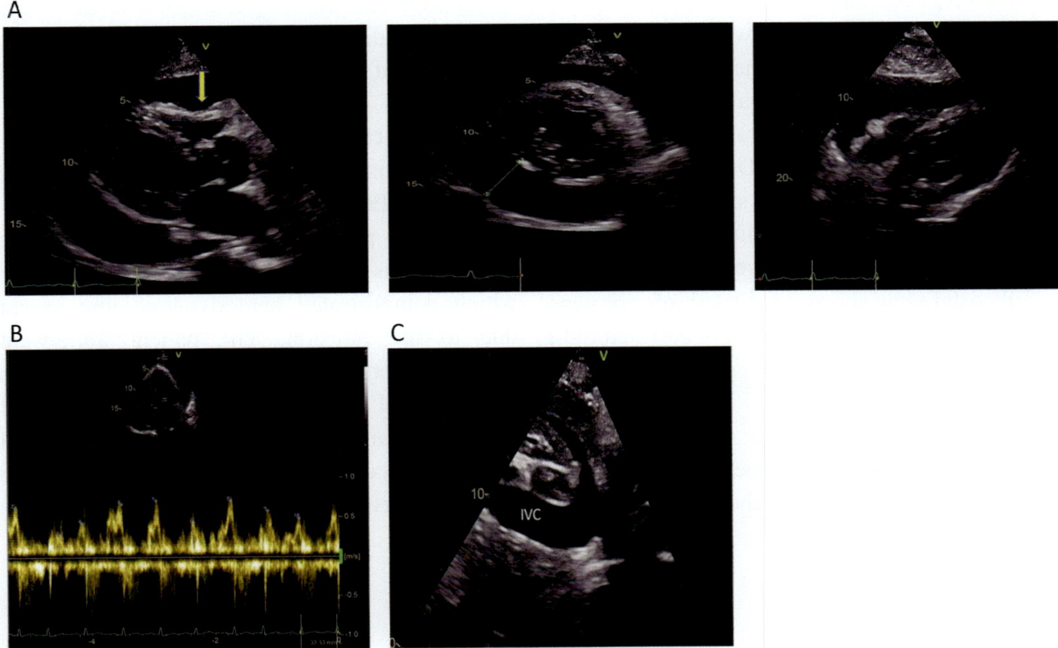

Parasternal and subcostal views showing significant pericardial effusion (top images, panel A). The arrow illustrates inversion of the RV free wall during diastole. The mitral valve inflow Doppler obtained in apical 4 chamber view (B) shows significant changes in flow velocities with inspiration. Subcostal view (C) showed a dilated inferior vena cava (IVC)

Echo Interpretation

Parasternal and subcostal views showing significant pericardial effusion. The arrow illustrates inversion of the RV free wall during diastole consistent with elevated intra pericardial pressure. The mitral valve inflow Doppler obtained in apical 4 chamber view shows significant changes in flow velocities with inspiration consistent with impaired diastolic filling as well.

Subcostal view showed a dilated inferior vena cava which is a non specific sign of elevated right sided filling pressures.

Echo Synthesis

The findings of significant pericardial effusion with diastolic collapse of the RV free wall, inspiratory flow velocity changes over the mitral valve and a dilated inferior vena cava is strongly suggestive of cardiac tamponade.

Cardiac Electrosonography Synthesis

In this patient, "electrosonography" revealed low voltage on ECG with electrical alternans. Suspected large pericardial effusion based on these findings was confirmed by echocardiography which demonstrated hemodynamic impairment due to the effusion. The patient underwent emergent pericardiocentesis with relief of his symptoms of shortness of breath. Pathology of the pericardial fluid was consistent with non small cell lung cancer and the patient was referred to the oncology service for further management.

3   Case 2

A 57 y.o. male with no significant past medical history presented to the ED with several months of palpitations. Over the 6 weeks prior to presentation he developed worsening shortness of breath, orthopnea and paroxysmal nocturnal dyspnea.

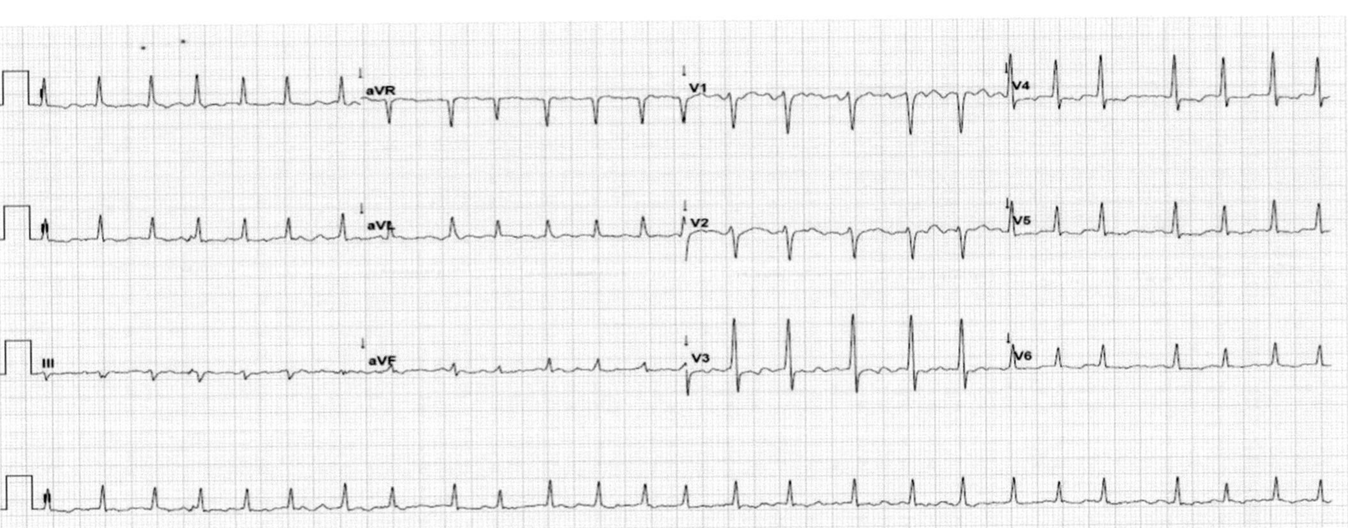

Additional Clinical History

Physical exam revealed irregularly irregular pulse, elevated JVP, bilateral rales at the bases

Additional information

CXR showed pulmonary congestion. NTProBNP was significantly elevated at 3453 pg/ml.

ECG Interpretation

Rhythm: Atrial fibrillation
Rate: 150 bpm
Intervals: PR not measurable due to AF, QRS 90 ms QTc 350 ms
Axis: Normal

Abnormalities on the ECG

Atrial fibrillation.

ST depression in V3 to V5

Nonspecific T wave changes

ECG Test Answers

18, 77.

ECG Synthesis

This patient has atrial fibrillation with a rapid ventricular rate.

ST depression in V3 to V5 may represent subendocardial ischemia, probably caused by the tachycardia. There are nonspecific T wave changes.

An interesting finding in this ECG is respiratory variation in QRS voltage. As opposed to respiratory variations in the RR interval in sinus rhythm (sinus arrhythmia), variation in voltage in not common. This is not to be confused with electrical alternans, where voltage changes happen consistently every other beat. Some have reported this finding to correlate with respiratory changes in blood pressure, which may hint at hypovolemia in an appropriate clinical setting.

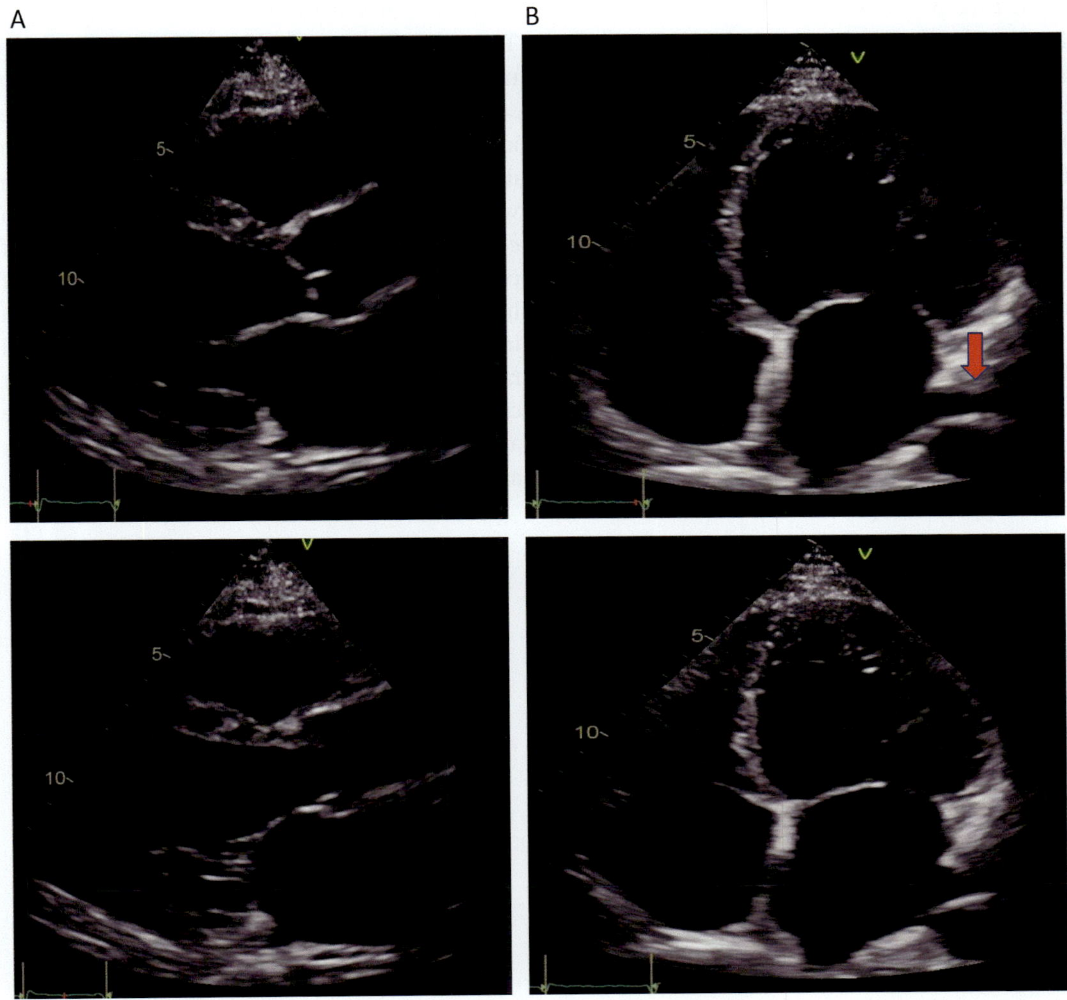

Parasternal long-axis (panel A) and apical 4 chamber views (panel B) demonstrate an enlarged left ventricle and left atrium with no significant difference in LV volumes between end diastolic images (upper) and end-systolic images (lower) consistent with diffuse, significant reduction in LV systolic function. In apical 4 chamber view a dilated pulmonary vein (indicated by arrow) is noted.

Echo Interpretation

Parasternal long-axis and apical 4 chamber views demonstrated an enlarged left ventricle and left atrium with no significant difference in LV volumes between end diastolic images (upper) and end-systolic images (lower) consistent with diffuse, significant reduction in LV systolic function. In apical 4 chamber view a dilated pulmonary vein (indicated by arrow) is noted.

Echo Synthesis

The enlarged and diffusely hypokinetic left ventricle is consistent with a non-ischemic cardiomyopathic process. The dilated left pulmonic vein supports the presence of elevated left sided filling pressures.

Cardiac Electrosonography Synthesis

The ECG findings in this patient demonstrated rapid atrial fibrillation which presumably began several months prior to presentation with the appearance of palpitations. The emergency echo demonstrated significant diffuse LV dysfunction with elevated left sided filling pressures which contributed to the clinical signs and symptoms of congestive heart failure. This constellation of findings suggested a diagnosis of tachycardia induced cardiomyopathy due to the untreated rapid atrial fibrillation. The patient underwent cardioversion and subsequent ablation of the atrial fibrillation with resolution of symptoms and improvement in ventricular function.

4 Case 3

A 62 y.o. male with a history of diabetes and smoking presented to the ED with shortness of breath and general weakness. 10 days prior to admission he had a prolonged episode of chest and back pain. He denied fever or cough

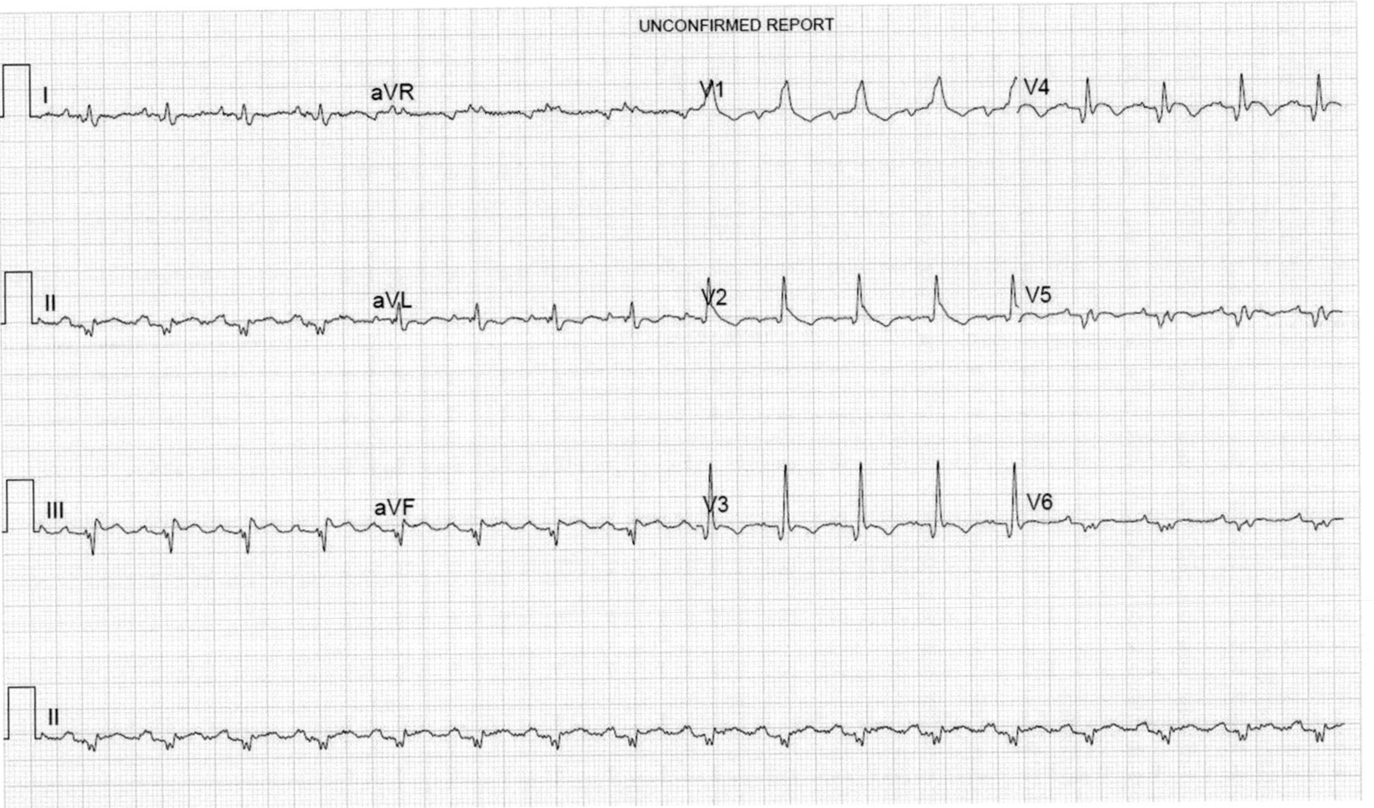

Additional Clinical History

Physical exam revealed diaphoresis with a blood pressure of 75/40 mmHg and poor capillary refill, crepitation at both lung bases. Decreased heart sounds

Additional information

CXR showed pulmonary congestion. High-sensitive troponin was 9922 with normal CPK

ECG Interpretation

Rhythm: Sinus
Rate: 100 bpm
Intervals: PR 190 ms, QRS 145 ms, QTC 410 ms
Axis: Left

Abnormalities on the ECG

Right bundle branch block

Q waves in inferior, anterior and lateral leads.

Low voltage in lateral leads 1, aVL, V5, V6.

ECG Test Answers

37, 57, 68, 70, 72, 79.

ECG Synthesis

The ECG suggests prior infarction of the inferior, anterior and lateral walls. Low voltage in some of these leads suggests significant loss of myocardium. However, the ECG does not fulfill formal criteria for limb lead or precordial lead low voltage, requiring a total voltage less than 5 mv for limb leads or 10 mv for the precordial leads. This may point to the fact that the reduced voltage is not related to an extra-cardiac cause such as pericardial effusion or pulmonary emphysema.

Right bundle branch block may be a result of previous anterior wall myocardial infarction. If this is the case, it indicates greater damage to the interventricular septum and a worse prognosis.

Left axis deviation in this case is not the result of left anterior fascicular (hemi) block since there is no initial r wave in lead II. Rather, it is a result of the inferior infarction.

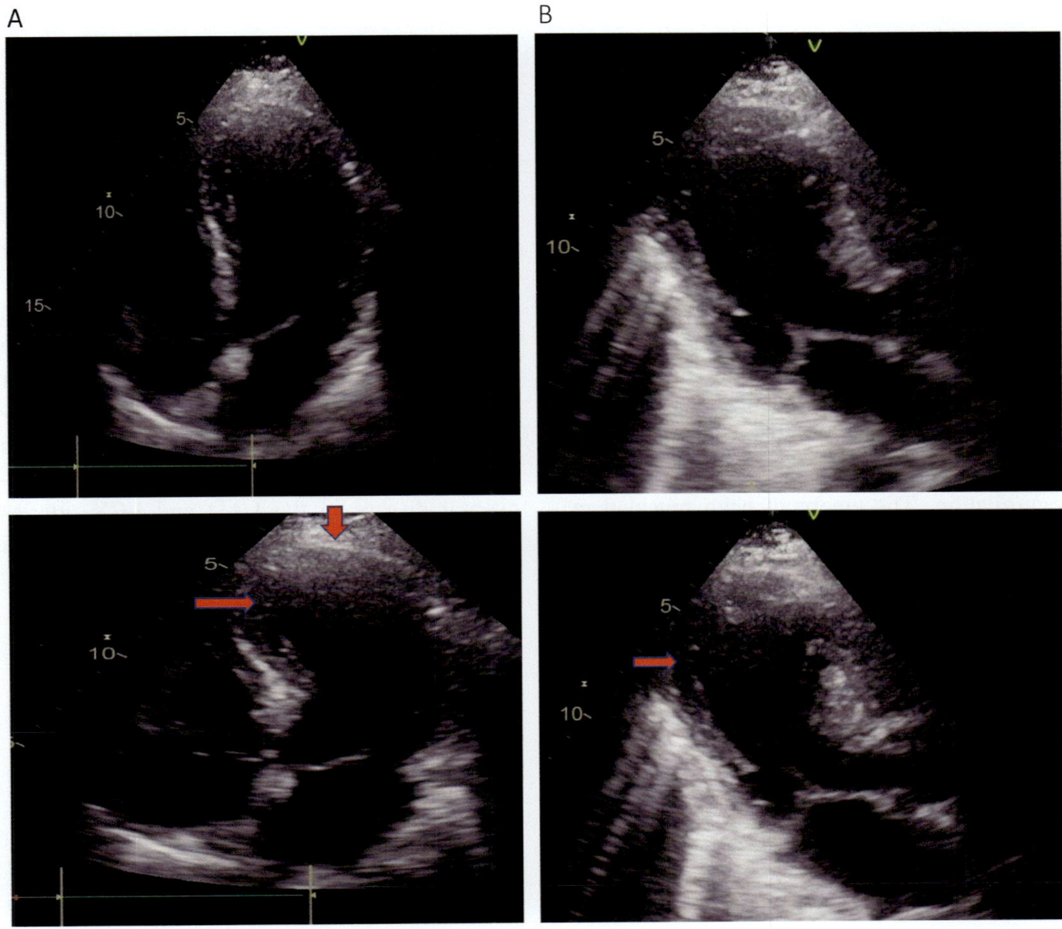

Parasternal long-axis (panel A) and apical 3 chamber views (panel B) (end diastolic images above and end systolic images below) reveal wall motion abnormalities of both posterolateral wall and the apex (indicated by arrows).

Echo interpretation

Parasternal long-axis and apical 3 chamber views (end diastolic images above and end systolic images below) revealed wall motion abnormalities of both posterolateral wall and the apex. No evidence of pericardial effusion or significant mitral regurgitation.

Echo Synthesis

Possible explanations for cardiogenic shock in the setting of myocardial infarction include significant left and/or right ventricular dysfunction or a mechanical complication including free wall rupture, ventricular septal defect or papillary muscle rupture causing severe mitral regurgitation. The emergent echo revealed evidence of multivessel coronary disease which suggested myocardial dysfunction as the primary mechanism of the hemodynamic compromise.

Cardiac Electrosonography Synthesis

The ECG findings in this patient were suggestive of a non acute inferolateral infarct with low voltage and right bundle branch block suggestive extensive myocardial dysfunction. The emergency echo demonstrated significant LV dysfunction in a pattern suggesting multivessel coronary artery disease, findings consistent with the ECG. Despite the relatively late arrival after the beginning of symptoms, given the hemodynamic instability an intraaortic balloon pump was placed. Emergent catheterization revealed significant disease in the LAD and LCX arteries which underwent stent placement with resolution of the cardiogenic shock.

5 Case 4

A 71 year old male presented with 4 weeks of worsening exertional shortness of breath, weight loss, and bilateral leg swelling.

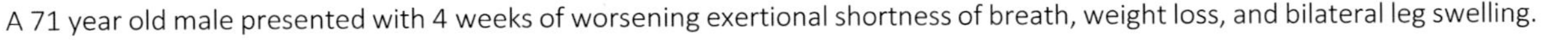

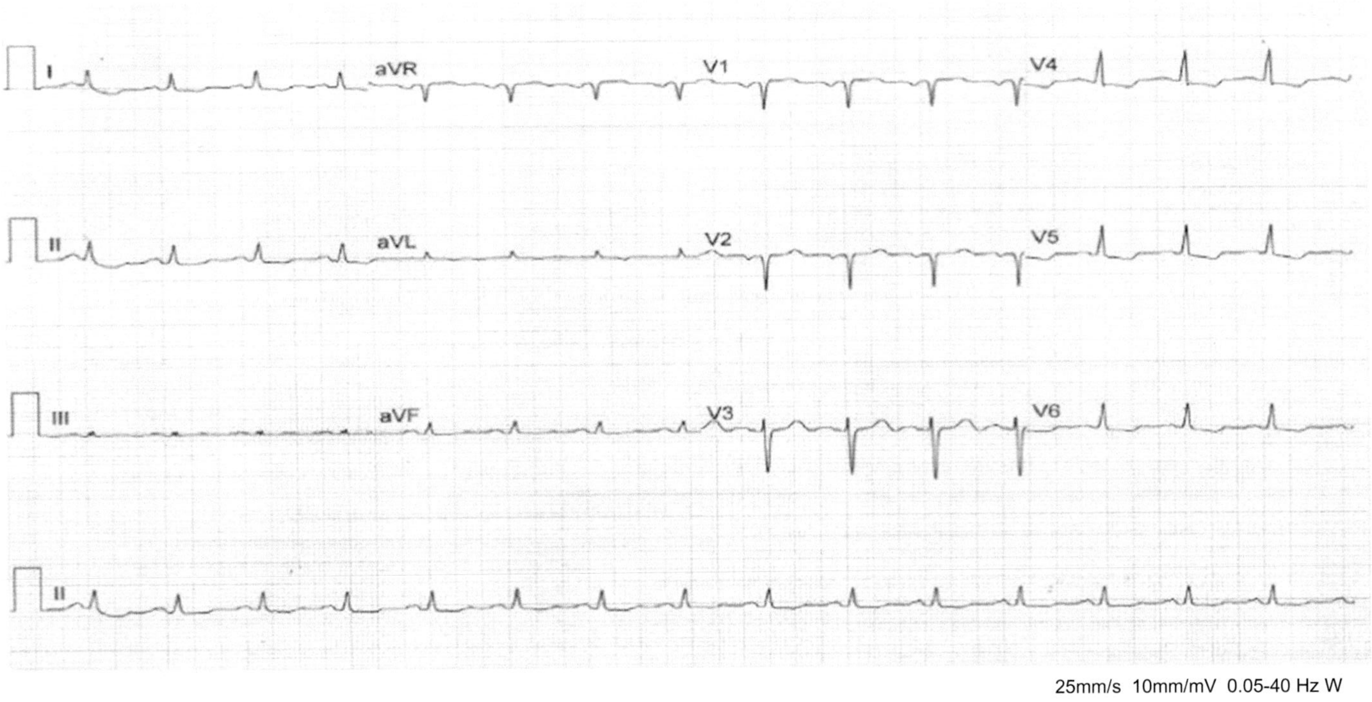

25mm/s 10mm/mV 0.05-40 Hz W

Additional Clinical History
He underwent bilateral carpal tunnel release surgery 3 years prior to his presentation. On physical examination jugular venous pressure was elevated to the angle of the jaw. Decreased breath sounds were noted at the lung bases. Heart sounds were decreased with no murmurs. Pitting edema of both lower extremities was noted.

Additional information
CXR revealed bilateral pleural effusions and a mildly enlarged cardiac silhouette

ECG Interpretation

Rhythm: Sinus
Rate: 95 bpm
Intervals: PR = 170 ms, QRS = 80 ms, QTC 452 ms.
Axis: Normal

Abnormalities on the ECG

- Low voltage in limb leads.
- Nonspecific ST-T abnormality.
- Q waves in V1, V2.

ECG Test Answers

7, 35, 52, 68, 77.

ECG Synthesis

This ECG shows sinus rhythm at 90 bpm, normal intervals and axis.

The main abnormalities are low limb lead voltage and Q waves in V1, V2.

The differential diagnosis of low voltage ECG includes conditions separating the myocardium from the body surface such as COPD (lung hyperinflation), obesity, pleural or pericardial effusion; and conditions where the heart muscle produces a weak electrical signal, including extensive scarring due to myocardial infarction and infiltrative or restrictive cardiomyopathies, especially amyloidosis.

The differential diagnosis of Q waves includes myocardial infarction and a variety of conditions causing a 'pseudo-infarct' pattern. When the Q waves appear in leads V1 and V2, the main differential is anteroseptal MI vs infiltrative cardiomyopathies. The extent of abnormal Q waves, limited to V1-V2, however, would render infarction less likely to account for the full clinical presentation.

The combination of low voltage ECG and prominent jugular venous distention is suggestive of possible pericardial effusion which must be ruled out immediately by echocardiography.

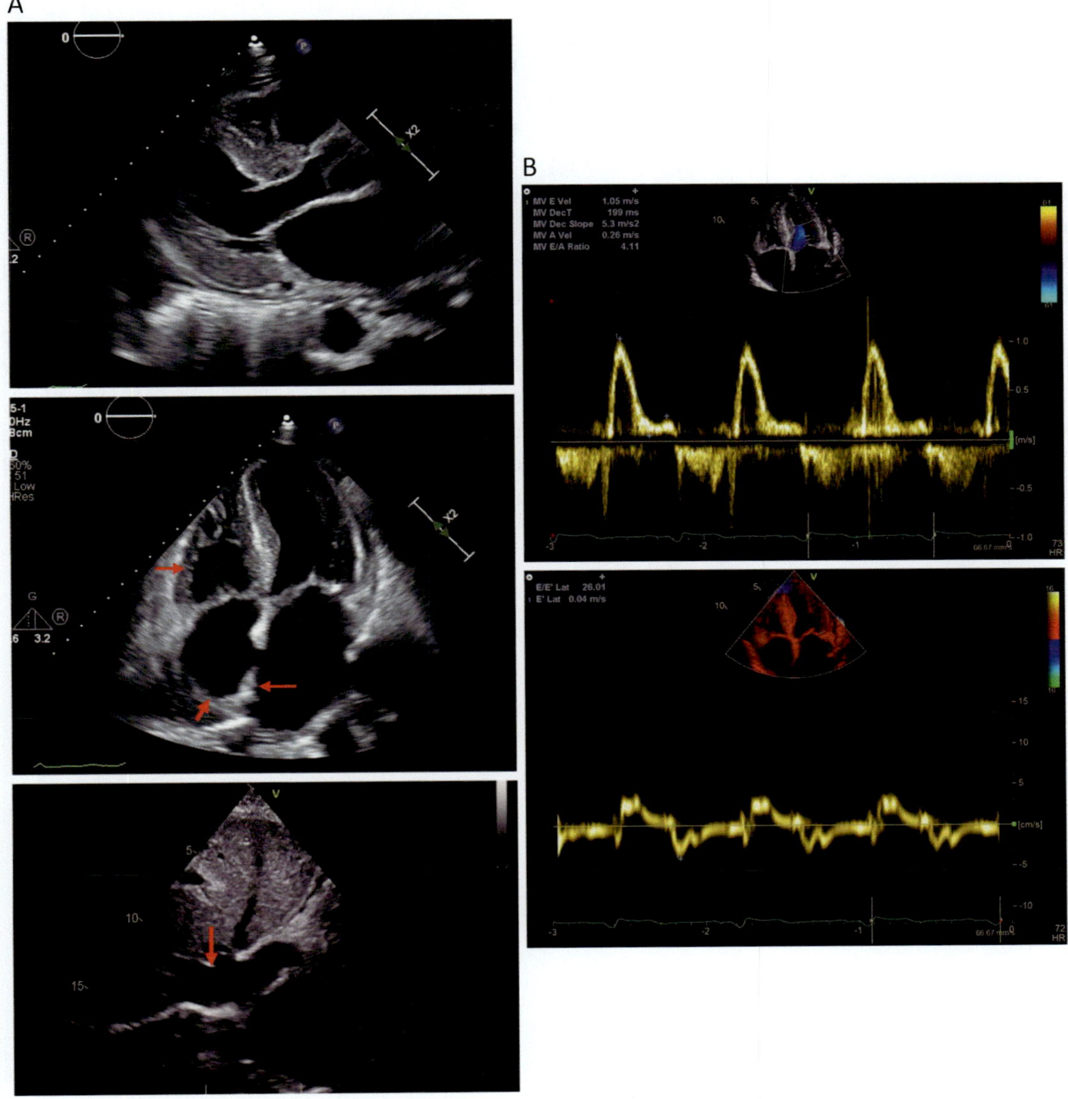

The echo shows concentric left ventricular wall thickening with thickening of the right ventricle, atrial wall and interatrial septum (panel A, arrows). A dilated inferior vena cava is seen on subcostal imaging. (Panel A bottom image, arrow). Doppler interrogation in apical 4 chamber view (Panel B) shows a restrictive filling pattern (high e:e' ratio) consistent with elevated LV filling pressures

Echo Interpretation

The echo shows concentric left ventricular wall thickening with thickening of other cardiac chambers including the right ventricle, atrial wall and interatrial septum. Doppler interrogation in apical 4 chamber view shows a tall e wave on mitral inflow Doppler with a small e' wave on mitral annular tissue Doppler imaging consistent with a restrictive filling pattern and elevated LV filling pressures.

A dilated inferior vena cava is seen on subcostal imaging.

Echo Synthesis

The findings of thickening of the RV, atria and interatrial septum in addition to thickening of the LV supports infiltrative cardiomyopathy.

The mitral Doppler and tissue Doppler findings and the dilated IVC suggest elevated left and right sided pressures.

Cardiac Electrosonography Synthesis

The constellation of findings noted on "electrosonography" in particular the thickened LV walls with low voltage on ECG in conjunction with the clinical history of mainly right sided congestive heart failure and bilateral carpal tunnel syndrome were highly suggestive of cardiac amyloidosis and the patient was admitted for evaluation. Workup including free light chains, cardiac MRI and nuclear scanning confirmed the diagnosis of transthyretin amyloidosis and appropriate treatment was begun.

6 Case 5

A 27 y.o. woman with no significant past medical history presented to the ED with several months of worsening shortness of breath as well as significant peripheral edema.

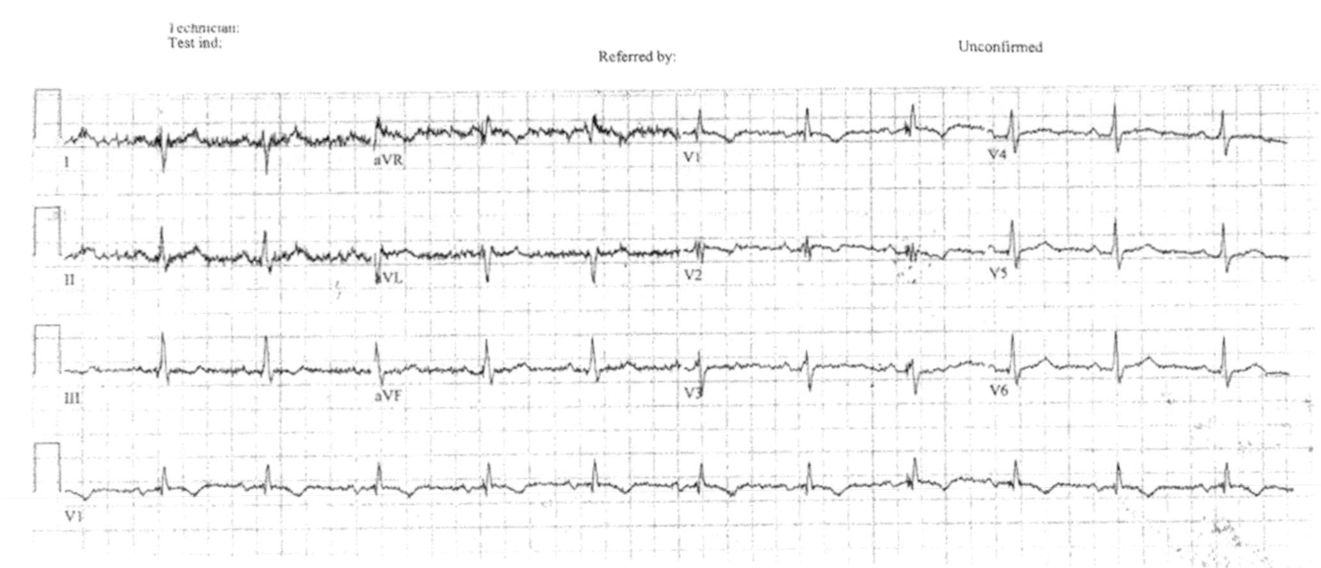

Additional Clinical History

Physical exam revealed mild tachypnea, decreased breath sounds at both lung bases, significant ascites as well as 3+ bilateral peripheral edema. There was a third heart sound which increased during inspiration

Additional information

CXR was unremarkable. High-sensitive troponin was mildly elevated

ECG Interpretation

Rhythm: Sinus
Rate: 60 bpm
Intervals: PR 200 ms, QRS 130 ms, QTC 360 ms
Axis: Right axis deviation

Abnormalities on the ECG

Right bundle branch block.

Right axis deviation.

ECG Test Answers

7, 38, 57.

ECG Synthesis

The main findings on this ECG are RBBB and right axis deviation.

The differential diagnosis includes conduction system disease; the right axis deviation may be a result of left posterior hemiblock as an additional manifestation of conduction disorder.

Another possibility is that one or both findings are due to right heart strain secondary to pulmonary disease, or congenital heart disease.

Conduction disease in itself should not cause symptoms of shortness of breath and signs of right heart failure. Therefore, the possibility of pulmonary disease or congenital heart disease is most likely and should be investigated by echocardiogram.

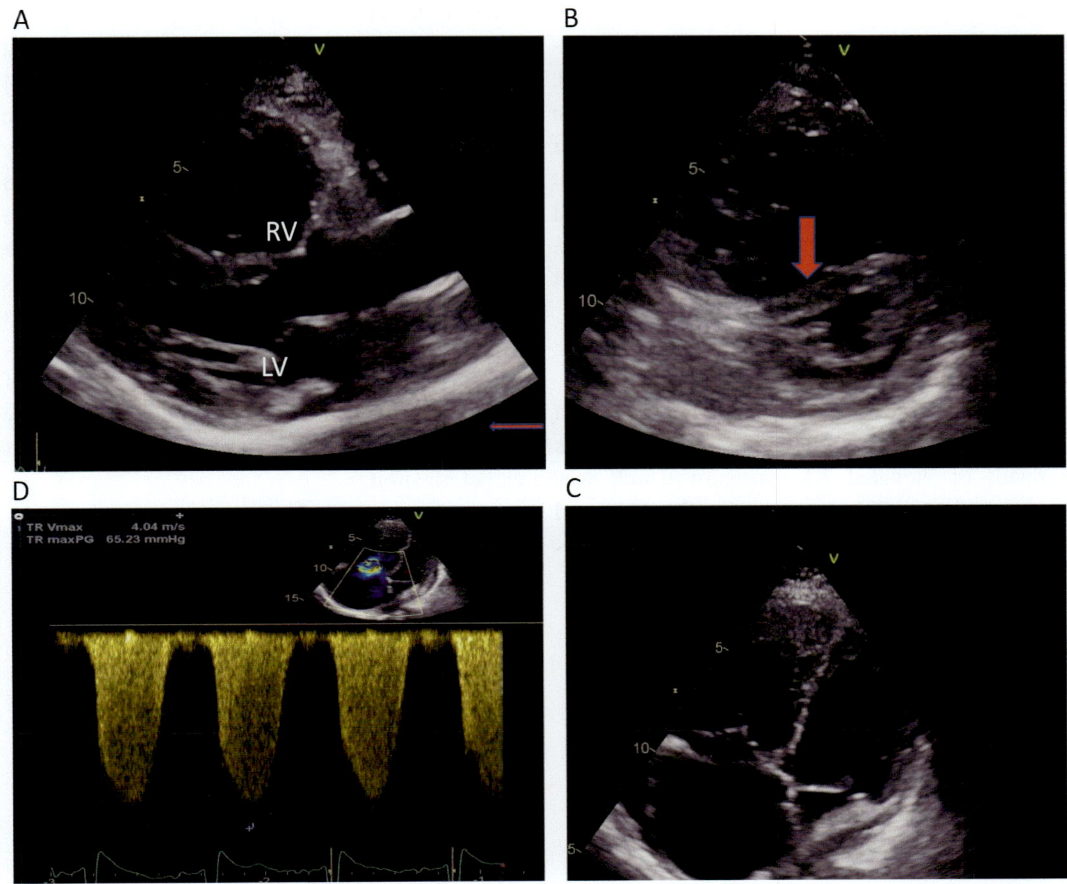

Parasternal long-axis (A) and short axis (B) views demonstrate a very enlarged right ventricle (RV). In short axis view flattening of the septum (indicated by arrow) is noted. Apical 4 chamber view (C) shows enlarged right atrium and right ventricle. Doppler interrogation (D) revealed significant pulmonary hypertension

Echo Interpretation

Parasternal long-axis and short axis views demonstrate a very enlarged right ventricle (RV). In short axis view flattening of the septum (indicated by arrow) is noted. Apical 4 chamber view shows enlarged right atrium and right ventricle which are significantly more dilated than the corresponding left sided chambers. Doppler interrogation of the tricuspid velocity jet revealed significant pulmonary hypertension.

Echo Synthesis

The enlarged right sided chambers are consistent with right heart strain. Flattening of the septum is a result of elevated RV pressure which was confirmed by the TR measurement. Structure and function of the left sided cardiac structures was normal.

Cardiac Electrosonography Synthesis

The ECG findings in this patient were consistent with right heart enlargement with the lack of tachycardia suggesting a chronic process. The emergency echo demonstrating pulmonary hypertension with enlargement of the RA and RV, was consistent with the ECG findings. The differential diagnosis is broad, however the young age of the patient who had no previous medical history, the chronicity of the symptoms symptoms, and the lack of left sided or congenital heart disease on echo was most suggestive of a diagnosis of primary or idiopathic pulmonary hypertension which was confirmed by right heart catheterization.

7 Case 6

65-years-old man with history of diabetes mellites and hypertension presented to the emergency department with three days of dyspnea and a nonproductive cough. He denied having chest pain.

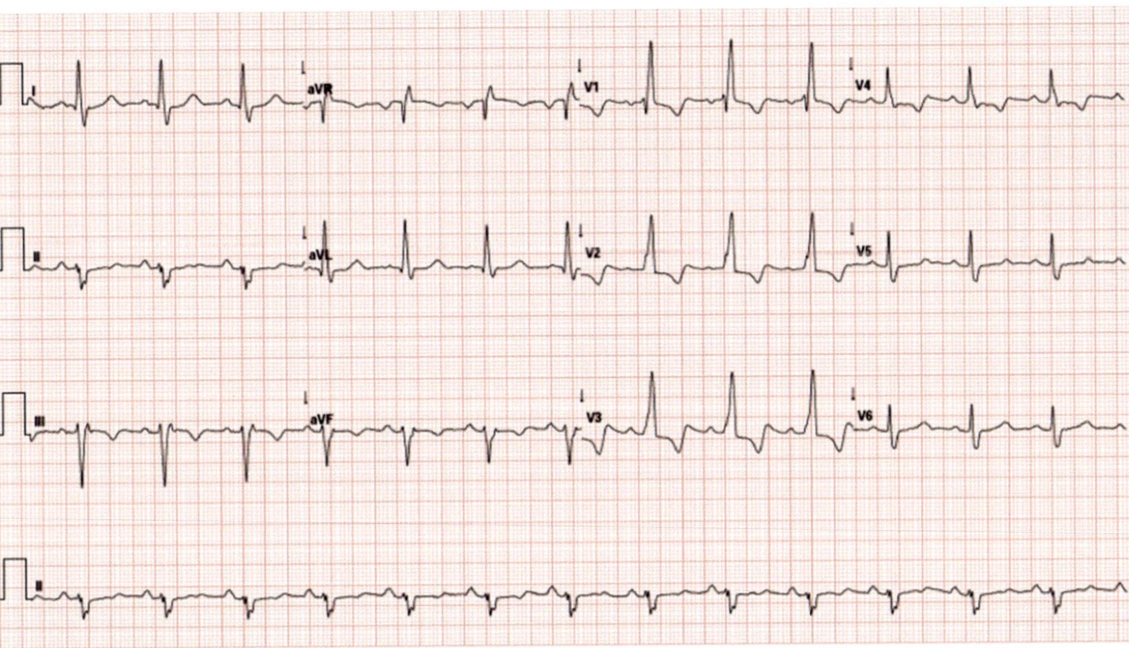

Additional Clinical History

On examination, his blood pressure was elevated to 180/100 mmHg, temperature was normal, and the oxygen saturation was 91% in room air. Laboratory workup showed a D-dimer of 8,000 ng/mL, and hsTnT was negative on two consecutive tests.

Additional information

Chest X-ray was normal. CT angiography demonstrated a segmental filling defect in the right upper lobe.

ECG Interpretation

Rhythm: Sinus
Rate: 90 bpm
Intervals: PR = 180 ms, QRS = 120 ms, QTc 452 ms.
Axis: − 45 (Left axis deviation)

Abnormalities on the ECG

- Right bundle branch block
- Left anterior hemiblock
- Nonspecific ST-T changes.

ECG Test Answers
7, 57, 59, 77.

ECG Synthesis

This patient has normal sinus rhythm with bifascicular block of right bundle branch block (RBBB) and left anterior hemiblock.

The differential diagnosis of a RBBB is wide, however, with the combination of left axis deviation the caregiver should consider atrial septal defect (primum type). Echocardiography is essential in this setting to define the next step in management.

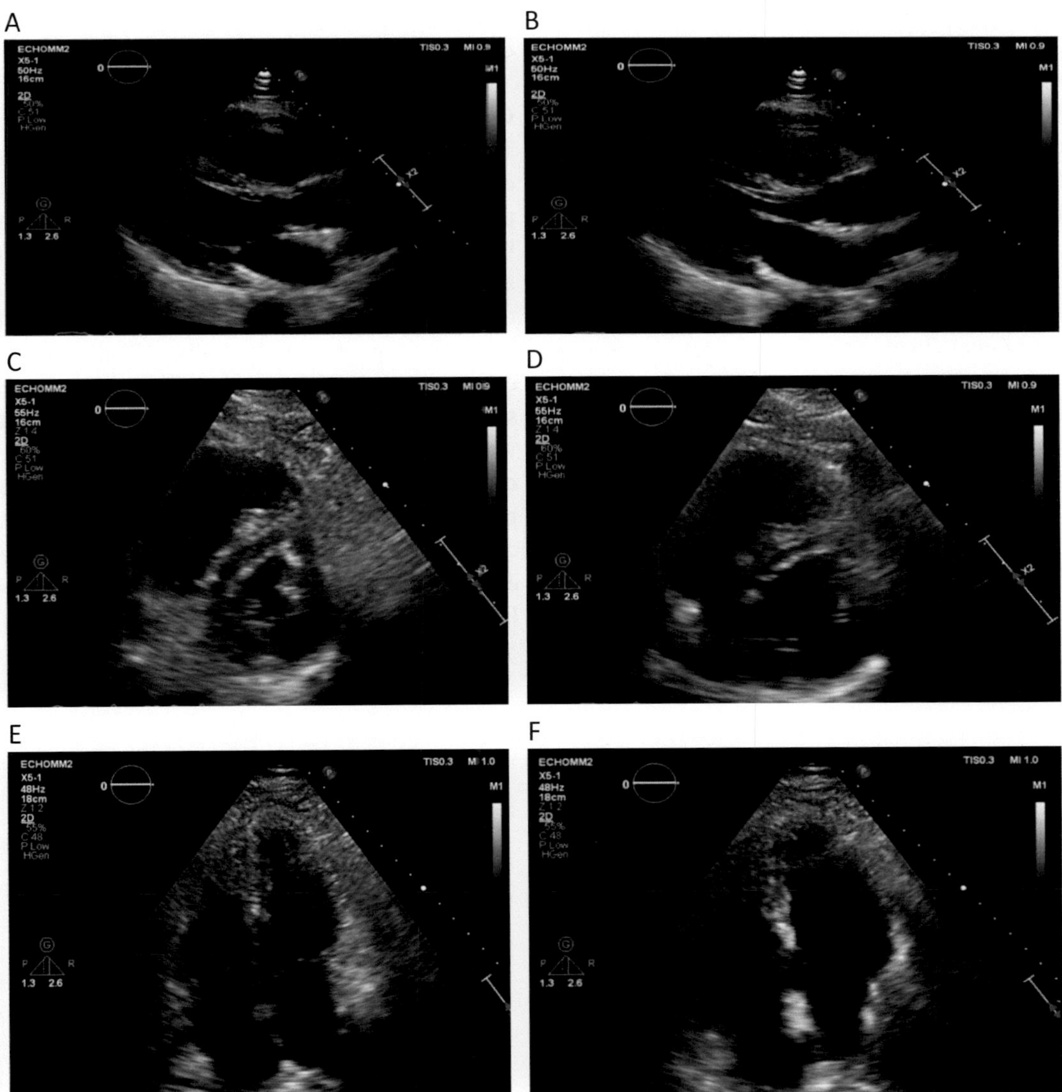

Transthoracic parasternal long axis imaging in systole (A) and diastole (B). Transthoracic parasternal short axis imaging in systole (C) and diastole (D). Apical 4-chamber imaging in systole (E) and diastole (F)

Echo Interpretation

Transthoracic parasternal long axis imaging in systole (A) and diastole (B) demonstrated normal LV systolic function. However, there is marked dilatation of the right ventricular outflow tract (RVOT) with decreased systolic function of the RVOT.

Transthoracic parasternal short axis imaging in systole (C) and diastole (D) confirmed the preserved LV systolic function. As in the parasternal long axis view there is marked dilatation of all segments of the right ventricle with septal flattening in systole and diastole suggesting pressure and volume overload. Apical 4-chamber imaging in systole (E) and diastole (F) confirmed the dilatation and decreased systolic function of the right ventricle.

Echo Synthesis

Echo images demonstrated preserved LV systolic function with a moderately dilated right ventricle and evidence of right- sided pressure and volume overload.

Cardiac Electrosonography Synthesis

This patient has a diagnosis of pulmonary embolism made on his CT angiography of the pulmonary arteries. His ECG demonstrated right bundle branch block pattern (RBBB) with left axis deviation. While RBBB is consistent with the clinical picture, left axis deviation is not common in pulmonary embolism. Transthoracic echocardiography demonstrated preserved LV systolic function with a moderately dilated right ventricle with evidence of pressure and volume overload, confirming the diagnosis. Since the patient's troponin levels were negative, he is considered an intermediate low risk pulmonary embolism and was treated with oral anticoagulation under close observation.

8 Case 7

A 57 year old male with a history of hypertension and active smoking presented with 3 days of worsening dyspnea, cough and pleuritic chest pain despite antibiotic therapy for presumed community acquired pneumonia

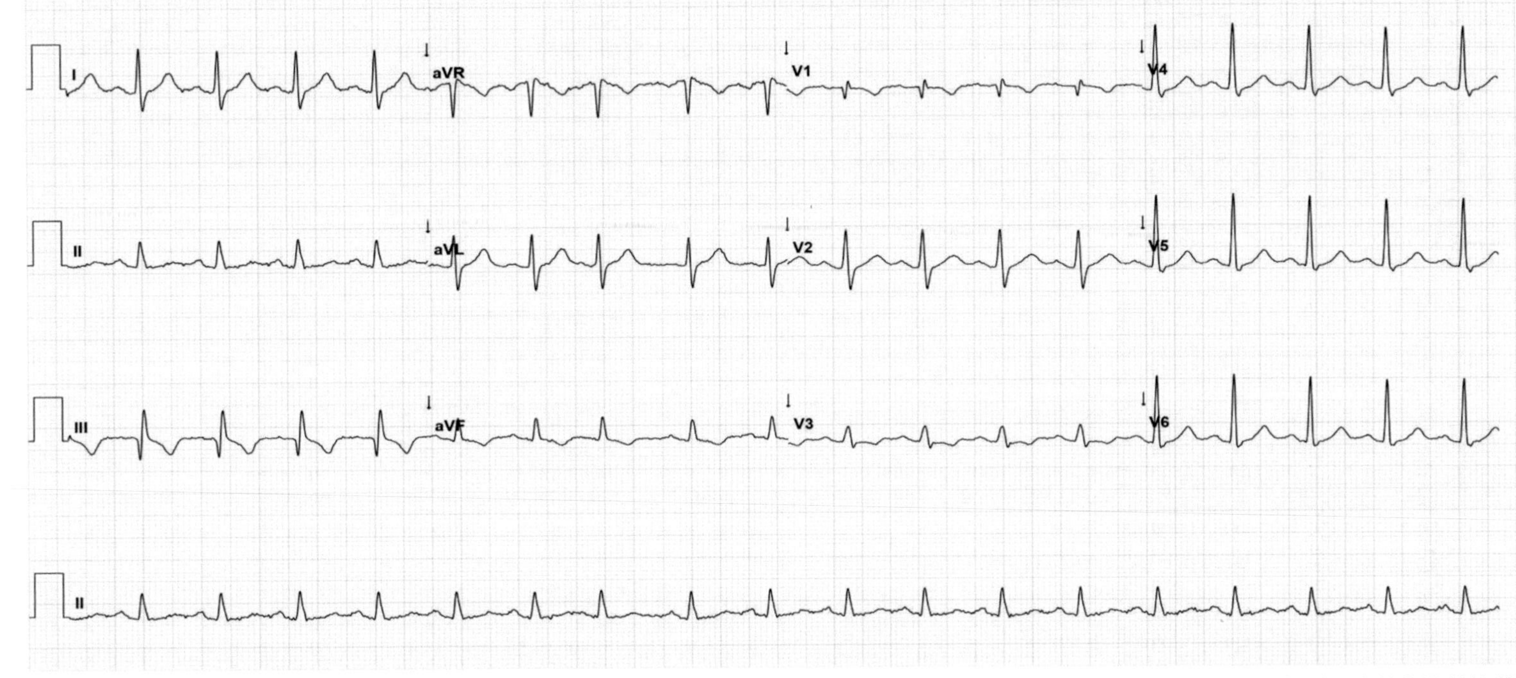

Additional Clinical History

Physical exam revealed mild tachypnea with a borderline blood pressure of 100/60

Additional information

CXR was unremarkable. High-sensitive troponin was elevated

ECG Interpretation

Rhythm: Sinus
Rate: 112 bpm
Intervals: PR 124 ms, QRS 90 ms, QTc 380 ms
Axis: Normal

Abnormalities on the ECG

Sinus tachycardia

An atrial premature beat is noted (7th beat on rhythm strip)

An s wave is present in lead I, with a q wave and inverted t wave in lead 3 A tall R wave is noted in V2 with an inverted t wave in lead 3.

ECG Test Answers

10, 13, 51

ECG Synthesis

The ECG shows signs of right ventricular strain including a tall R wave in V2, as well as the classic triad of 'S1Q3T3', which is quite specific for pulmonary embolism.

Sinus tachycardia is the most sensitive sign of pulmonary embolism, however it is not specific. The presence of sinus tachycardia suggests significant hypoxia and/or hemodynamic impairment. The atrial premature beat is non specific.

The combination of these signs with the clinical history should prompt an immediate workup for PE, including an echocardiogram.

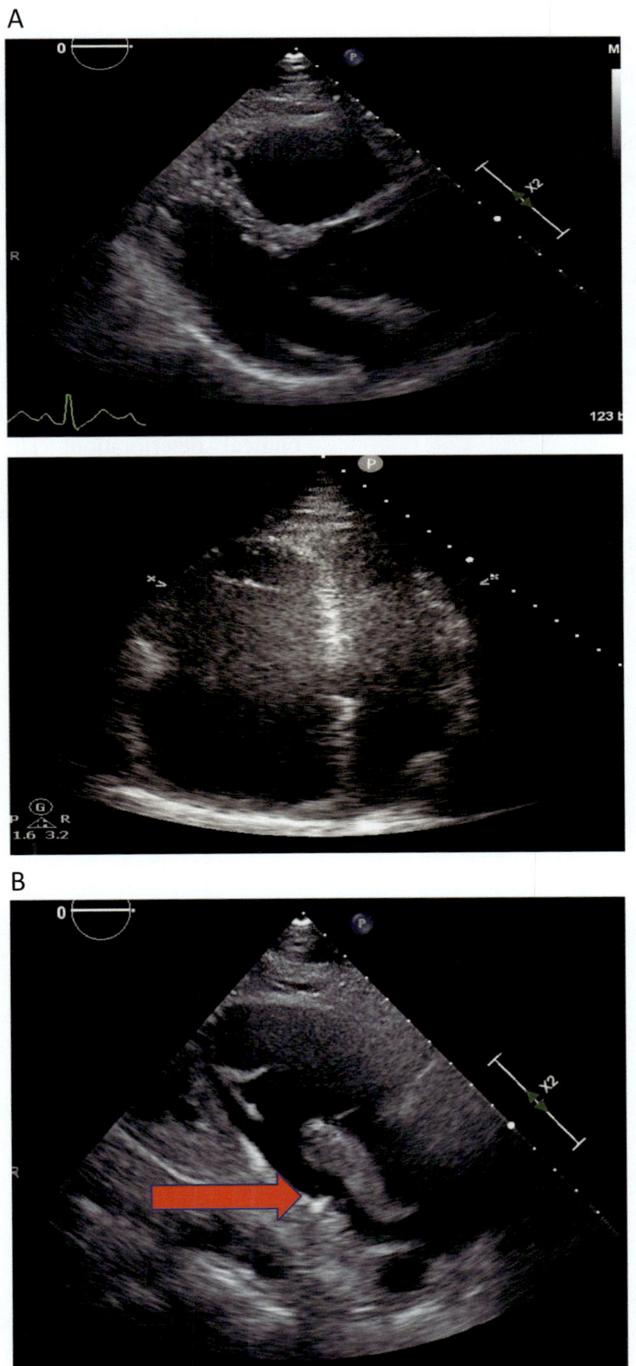

In Panel A, parasternal long-axis view demonstrates an enlarged right ventricle (RV (top image)). Apical 4 chamber view (bottom image) shows an enlarged right atrium and right ventricle. In panel B the parasternal long axis RV inlet view shows a large echodensity (arrow) which protrudes from the right atrium through the tricuspid valve and into the RV

Echo Interpretation

Parasternal long-axis view demonstrates an enlarged right ventricle (RV). Apical 4 chamber view shows enlarged right atrium and right ventricle which are significantly more dilated than the corresponding left sided chambers. The RV free wall was significantly hypokinetic with sparing of the apex. The lower image of parasternal long axis RV inlet view shows a large echodensity (arrow) which protrudes from the right atrium through the tricuspid valve and into the RV. Pulmonary pressures were not significantly elevated.

Echo Synthesis

The enlarged right sided chambers are consistent with right heart strain. The pattern of RV dysfunction is highly suggestive of pulmonary embolism. The echodensity in the right side is most likely an intracardiac thrombus in situ.

Cardiac Electrosonography Synthesis

The ECG findings in this patient were consistent with acute pulmonary embolism. This finding was confirmed by the emergency echo demonstrating enlargement of the RA and RV and hypokinesis of the RV free wall with apical sparing. Elevated troponin is also consistent with hemodynamic impairment. The finding of right sided thrombus has grave clinical implications as it may easily embolize to the lungs causing further clinical deterioration. The patient underwent emergent thrombolysis with gradual resolution of both his clinical symptoms and echocardiographic findings.

9 Case 8

A 64 y.o. female with a history of hypertension and hyperlipidemia presented to the ED with one week of weakness, dizziness and shortness of breath

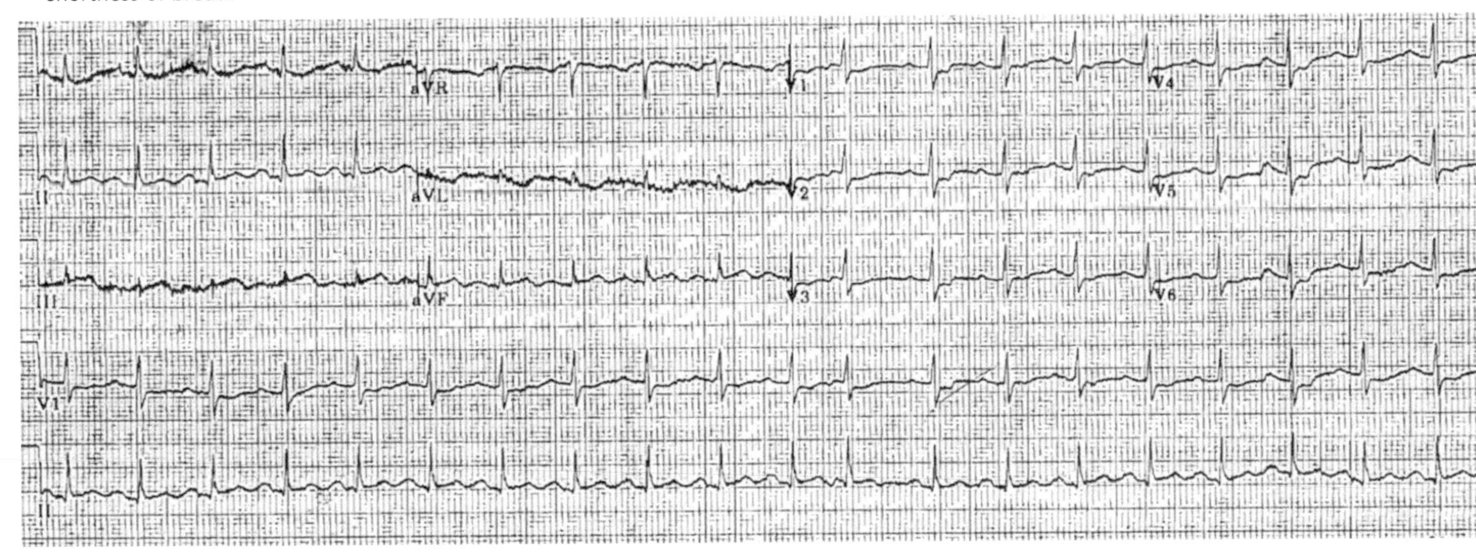

Additional Clinical History
Physical exam revealed tachycardia with a blood pressure of 100/60 mmHg. JVP was elevated, crepitations at the lung bases. A soft 3\6 systolic murmur was heard at the apex
Additional information
CPK 247   u/L, Trop HS 139 ng/L. Mild congestion on CXR.

ECG Interpretation

Rhythm: Sinus
Rate: 136 bpm
Intervals: PR = 200 ms, QRS = 80 ms, QTC = 391 ms
Axis: Normal

Abnormalities on the ECG

Sinus tachycardia

ST elevation in 2, 3, aVF

ST depression in V1 to V6.

On first impression, there seems to be a very tall R wave in V1, possibly suggesting RV hypertrophy. However this R wave is taller than one would expect to see even in cases of RVH. Moreover, if there is severe RVH, right axis deviation may be expected, absent in this ECG. Careful observation of the QRS complex in precordial leads reveals that they seem identical. This is a most unusual finding which suggests a technical issue.

ECG Test Answers
10, 71, 79.

ECG Synthesis

The patient has sinus tachycardia which is appropriate for her clinical condition.

ST elevation of > 1 mm in 2, 3 and aVF, combined with ST depression in precordial leads, is diagnostic of inferior wall myocardial infarction. The QRS, and therefore ST and T segments in precordial leads is difficult to understand; however, there is ST depression and T wave inversion which are also typical of inferior wall MI. It is not known whether the ST depressions represent distant ischemia of the anterior wall, involvement of the posterior wall in the infarction, or merely 'reciprocal' changes representing the same inferior wall injury seen in leads II, III and aVF as 'seen' by the chest leads.

In cases of inferior wall myocardial infarction, in addition to performing an echocardiogram, ECG electrodes should be placed to record posterior and right sided chest leads.

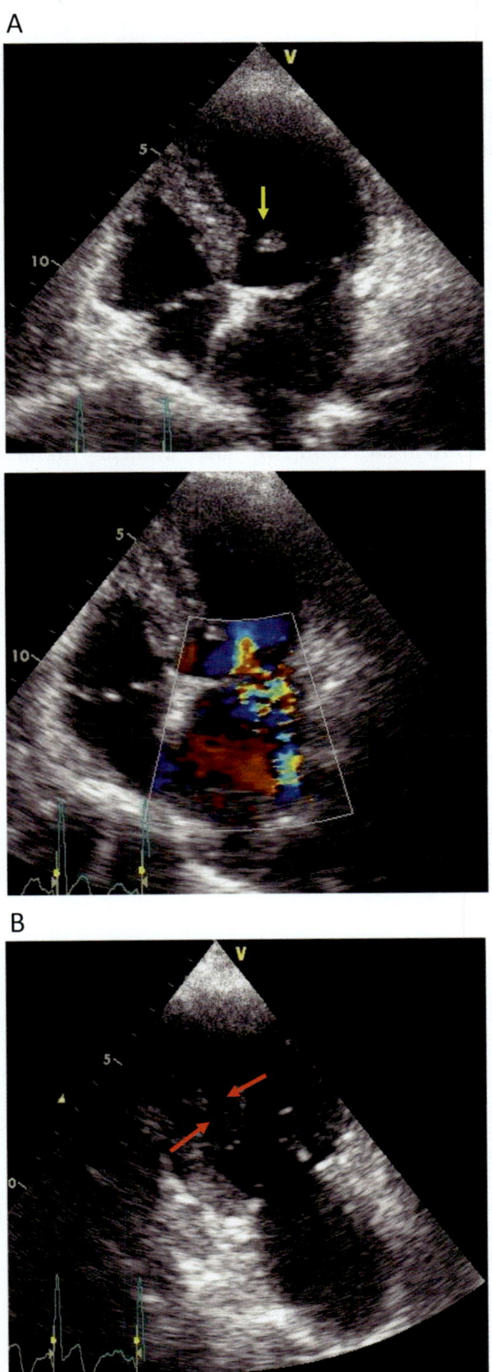

Apical 4 chamber views in panel A show an echodensity in the LV cavity (yellow arrow, top image) which appears attached to the subvalvular apparatus of the mitral valve. Color Doppler imaging shows a large, posteriorly directed jet of mitral regurgitation. Apical 2 chamber view in panel B revealed a clearly transected papillary (red arrows)

Echo Interpretation

Apical 4 chamber view shows an echodensity in the LV cavity (yellow arrow) which appears attached to the subvalvular apparatus of the mitral valve. Color Doppler imaging shows a large, posteriorly directed jet of mitral regurgitation. Apical 2 chamber view revealed a clearly transected papillary muscle with the red arrows pointing to the edges of papillary muscle with an echogenic space separating them.

Echo Synthesis

Possible explanations for hemodynamic impairment and congestive heart failure in the setting of myocardial infarction include significant left and /or right ventricular dysfunction or a mechanical complication including free wall rupture, ventricular septal defect or papillary muscle rupture causing severe mitral regurgitation. The emergent echo revealed evidence of severe mitral regurgitation due to a torn papillary muscle.

Cardiac Electrosonography Synthesis

The clinical history and ECG findings in this patient were suggestive of a subacute inferoposterior infarct. The physical exam was consistent with congestive heart failure with a systolic murmur. The emergency echo demonstrated a torn posteromedial papillary muscle with acute severe mitral regurgitation explaining the clinical findings. An intraaortic balloon pump was placed and the patient was referred to cardiothoracic surgery for emergent repair of the mitral valve.

10 Case 9

57 year old male with no significant past medical history presented with 4 weeks of worsening exertional dyspnea

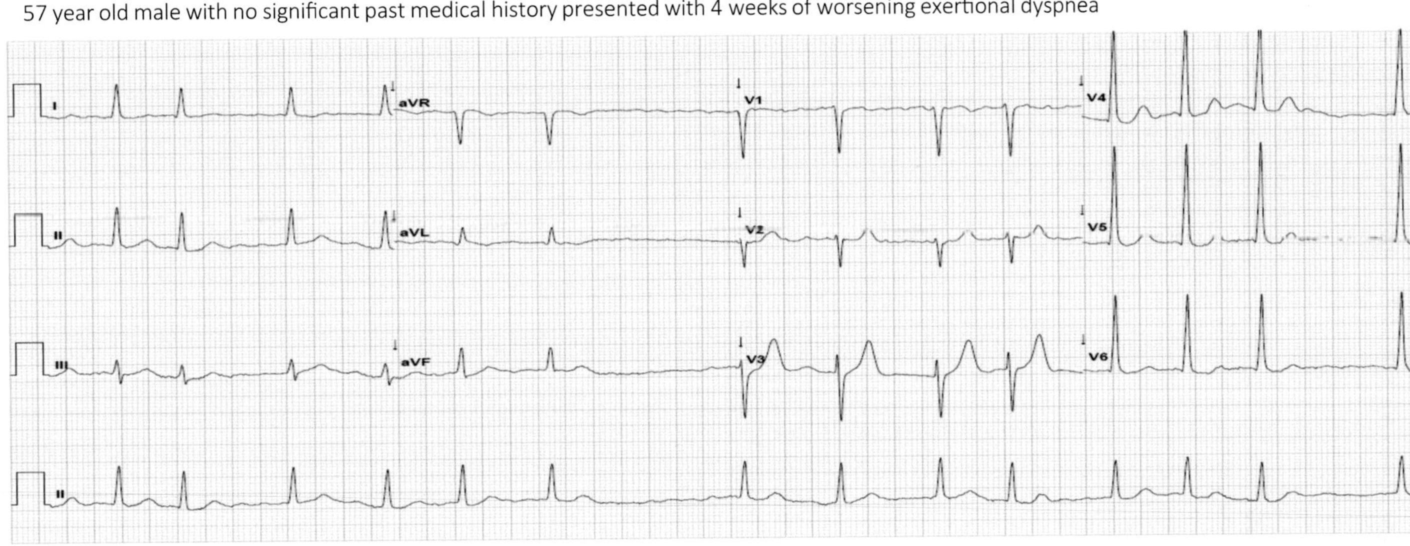

Additional clinical history

The patient reported being told of a heart mumur on routine physical examination performed 8 years earlier. On physical examination decreased breath sounds noted at the lung bases. A 3\6 holosystolic murmur was heard at the apex.

Additional information

CXR revealed signs of congestion and an enlarged cardiac silhouette

ECG Interpretation

Rhythm: Atrial fibrillation
Rate: 83 bpm
Intervals: PR not measurable due to AF, QRS 97 ms, QTC 381 ms
Axis: Normal

Abnormalities on the ECG

Atrial fibrillation

Minor ST segment changes.

ECG Test Answers

18, 77.

ECG Synthesis

The patient is in atrial fibrillation. Having presented with symptoms of dyspnea, the possibility of symptomatic AF presenting as dyspnea is obvious. However, the ventricular rate is not rapid. It would not be common for well rate-controlled atrial fibrillation to cause severe and worsening dyspnea in the absence of underlying structural heart disease. This is clearly supported by the finding of a murmur on physical examination. Ventricular systolic function, atrial size, valvular anatomy and function and diastolic filling pressure should be promptly assessed by echocardiography.

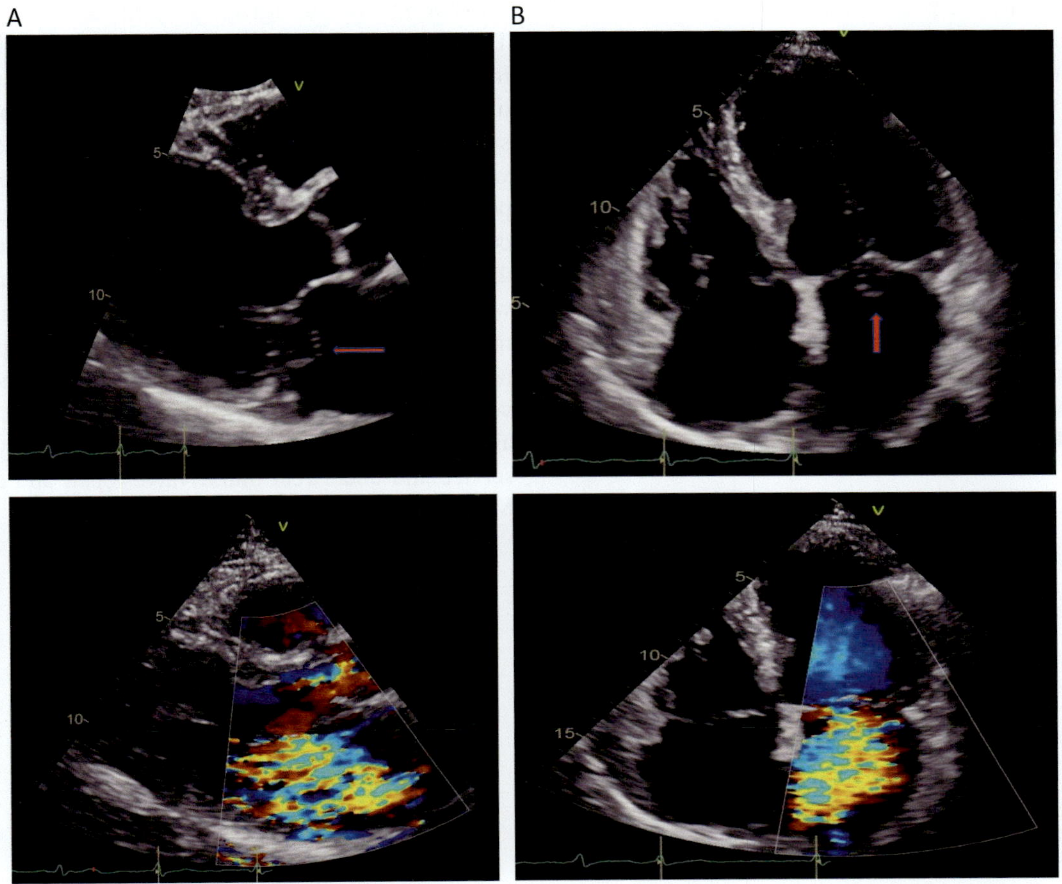

Parasternal long-axis view (A) and apical 4 chamber view (B) showing flail posterior mitral valve leaflet (top images, arrows) and severe mitral regurgitation. On color Doppler (bottom images)

Echo Interpretation

Parasternal long-axis view (A) and apical 4 chamber view (B) showing flail posterior mitral valve leaflet (top images) and severe mitral regurgitation on color Doppler images (bottom images). The left ventricle and left atrium appear dilated.

Echo Synthesis

The findings are consistent with degenerative mitral regurgitation due to severe mitral valve prolapse. The dilated cardiac chambers including the left ventricle and left atrium suggest relatively chronic MR.

Cardiac Electrosonography Synthesis

The presence of atrial fibrillation on the ECG in this patient with dyspnea pointed a cardiac cause of his complaints. As noted, the presence of symptoms despite a relatively well-controlled ventricular rate suggested additional cardiac pathology. In this case, the echo findings demonstrated that the atrial fibrillation noted on the ECG was secondary to an enlarged left atrium with elevated pressure as a results of significant mitral valve disease. Use of emergent echo diagnosed the underlying anatomic disorder and prevented needless clinical focus on the arrhythmia alone The patient was admitted to cardiac surgery service and underwent mitral valve repair and a MAZE procedure with clinical improvement.

11 Case 10

An 83 year old female with a history of hypertension and obesity presented to the emergency department with 4 weeks of worsening exertional shortness of breath and bilateral leg swelling.

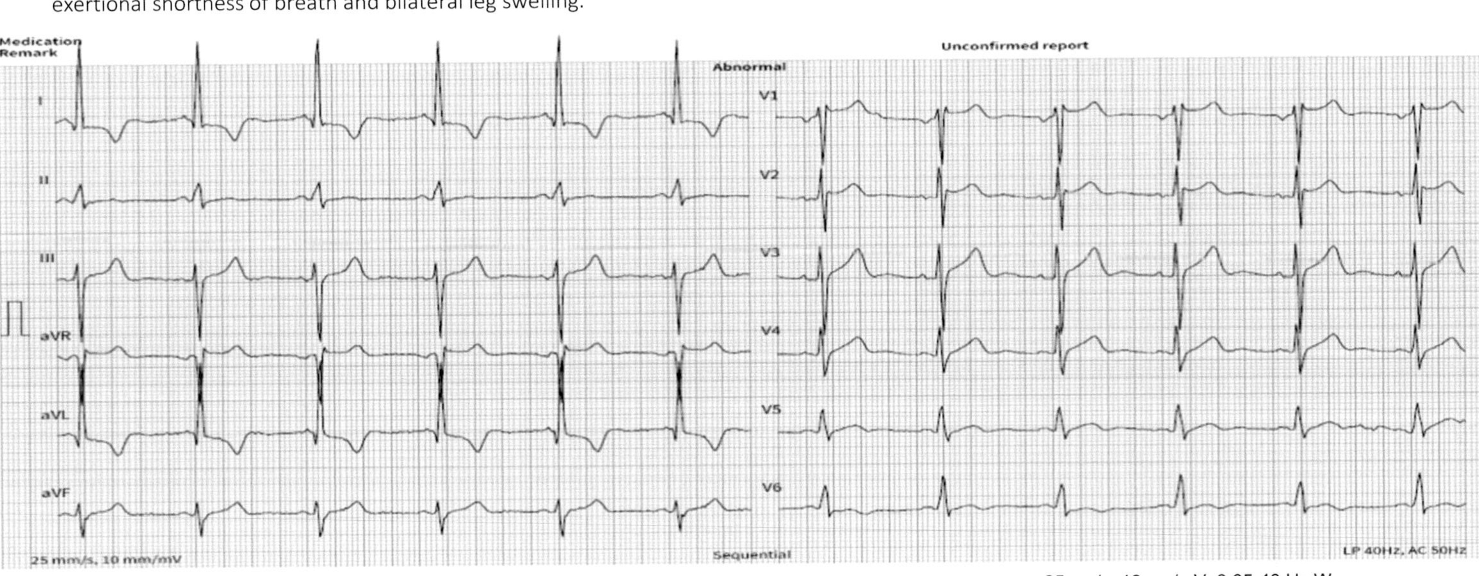

25mm/s 10mm/mV 0.05-40 Hz W

Additional Clinical History

On physical examination BP was 167\79, jugular venous pressure was elevated. Bilateral crepitations were noted at the lung bases. A fourth heart sound was noted

Additional information

CXR revealed a "boot-shaped heart" and pulmonary congestion. Troponin was normal while pro-BNP was elevated at 1,251 mg/dl

ECG Interpretation

Rhythm: Sinus
Rate: 70 bpm
Intervals: PR = 134 ms, QRS = 100 ms, QTC 432 ms
Axis: Normal

Abnormalities on the ECG

Incomplete right bundle branch block

Left atrial enlargement

Left ventricular hypertrophy with strain pattern

ECG Test Answers

6, 7, 40, 81.

ECG Synthesis

This ECG shows sinus rhythm at 90 bpm, with evidence of left atrial enlargement (with a prominent negative deflection of the p wave in lead V1). In addition high voltage is noted in lead 1 and AVL with mild ST depression and inverted t waves in the same leads. This finding is most consistent with left ventricular hypertrophy, a finding supported by the probable left atrial enlargement. The cause of the hypertrophy in this elderly female is most probably hypertension although valve disease such as aortic stenosis cannot be excluded. Ischemia is less likely but cannot be ruled out with certainty and an emergent echo was performed to assess left ventricular structure and function.

A

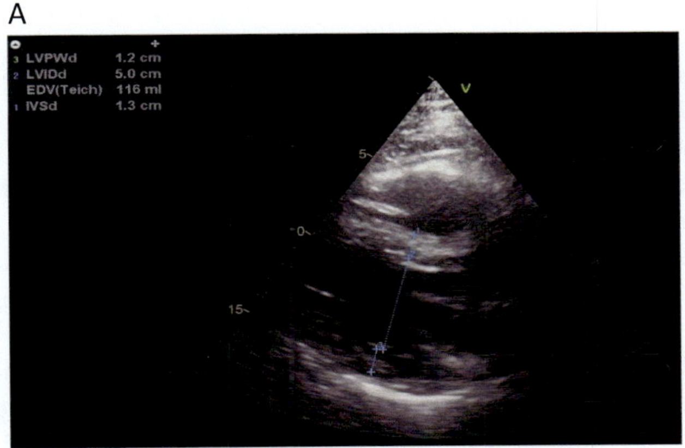

B

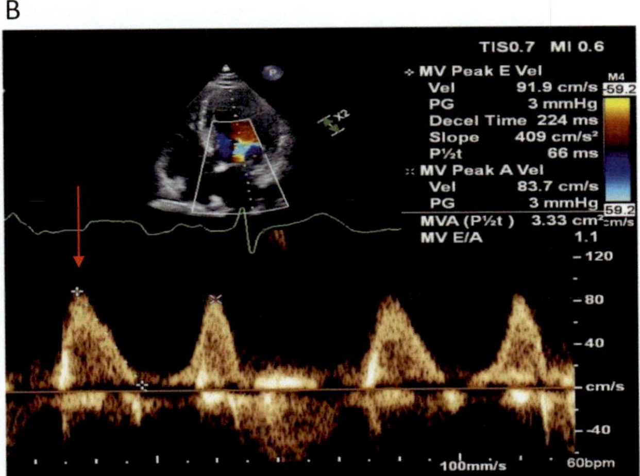

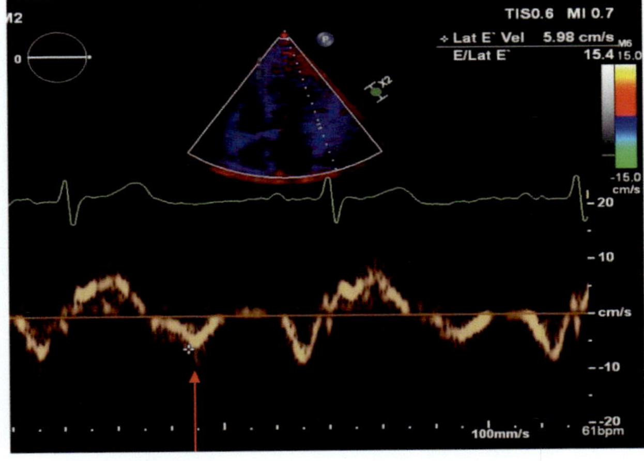

The echo showed evidence of concentric left ventricular hypertrophy (panel A) with normal ejection fraction. Mitral inflow and tissue Doppler in the apical 4 chamber view (panel B) showed a relatively tall e wave (top image, arrow) and a very small e' (bottom image arrow) leading to an elevated E: e'

Echo Interpretation

The echo showed evidence of concentric left ventricular hypertrophy (LVH) (panel A) with normal ejection fraction. In addition, there was a mildly dilated left atrium and mild pulmonary hypertension. Mitral inflow and tissue Doppler in the apical 4 chamber view (panel B) showed a relatively tall e wave (top image, arrow) which can either be a normal finding or a finding consistent with elevated filling pressures ("pseudonormal"). The tissue Doppler showed a very small e' (bottom image arrow) leading to an elevated E: e' consistent with elevated filling pressures.

Echo Synthesis

The findings of concentric LVH with normal systolic function, a dilated left atrium with pulmonary hypertension and a low tissue Doppler e' with an elevated E:e' are all consistent with elevated LV filling pressures due to impaired diastolic filling.

Cardiac Electrosonography Synthesis

The ECG showed signs of LVH in this elderly, hypertensive female, a diagnosis which was confirmed by echocardiography which did show any evidence of ischemic heart disease. The clinical picture including the elevated BNP and the echo findings noted support a diagnosis of heart failure with preserved ejection fraction as the cause of the patients symptoms. She was treated with diuretics and anti hypertensive therapy with clinical improvement.

12 Case 11

A 67 year old woman presented to the ED with several weeks of dyspnea on exertion.

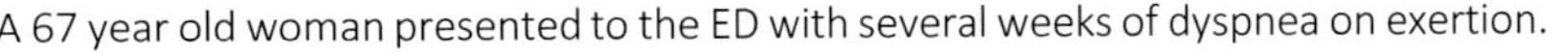

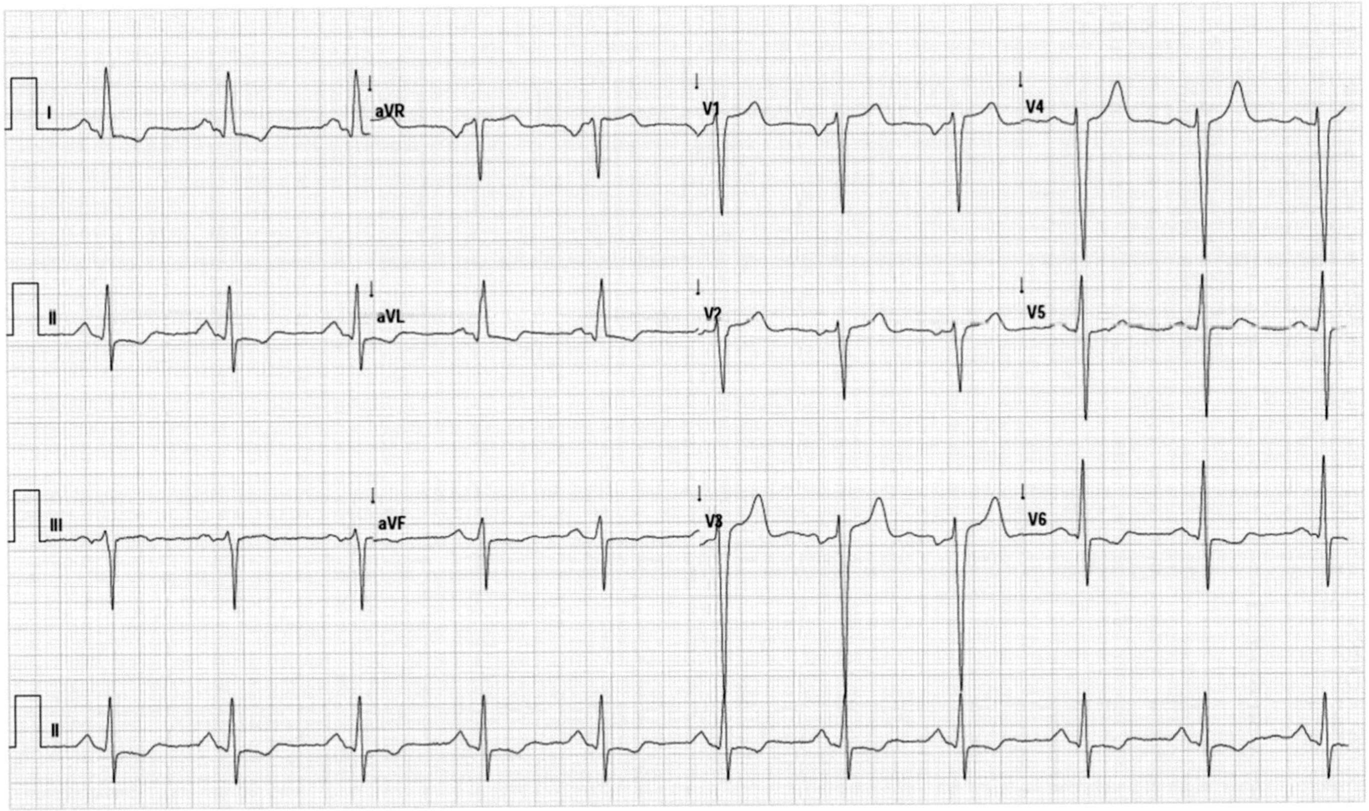

Additional Clinical History:

The patient reports hypertension controlled with ARB and hyperlipidemia treated with statin. Physical examination notable for no significant jugular venous distention, 2/6 systolic ejection murmur across the precordium and holosystolic murmur at the apex. Lungs are clear.

ECG Interpretation

Rhythm: Sinus rhythm
Rate: 64 bpm
Intervals: PR 199 ms, QRS 117 ms, QTc 442 ms
Axis: − 23°

Abnormalities on the ECG

- Left atrial enlargement
- Left ventricular hypertrophy with QRS widening and repolarization abnormalities.

ECG Test Answers

6, 7, 40, 64, 81.

ECG Synthesis

The ECG in this patient is notable for marked left ventricular hypertrophy (LVH) accompanied by QRS widening and repolarization abnormalities. Prolongation of the QRS duration may result from increased thickness of the left ventricle wall and intramural fibrosis, which distorts and prolongs transmural impulse propagation. The presence of ST-T abnormalities may be associated with greater impairment of systolic and diastolic mechanics in HCM, and more interstitial fibrosis. The left atrial (LA) enlargement is presumably secondary to elevated LA pressures due to the LVH.

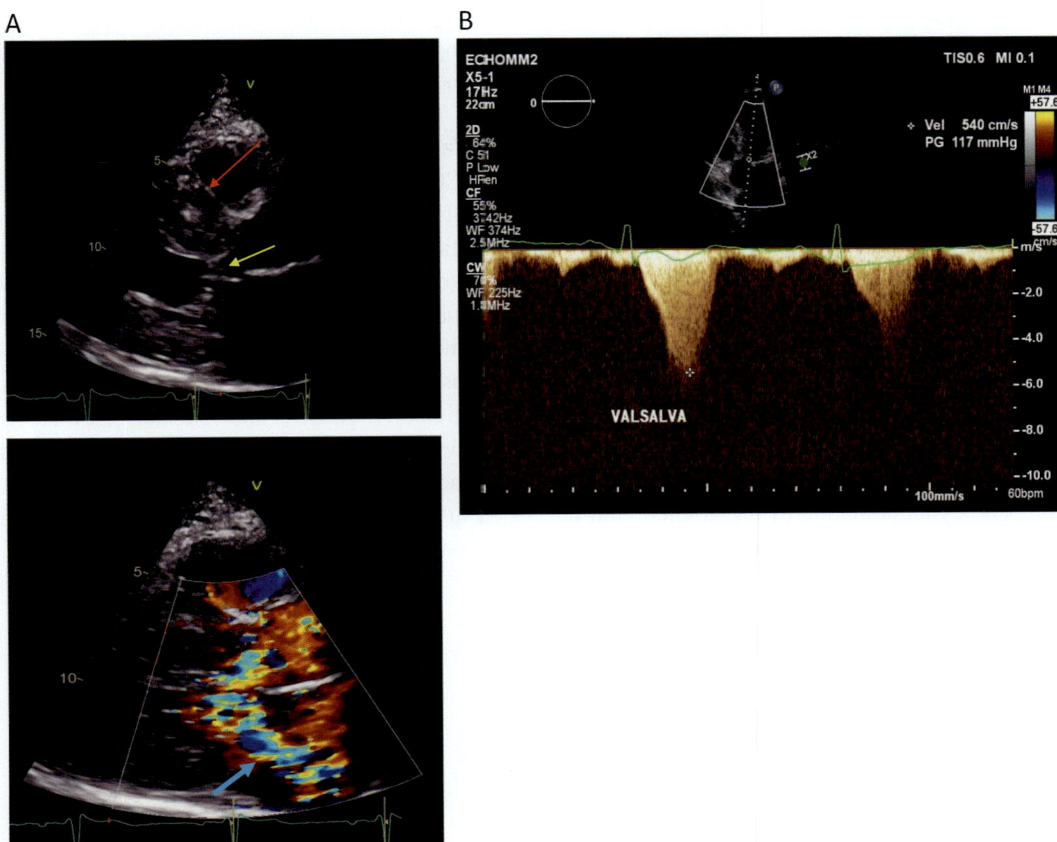

Panel A showing with the top image showing parasternal long axis view with septal hypertrophy (red arrow) and left ventricular outflow tract obstruction (LVOTO) (yellow arrow). The bottom image shows the resulting large color flow jet (blue arrow) indicative of mitral regurgitation. Panel B shows the large LVOTO with Valsalva on continuous Doppler imaging from the apical 5 chamber view

Echo Interpretation

The echocardiogram is notable for asymmetric hypertrophy, and systolic anterior motion of the mitral leaflets, leading to LV outflow tract obstruction and severe mitral regurgitation. Left atrial enlargement is noted as well. In apical 5 chamber view, a large pressure gradient with performance of a Valsalva maneuver is seen.

Echo Synthesis

This echocardiogram suggests that the symptoms reported by the patient are related to hypertrophic obstructive cardiomyopathy, with significant dynamic obstruction leading both to an outflow tract gradient and mitral regurgitation. The dynamic nature of the gradient and the mitral regurgitation suggest that she may benefit from pharmacologic therapy to reduce the hyperdynamic systolic function and the accompanying systolic anterior motion of the mitral leaflets.

Cardiac Electrosonography Synthesis

The ECG and echo findings suggest that this patient is at increased risk of the long term complications of hypertrophic obstructive cardiomyopathy. The presence of QRS prolongation and marked repolarization abnormalitiessuggest that there is significant underlying myocardial fibrosis and increased risk of heart failure. LA dilatation on both ECG and echo suggest that she has chronically elevated left sided pressures and is at increased risk of atrial fibrillation and stroke. Careful risk stratification and follow up are warranted for this patient.

13   Case 12

31 year old woman with dyspnea on exertion and palpitations.

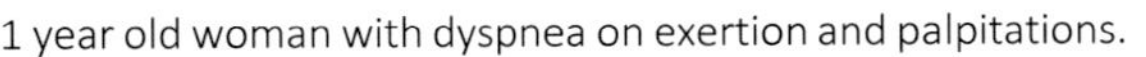

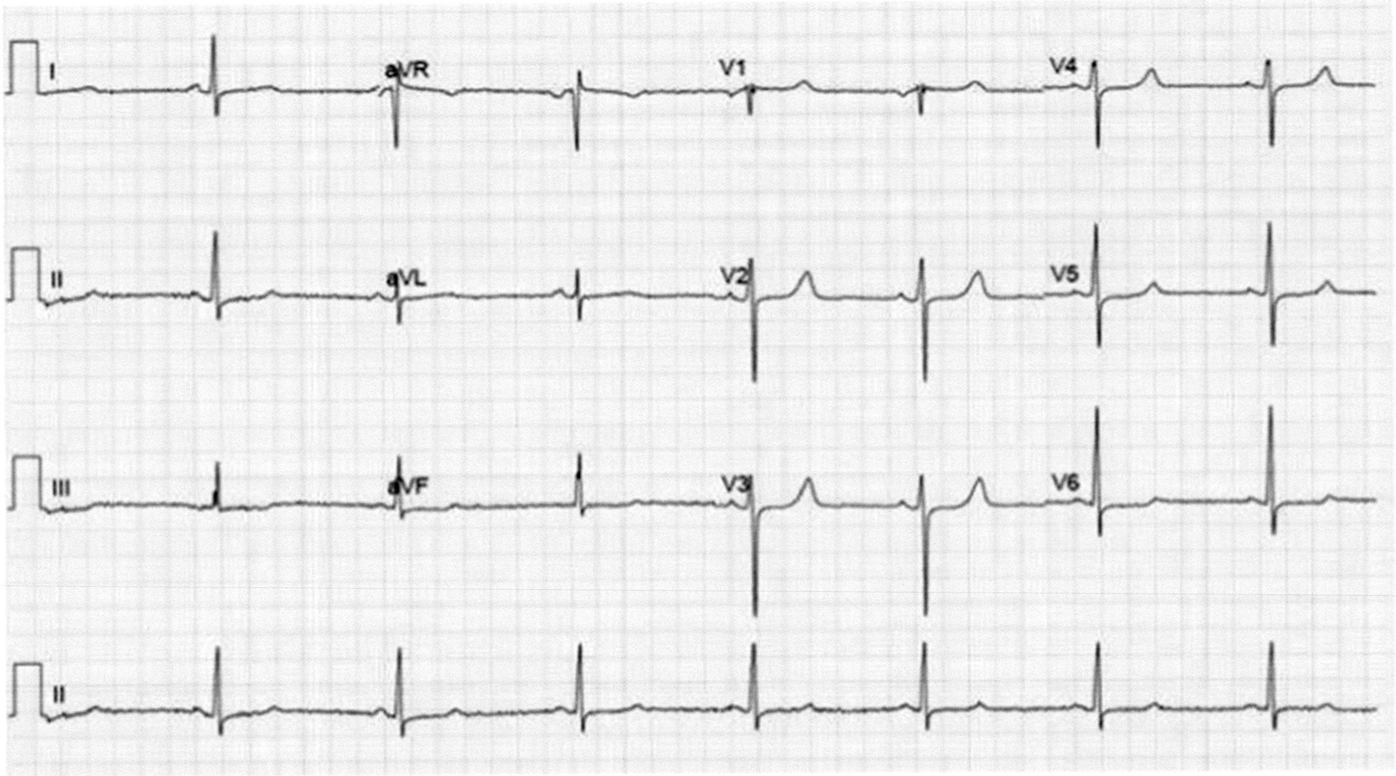

Additional Clinical History

The patient reports reduced exercise tolerance since high school. Physical examination was notable for s4 and soft systolic ejection murmur that did not change with Valsalva maneuver. Chest x-ray with cardiomegaly but no congestion.

ECG Interpretation

Rhythm: Sinus bradycardia
Rate: 45 bpm
Intervals: PR 166 ms, QRS 100 ms, QTc 500 ms
Axis: 59

Abnormalities on the ECG

- Sinus bradycardia
- Left ventricular hypertrophy
- Prolonged QT
- Inferolateral T-wave changes

ECG Test Answers

9, 40, 54, 81, 82.

ECG Synthesis

The ECG in this patient is notable for left ventricular hypertrophy, and in addition, QT prolongation and QRS fragmentation. QT prolongation can be present in 1 out of 8 patients with HCM and may be reflective of the degree of cardiac hypertrophy and left ventricular outflow tract obstruction. QRS fragmentation is present when there are various RSR' patterns, including notching in the R or S wave or presence of > 1 additional R in 2 or more beats of a non-aVR lead. In some cases hypertrophic cardiomyopathy is characterized by myocyte hypertrophy, interstitial fibrosis and myofibrillar disarray. These findings suggest that there may be significant underlying interstitial fibrosis and pro-arrhythmic substrate.

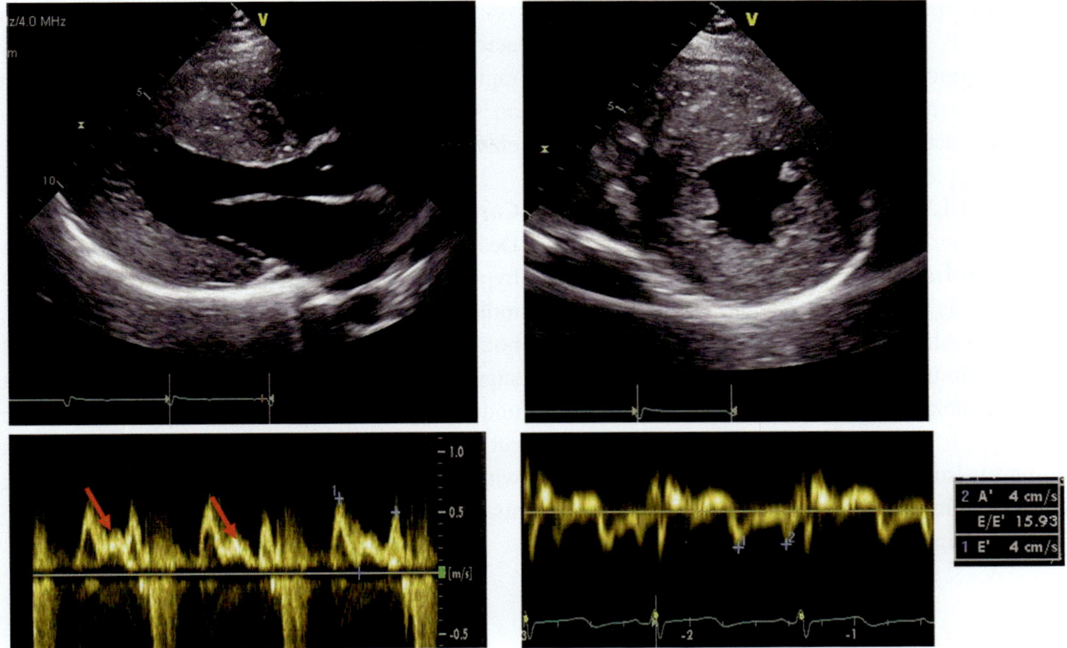

Parasternal views (top images) demonstrate marked concentric left ventricular hypertrophy. The transmitral and tissue Doppler (bottom images) are suggestive of significant LV diastolic dysfunction

Echo Interpretation

Parasternal views (top images) demonstrate marked concentric left ventricular hypertrophy. There was no systolic anterior motion or LV outflow tract obstruction. The transmitral and tissue Doppler (bottom images) are suggestive of significant LV diastolic dysfunction.

Echo Synthesis

This echo is suggestive of significant concentric left ventricular hypertrophy. Despite a relatively low transmitral E wave velocity, the markedly reduced lateral tissue Doppler e' wave of leads to an E/e' of 15.9 which suggests elevated LV filling pressure. In addition, there is a mitral "L" wave seen in in the transmitral Doppler (arrow). This is thought to represent continued pulmonary vein mid diastolic flow through the left atrium across the mitral valve into the LV after early rapid filling. Presence of an L wave together with an elevated E/e' is indicative of significantly elevated LV filling pressures.

Cardiac Electrosonography synthesis

Despite the young age of this patient with hypertrophic cardiomyopathy, there are several indicators of advanced disease and increased risk, both on ECG and echocardiogram. The ECG suggests that the patient may have significant underlying fibrosis and arrhythmic risk and the echo also is suggestive of an advanced process with increased LV filling pressure. Further risk stratification and careful follow up are advised.

14   Case 13

A 75 y/o female was brought by ambulance to the emergency department after surviving an acute respiratory arrest requiring intubation in the field.

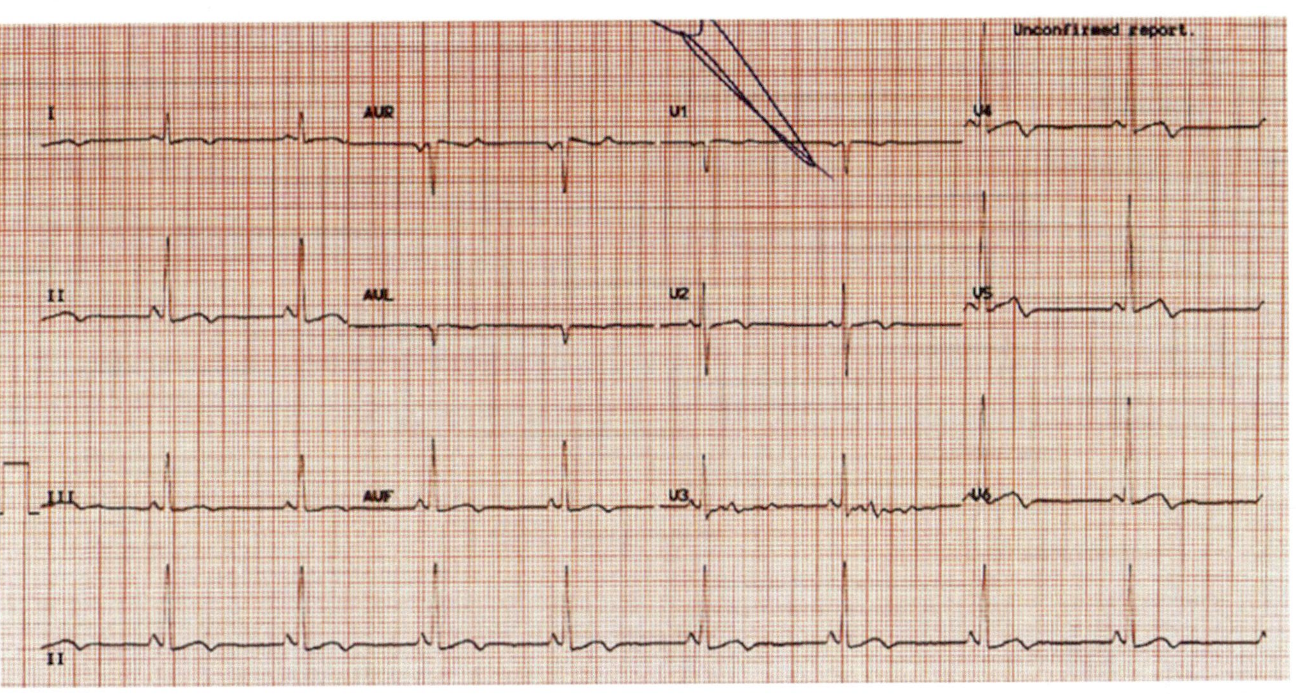

Additional Clinical Information

On arrival to the ED, her BP was 212/98 mmHg and HR was 56 bpm. Physical exam was remarkable for bibasilar rales and 3/6 systolic murmur best heard in the left sternal border.

ECG Interpretation

Rhythm: Sinus bradycardia
Rate: 56 bpm
Intervals: PR 110 ms, QRS 60 ms, QTc 440 ms
Axis: Normal

Abnormalities on the ECG

- Sinus bradycardia
- Short PR interval
- ST and T wave abnormalities.

ECG Test Answers
9, 81.

ECG Synthesis
The ECG in this patient is notable for profound ST segment and T wave abnormalities in multiple leads. The diffuse nature of the changes suggests primary myocardial pathology; however, diffuse ischemia could not be excluded. Given the patients unstable clinical condition and the uncertain etiology of the ECG changes, emergent echocardiography was performed.

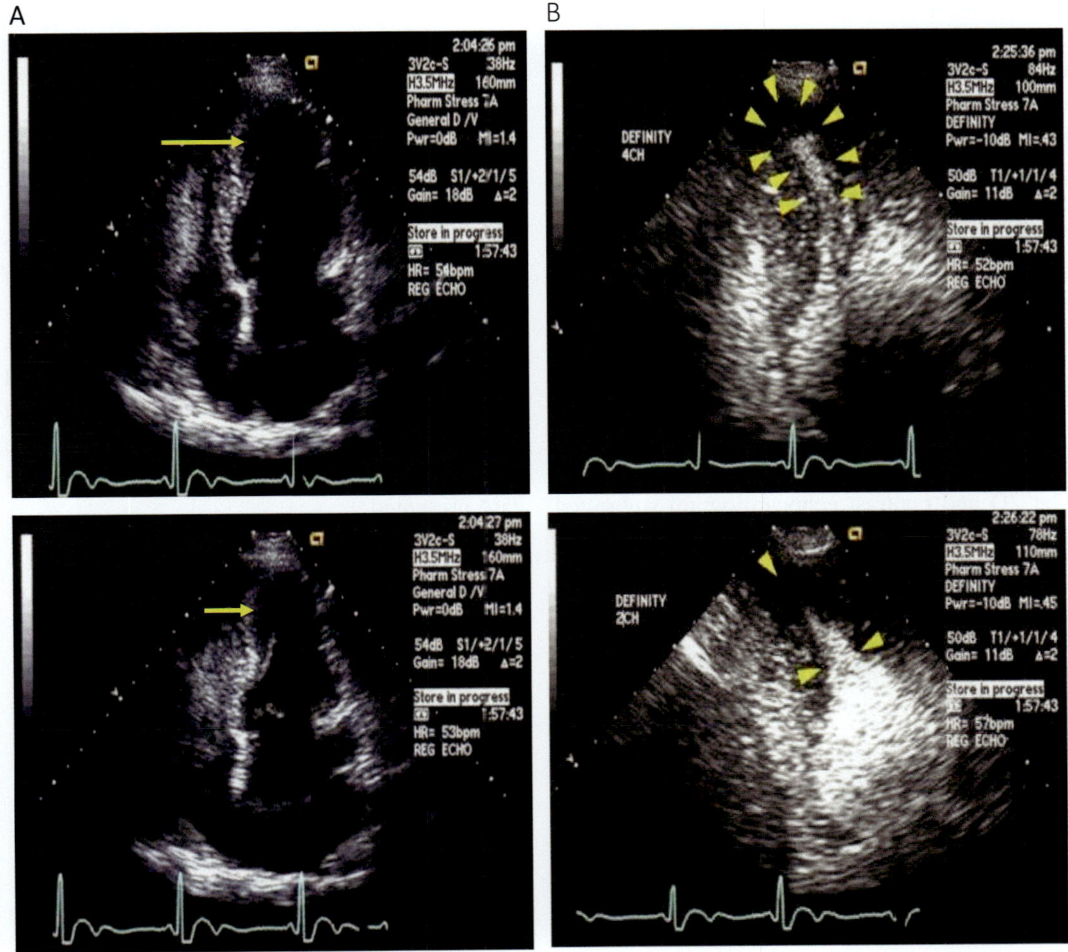

The initial 2D echocardiogram (panel A) was notable for suspected significant apical ballooning (arrows) seen on apical 4 chamber views at end diastole (upper image) and end-systole (lower image). As the patient was intubated, study quality was impaired and an intravenous imaging enhancing agent ("contrast") was injected (panel B)

Echo Interpretation

The initial 2D echocardiogram (panel A) was notable for suspected significant apical ballooning (arrows) as seen in patients with stress induced cardiomyopathy (Takotsubu). As the patient was intubated, study quality was impaired and an intravenous imaging enhancing agent ("contrast") was injected (panel B). The contrast study delineates the endocardium enabling a more definitive diagnosis of apical hypertrophy. The contrast "remains" in the area of the apex during systole and diastole (arrows) confirming the presence of apical obstructive hypertrophy.

Echo Synthesis

The 2D and contrast echocardiogram suggested that the underlying pathology in this patient with apical hypertrophic cardiomyopathy. The "spade-like" pattern of the contrast in the images in panel B is a common finding in this disease.

Cardiac Electrosonography Synthesis

The patient had a respiratory arrest of uncertain etiology. The ECG findings pointed to a diffuse myocardial disease process and the diagnosis of apical hypertrophic cardiomyopathy was established using contrast enhancing agents. Frequently echo imaging is challenging in intubated patients or those with chronic lung disease and the use of contrast can contribute significantly to an accurate diagnosis and management as in the case presented.

References

Adler Y, et al. ESC guidelines for the diagnosis and management of pericardial diseases. Eur Heart J. 2015;36:2921–64.

Dabbouseh et al. Role of echocardiography in managing acute pulmonary embolism. Heart. 2019;105.

Galie, et al. ESC/ERS guidelines for the diagnosis and treatment of pulmonary hypertension. Eur Heart J. 2016;37:67–119.

Garcia-Pavia P, et al. Diagnosis and treatment of cardiac amyloidosis. Eur Heart J. 2021;42:1554–68.

Gong FF, et al. Mechanical complications of acute myocardial infarction: a review. JAMA Cardiol. 2021;6:341–9.

Grigoni F, et al. Long term implications of atrial fibrillation in patients with degenerative mitral regurgitation. J Am Coll Cardiol. 2019;73:264–74.

Ha JW, Oh JK, Redfield MM, Ujino K, Seward JB, Tajik AJ. Triphasic mitral inflow velocity with middiastolic filling: clinical implications and associated echocardiographic findings. J Am Soc Echocardiogr. 2004;17:428–31.

Huang G, et al. Apical variant hypertrophic cardiomyopathy "multimodality imaging evaluation." Int J Cardiovasc Imaging. 2020;36(3):553–61.

Huizar JF, et al. Arrhythmia induced cardiomyopathy: JACC State of the art review. J Am Coll Cardiol. 2019;73:2328–44.

Masiero, et al. When to achieve complete revascularization in infarct-related cardiogenic shock. J Clin Med. 2022;11:3116.

Ommen SR, Mital S, Burke MA, Day SM, Deswal A, Elliott P, Evanovich LL, Hung J, Joglar JA, Kantor P, Kimmelstiel C, Kittleson M, Link MS, Maron MS, Martinez MW, Miyake CY, Schaff HV, Semsarian C, Sorajja P. 2020 AHA/ACC guideline for the diagnosis and treatment of patients with hypertrophic cardiomyopathy: a report of the American College of Cardiology/American Heart Association Joint Committee on Clinical Practice Guidelines. Circulation. 2020;142. https://doi.org/10.1161/CIR.000000000000 0937

Ommen SR, et al. 2020 AHA/ACC guideline for the diagnosis and treatment of patients with hypertrophic cardiomyopathy: a report of the American College of Cardiology/American Heart Association Joint Committee on Clinical Practice Guidelines. Circulation. 2020;142. https://doi.org/10.1161/CIR.000000000000 0937

Rahamim E, et al. Illustrative cases of multimodality imaging in the diagnosis and management of pulmonary embolism. In: Herzog E, editor., et al., Pulmonary Embolism. Springer; 2022. p. 269–87.

Redfield MM, Borlaug BA. Heart failure with preserved ejection fraction: a review. JAMA. 2023;14:827–38.

Clinical Cases of Electrosonography in Patients with Syncope and Palpitations

Yair Elitzur, Mohammad Mowaswes,
Batel Nisan, Habib Hilo, Eldad Rachamim,
Eyal Herzog, and David Leibowitz

Abstract

In this chapter we present 14 cases of patients who presented to health care systems with syncope, pre-syncope or palpitations. The cases illustrate the systematic electrosonography diagnostic approach. We include cases of patients with a variety of cardiac arrhythmias with and without concomitant cardiac structural abnormalities.

Keywords

Electrocardiogram · ECG · Electrosonography · Palpitations · Syncope · Pre-syncope · Arrythmia

Y. Elitzur (✉) · M. Mowaswes · B. Nisan · H. Hilo ·
E. Rachamim · E. Herzog · D. Leibowitz
The Heart Institute, Department of Cardiology,
Hadassah Medical Center, Hebrew University
of Jerusalem, Jerusalem, Israel
e-mail: elitzur1@hadassah.org.il

1 Case 1

: A 67 year old male with a remote history of myocardial infarction and known congestive heart failure
a 2 day history of fatigue, diaphoresis and dizziness

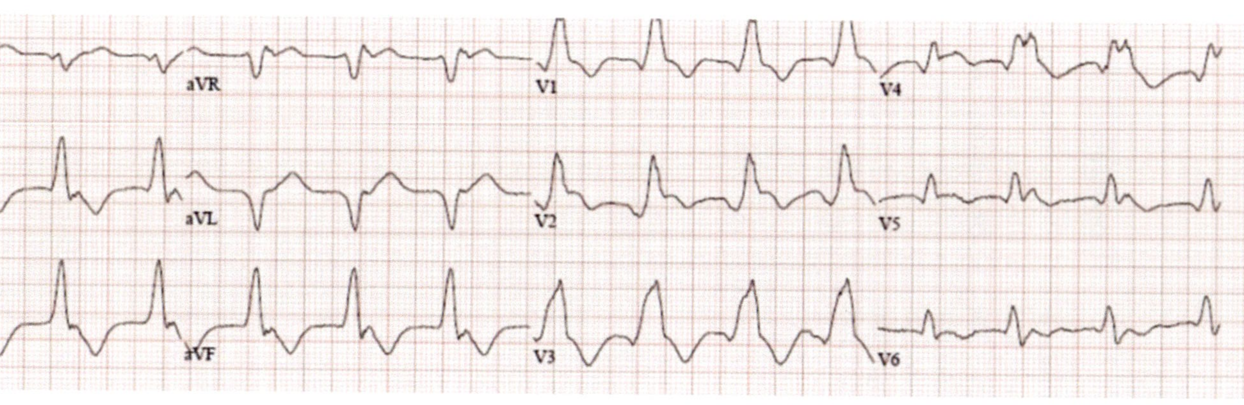

istory
have exertional dyspnea and orthopnea. He has an implanted ICD. Eight months previously he has had an ablation procedure for a previous case of

ECG Interpretation

Rhythm: idioventricular rhythm

Rate: 100 BPM.

Intervals: QRS 320 ms.

Axis: right axis deviation.

Abnormalities on the ECG

- Very wide QRS complexes
- Positive precordial lead concordance
- Time to first deflection in II > 40 ms
- Right axis deviation

ECG Test Answers
25, 38.

ECG Synthesis
This patient has a 'slow VT', or idioventricular rhythm. The term 'slow VT' is not appropriate, since the rate is less than 100 BPM, therefore this is formally not a tachycardia. However, in the context of previous myocardial infarction, clinical heart failure and recent onset of extreme fatigue, this rhythm should be viewed as VT.

Echo Images

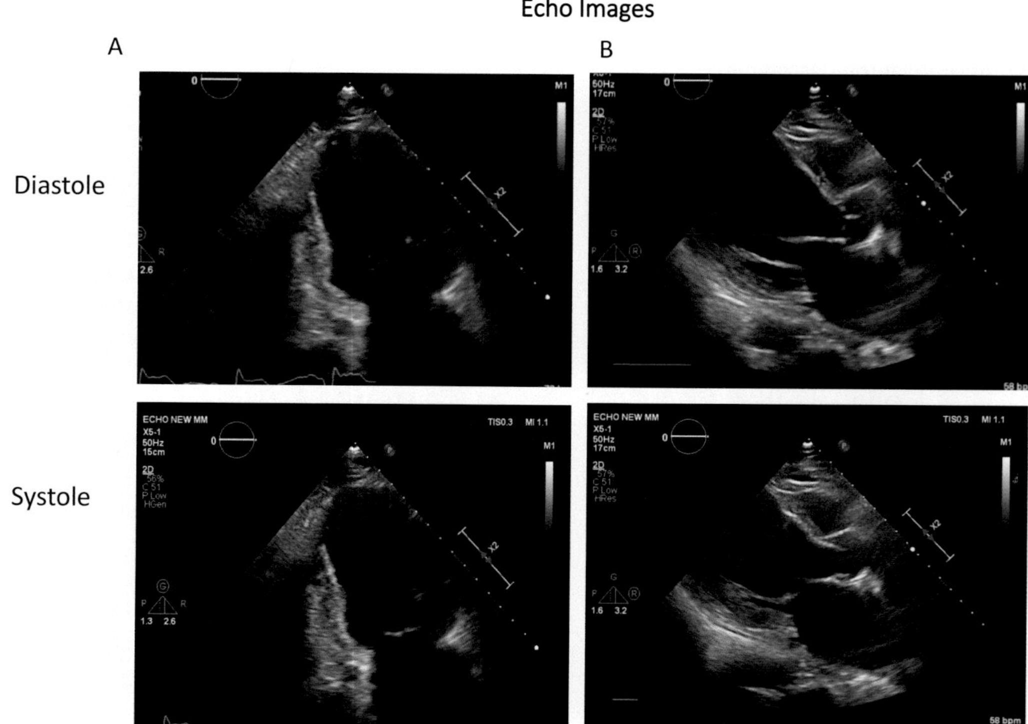

Echo interpretation

Apical two chamber (A) and parasternal long axis(B) views in systole (closed mitral valve) and diastole (open mitral valve) demonstrate a severely dilated left ventricle, with anterior, anteroseptal, apical and inferior akinesia.

Echo Synthesis

The echocardiogram shows significantly reduced left ventricular function. From the images the cause of the cardiomyopathy is not clear, and may be ischemic or non ischemic. The inferior wall in the two chamber view is somewhat echobright, possibly suggestive of ischemic scarring from old myocardial infarction.

Cardiac Electrosonography Synthesis

In this heart failure patient presenting with recent onset of fatigue and dizziness, the reason for deterioration is sustained monomorphic ventricular tachycardia resulting from extensive myocardial scarring.

The unusually wide and abnormal QRS complexes the fact that no P waves are visible should prompt checking of electrolye concentrations, although not all features of hyperkalemia are present (e.g. T waves are shallow).

This patient has had a previous VT ablation and ICD implantation. An important consideration is the reason for his ICD not delivering a therapeutic shock to terminate this episode. The reason for this is probably the slow rate of the arrhythmia. Implanted defibrillators are programmed to detect actionable VT above a certain rate. If this rate is programmed too low, inappropriate shock may result from erroneous interpretation of a modestly rapid rhythm, such as sinus tachycardia or SVT, as dangerous ventricular arrhythmia. Various discriminatory algorithms exist to help differentiate truly dangerous VT or VF from other rapid, benign rhythms. In this case, due to the slow rate, arrhythmia was not detected by the ICD. The patient underwent a second procedure of mapping and ablation of VT and had his ICD appropriately programmed using different discriminators.

2 Case 2

A 74 year old female with a history of hypertension and diabetes presented with dizziness and near-syncope.

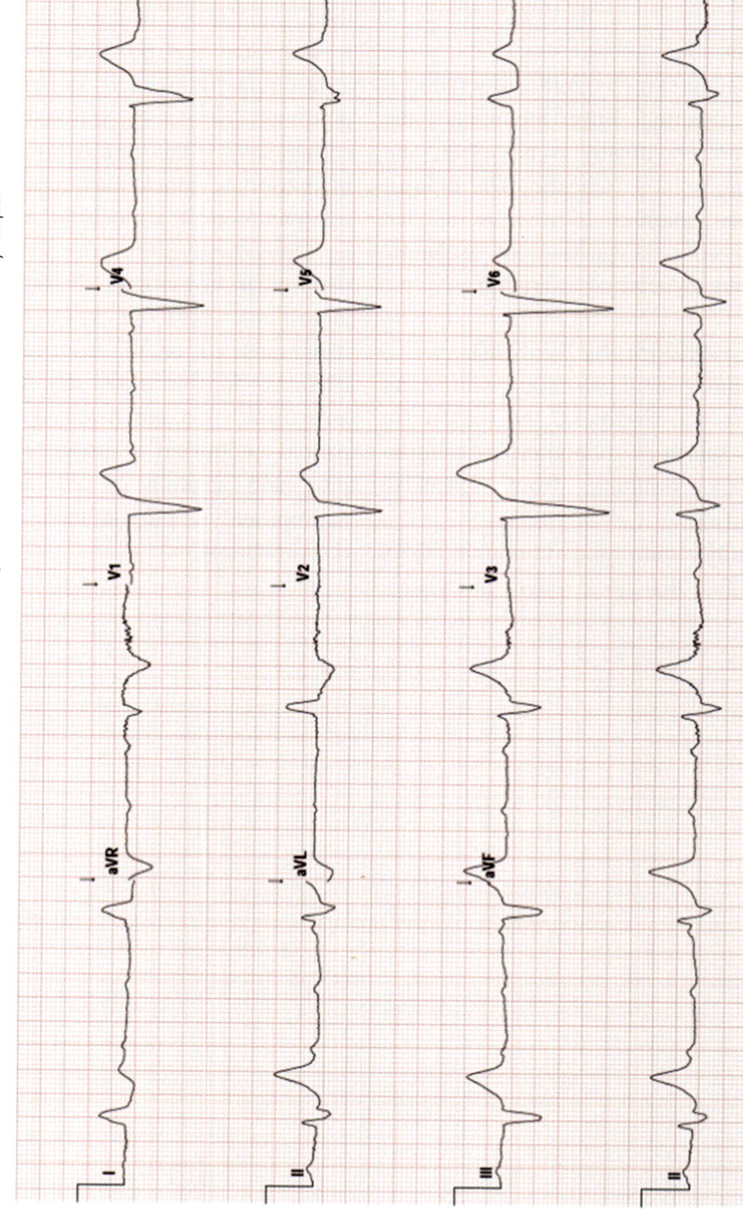

Additional Clinical History

The patient had breast cancer treated with radiation many years prior to presentation

Physical exam was significant for BP of 80/40 with cold, clammy extremities. Cardiac exam revealed a 3\6 systolic murmur at the base. Electrolytes were normal.

ECG Interpretation

Rhythm: Sinus rhythm with complete atrioventricular block.

Rate: 34 BPM.

Intervals: PR interval not measurable due to AV dissociation. QRS 190 ms. QTc = 480 ms.

Axis: Normal.

Abnormalities on the ECG

Complete (3rd degree) atrioventricular block (CAVB). Wide-QRS slow escape rhythm. This may be a purely ventricular escape rhythm, or a more proximal escape with pre-existing left bundle branch block.

ECG Test Answers

7, 32, 61.

ECG Synthesis

The ECG shows complete atrioventricular block with with no correlation between the p waves and the QRS complexes. The intervals between the p waves are constant and the intervals between the QRS complexes are constant, with no connection between the two. The QRS complexes are relatively wide and probably represent a ventricular escape rhythm.

This finding could easily explain the patient's symptoms. The differential diagnosis of complete AV block is wide; common causes include degenerative disease of the conduction system, medical therapy such as beta blockers, electrolyte abnormalities or acute ischemia. Emergent echocardiography is indicated to assess for the presence of concomitant heart disease and to guide the choice of appropriate pacemaker.

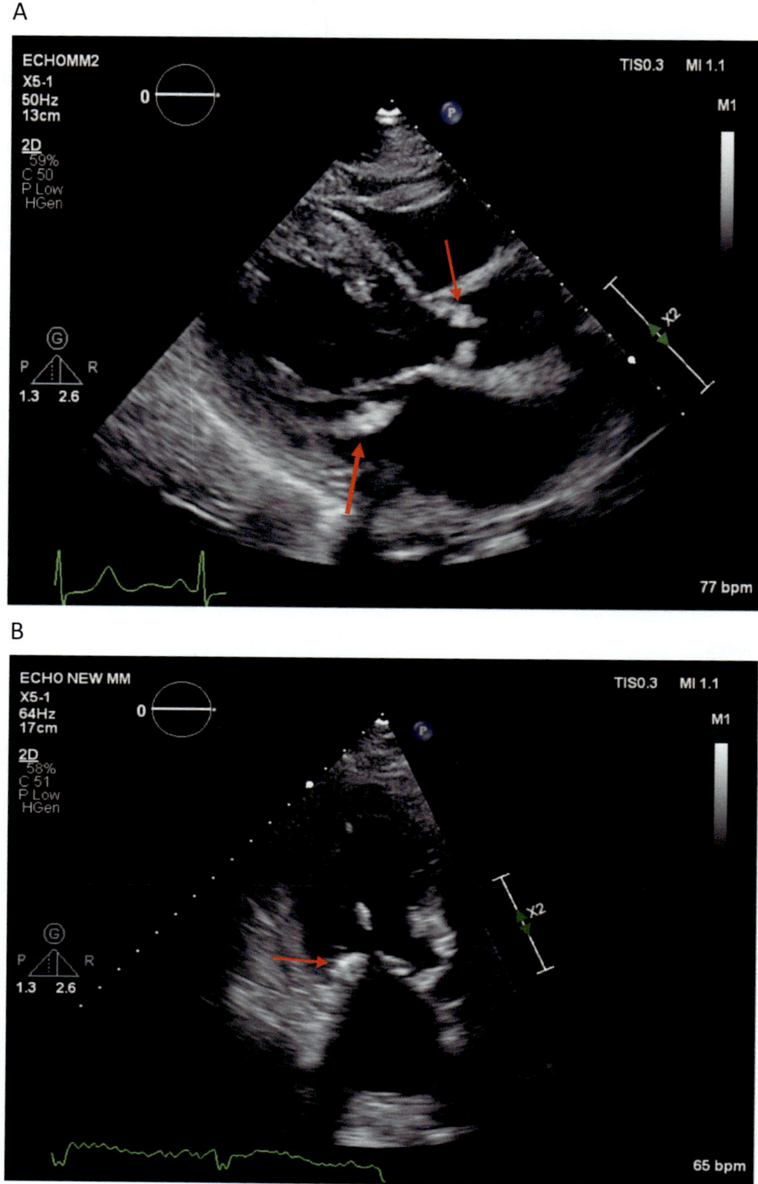

Parasternal long axis (A) and apical three chamber views (B) show a dilated left atrium with significant calcification of the mitral valve annulus and the aortic valve (arrows).

Echo interpretation

Parasternal long axis (A) and apical three chamber views (B) show a dilated left atrium with significant calcification of the mitral valve annulus and the aortic valve (arrows). Ventricular function was normal with no evidence of regional wall motion abnormalities.

Echo Synthesis

The mitral valve annulus and aortic valve are significantly calcified. This may be idiopathic and related to the patient's age or may be a result of chest wall irradiation she received in the past. This advanced calcification may also be seen in patients with chronic renal disease. The normal ventricular function rules out acute ischemia as a cause of the heart block.

Cardiac Electrosonography Synthesis

This patient has complete (3rd degree) AV block leading to near-syncope and dizziness. The echo revealed calcification of the mitral and aortic valves, probably due to previous radiation therapy which may have affected the conduction system as well. She has a slow, wide-complex ventricular escape rhythm, is hemodynamically unstable and needs emergent temporary pacemaker implantation followed by a permanent pacemaker.

3 Case 3

A 79 y/o female with a medical history positive for hypertension and paroxysmal atrial fibrillation (PAF) presented with recurrent episodes of palpitation in the last month.

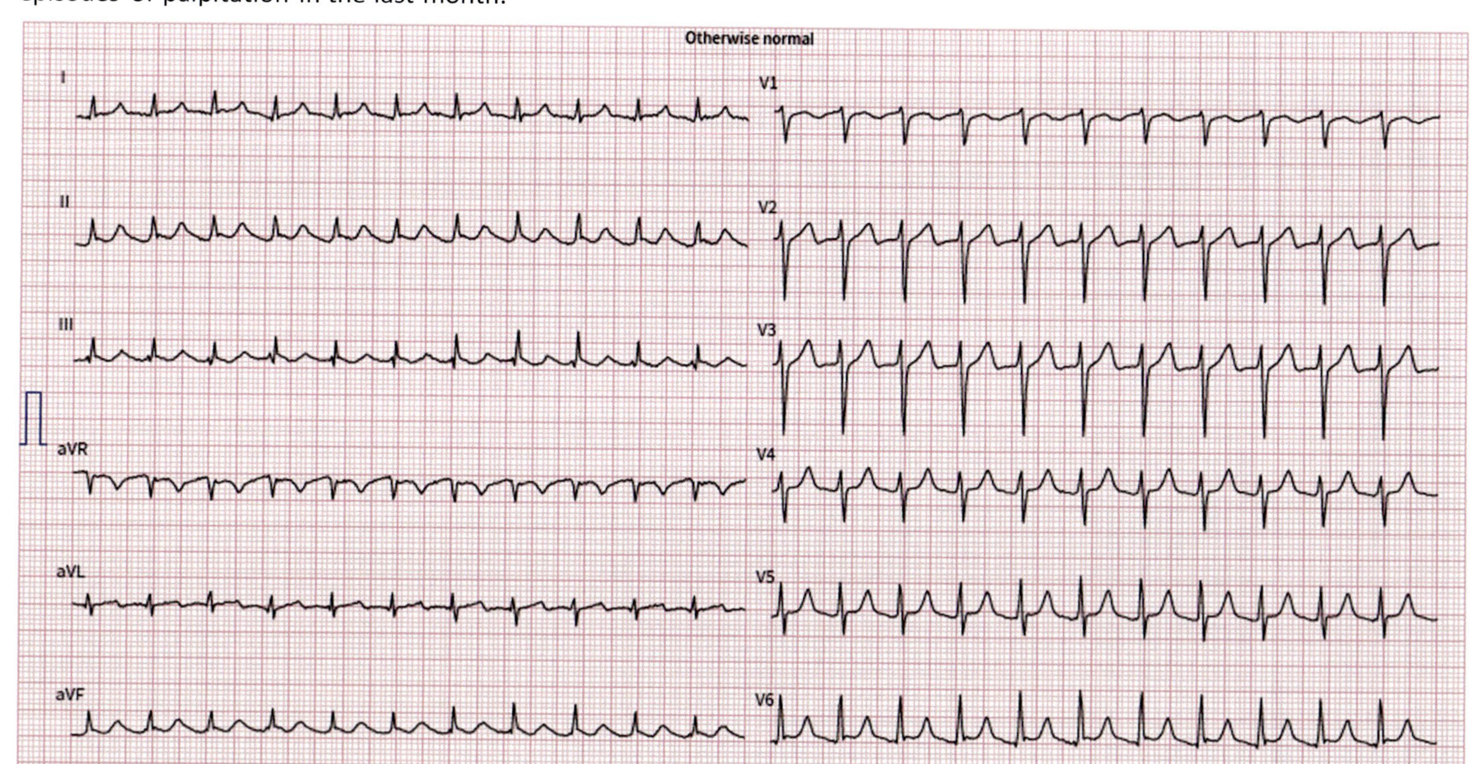

Additional clinical information

Physical exam revealed tachycardia of about 150 bpm, regular pulse. Medical treatment included propafenone, apixaban and a beta blocker.

ECG Interpretation

Rhythm: Atrial flutter

RATE: 150 BPM.

Intervals: PR not measured due to atrial flutter, QRS 79 ms, QTc 340 ms

Axis: Normal.

Abnormalities on ECG

Atrial flutter (Flutter waves seen in II, III, avF).

ECG Test Answers

17

ECG Synthesis

This patient presented with supraventricular tachycardia (SVT) while taking IC antiarrhythmic drugs. The differential diagnosis of SVT includes sinus tachycardia, atrial tachyarrhythmias including atrial fibrillation and atrial flutter, and reentrant rhythms such as AV nodal reentry or arrhythmia related to prexcitation syndromes. The heart rate of 150 is suggestive of atrial flutter. This is due to the fact that the atrial rate is generally around 300 bpm and the AV node is not capable of conducting at such a high rate. Therefore the atrial rhythm is conducted in a 2:1 ratio and the effective heart rate is 150 bpm. Negative p waves in a "sawtooth" pattern are noted in leads 2,3,F, a finding diagnostic of atrial flutter.

Typical atrial flutter is a reentrant rhythm of the right atrium. In this case the atrial rhythm is probably related to use of propafenone, a 1C agent, which regularizes the atrial fibrillation the patient has had in the past. Echocardiography is important to assess for structural abnormalities contributing to the patients arrhythmias and to evaluate left ventricular systolic function.

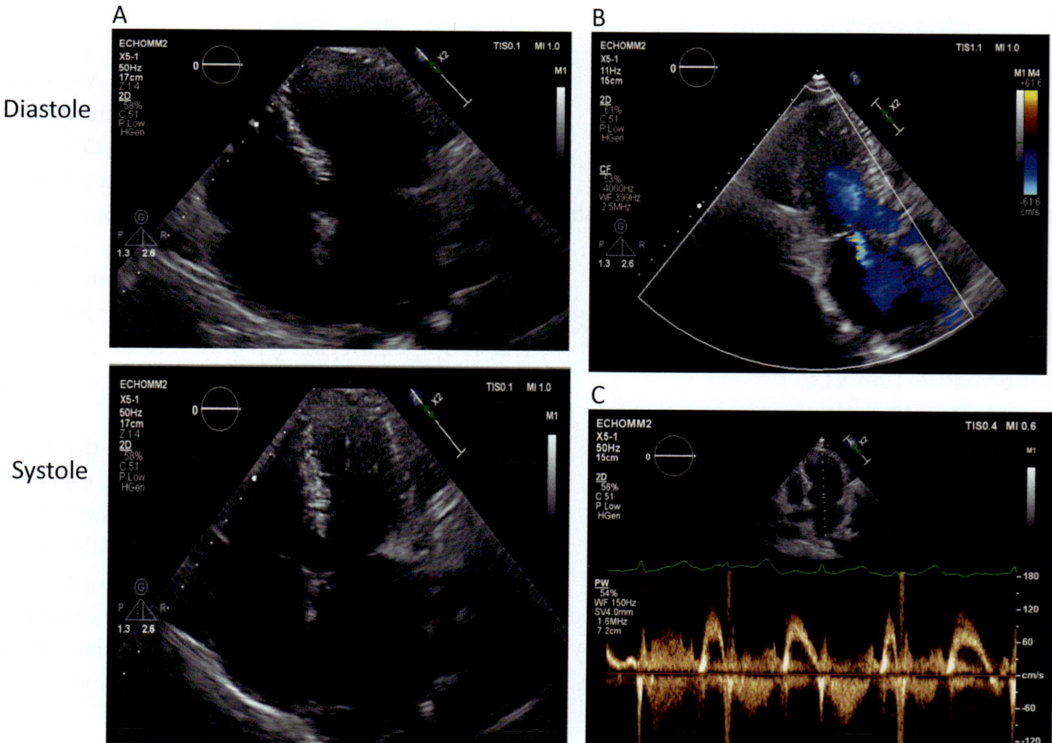

Apical four chamber view demonstrates enlarged left and right atria (panel A). Comparison of LV chamber size in diastole (top, mitral valve open) and systole shows normal LV systolic function. Apical three chamber view with color Doppler demonstrates moderate mitral regurgitation (panel B). Pulsed wave interrogation of the mitral valve (panel C) shows variable E waves with the absence of A waves due to atrial arrhythmia.

Echo Interpretation

Apical four chamber view demonstrates enlarged left and right atria (panel A). Comparison of LV chamber size in diastole (top, mitral valve open) and systole shows normal LV systolic function. Apical three chamber view with color Doppler demonstrates moderate mitral regurgitation (panel B). Pulsed wave interrogation of the mitral valve (panel C) shows variable E waves with the absence of A waves due to atrial arrhythmia during the echo examination.

Echo Synthesis

Echocardiography in this patient shows normal LV function, significant mitral regurgitation, left atrial enlargement and atrial fibrillation.

Cardiac Electrosonography Synthesis

Echocardiography and ECG point to a combination of mitral regurgitation, left atrial enlargement and atrial fibrillation/flutter. This combination is not uncommon as atrial arrhythmias may be idiopathic but are frequently associated with diseases of the left ventricle or left sided valves causing elevated left atrial pressure.

The patient was treated with propafenone, a class IC antiarrhythmic medication, and a beta blocker to relieve her atrial fibrillation symptoms. However, propafenone turned the fibrillation to an atypical flutter with more regular atrial activity, paradoxically causing worsening of the patient's symptoms.

4 Case 4

An 84 year old female with a history of atrial fibrillation presented to the ED with complaints of fatigue.

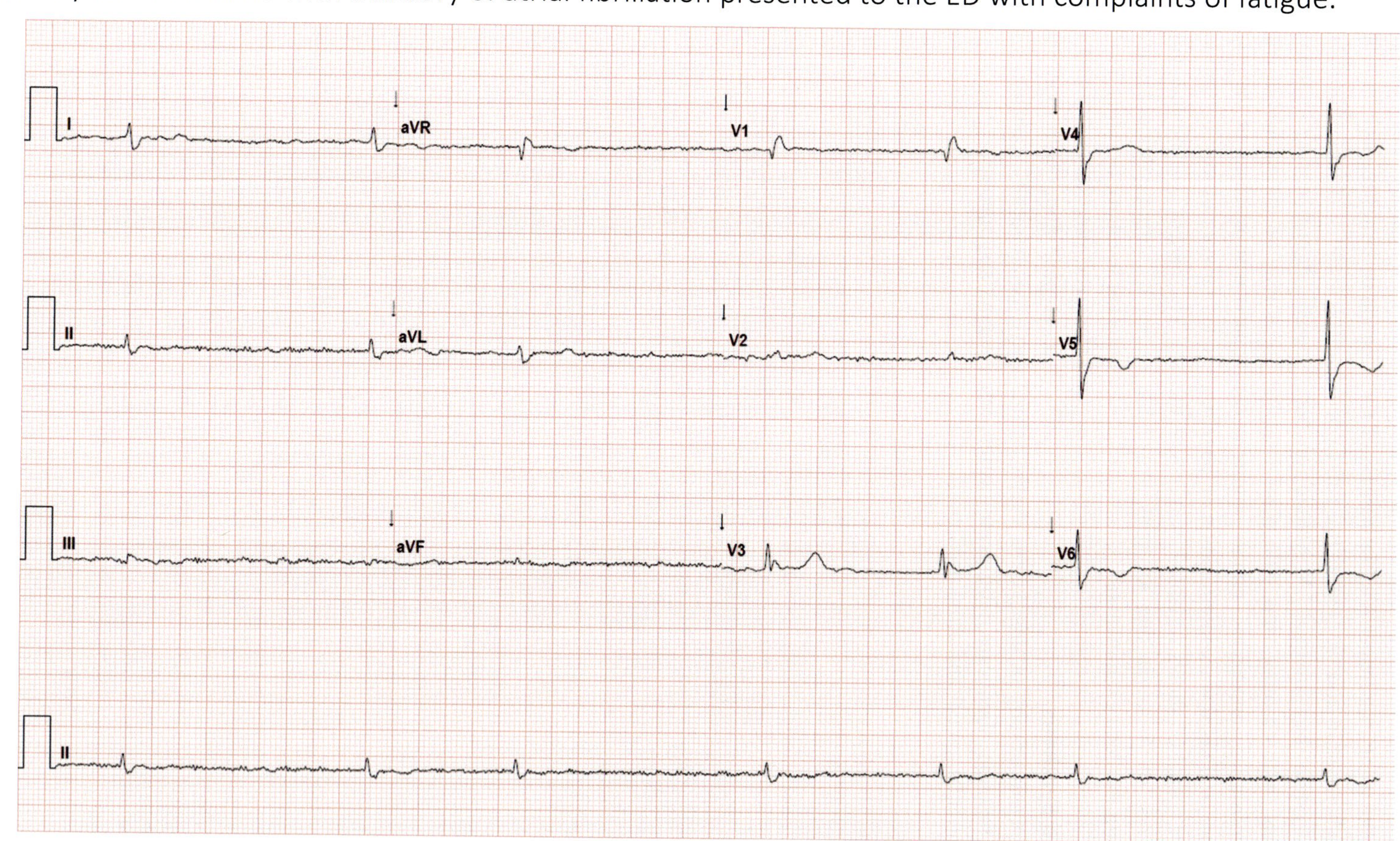

This patient was receiving beta blocker therapy for rate control of her atrial fibrillation.

ECG Interpretation

Rhythm: Atrial fibrillation

Rate: 40 BPM.

Intervals: PR not measurable due to AF, QRS 130 ms, QTc = 413 ms.

Axis: Normal.

Abnormalities on the ECG

- Atrial fibrillation
- Bradycardia
- RBBB
- Low voltage in limb leads.
- T wave inversion in V5 and V6.

ECG Test Answers

18, 57, 77

ECG Synthesis

The patient has an irregularly irregular rate and no p waves, consistent with atrial fibrillation. She also has RBBB, a possible sign of abnormal conduction. Beta blocker therapy probably plays a part in her bradycardia. However, additional factors such as age-related conduction disease may be considered. Low voltage in limb leads with impaired AV conduction should raise the possibility of infiltrative disease such as cardiac amyloidosis, as well as a pericardial effusion. Inverted T waves in V5 and V6 are a non specific finding. In a patient with atrial fibrillation, this may suggest use of digoxin; however, T wave inversions with digitalis use are typically accompanied by downsloping ST segment depression, absent in this tracing. Urgent echo is necessary to rule out structural causes for the ECG abnormalities.

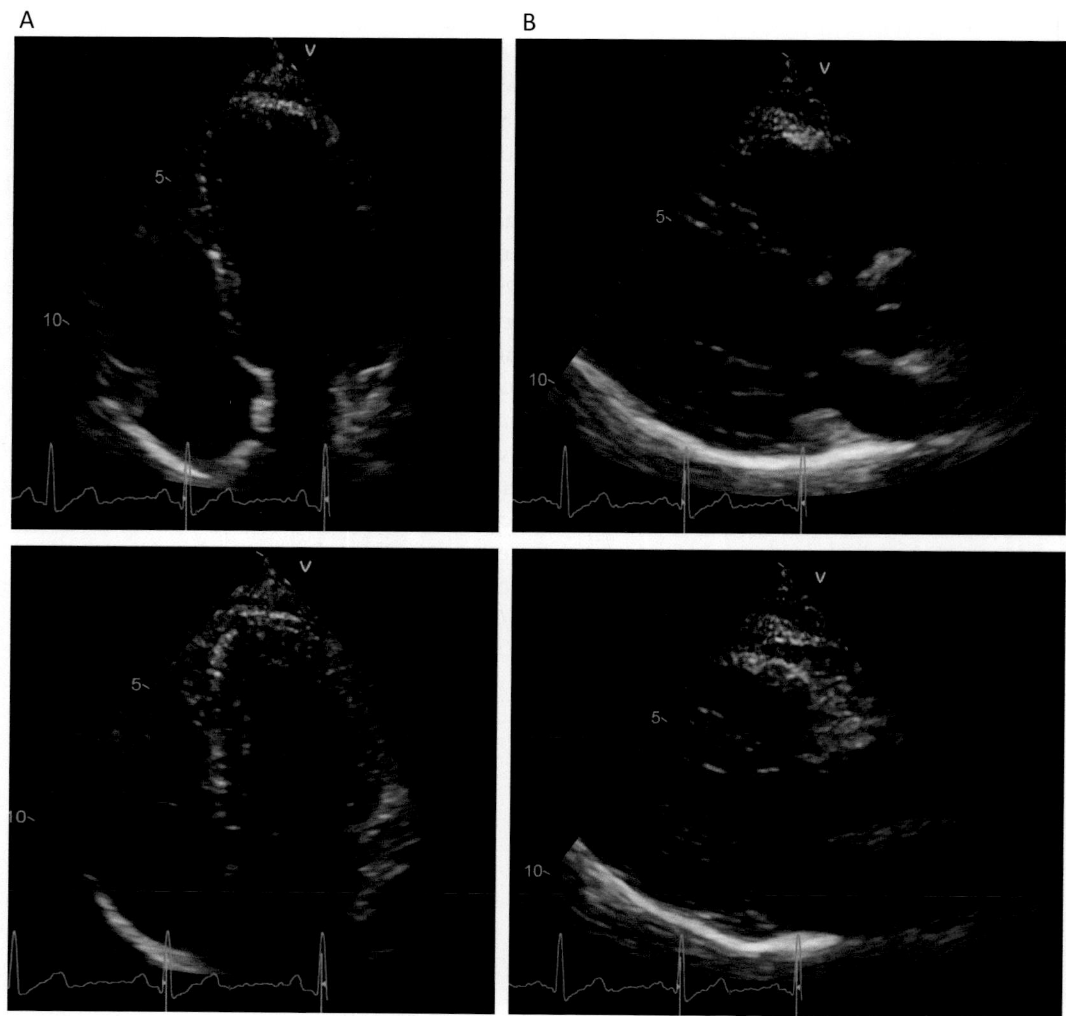

Apical four chamber (A) and parasternal long axis views (B) show normal left ventricular size and function, and a mildly dilated left atrium

Echo interpretation

Apical four chamber views (panel A, end diastolic top image, end systolic bottom image) and parasternal long axis views (panel B, end diastolic top image, end systolic bottom image) show normal left ventricular (LV) size and function, and a dilated left atrium.

Echo Synthesis

The mildly dilated atrium may provide a substrate for atrial arrhythmias such as atrial fibrillation. However, atrial fibrillation may also be a cause, not a result, of a dilated atrium. Left ventricular function was normal and no signs of pericardial effusion were noted.

Cardiac Electrosonography Synthesis

This patient presented with weakness and fatigue resulting from bradycardia due to atrial fibrillation with a slow ventricular response. There were no echocardiographic signs of abnormal LV function or pericardial effusion, ruling out structural causes for the additional ECG abnormalities (low voltage, t wave inversions) noted. Beta blocker therapy was withheld, however the bradycardia persisted and the patient eventually had a permanent pacemaker implanted.

5 Case 5

Clinical History

Clinical History: A 90 year old female with several syncopal events in the last 24 hours. She has sustained facial trauma and a hip fracture.

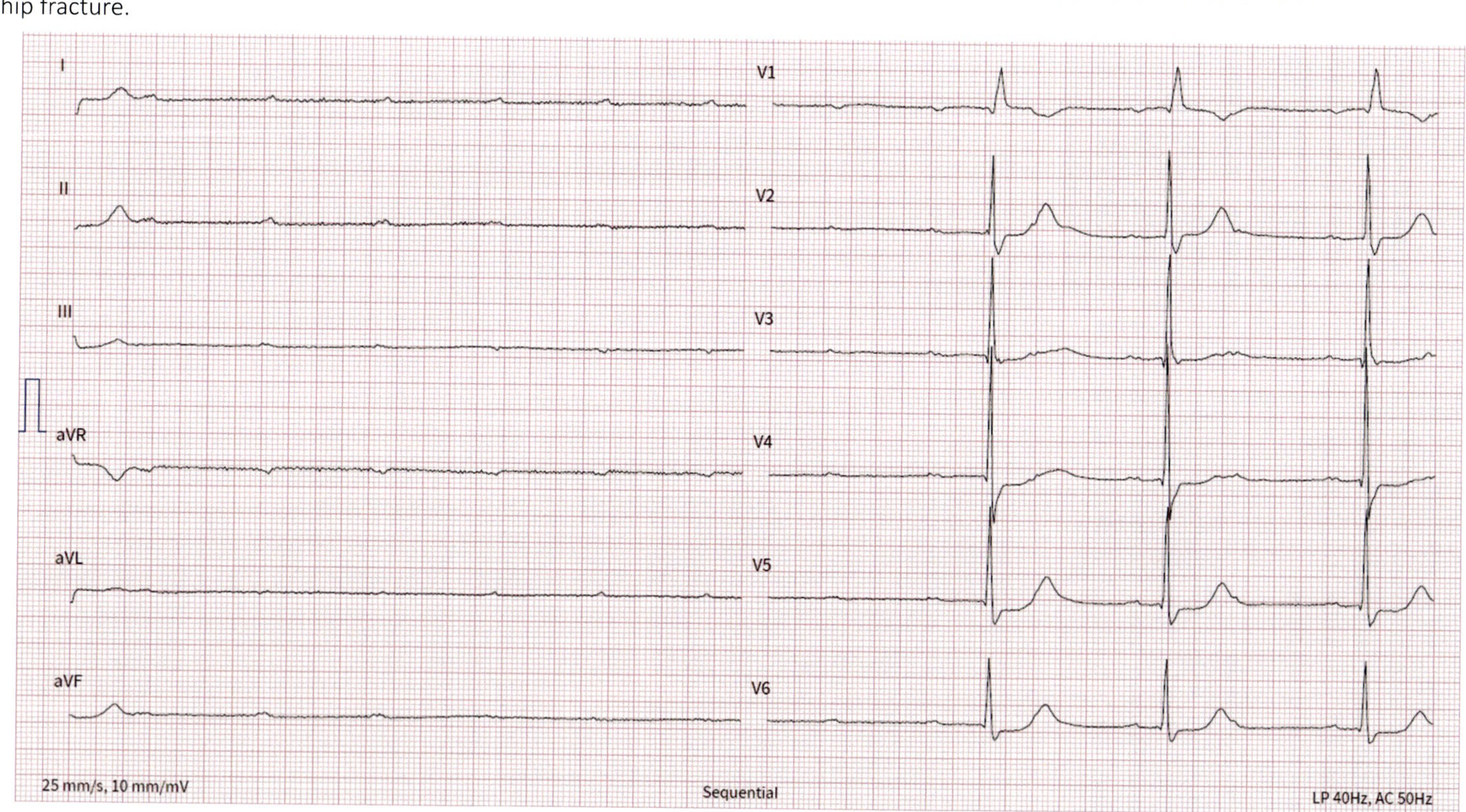

ECG Interpretation

Rhythm: The first part of the ECG shows sinus rhythm with complete AV block and no escape rhythm. In the second part AV conduction resumes with 2:1 AV block.

Rate: –

Intervals: QRS 130 ms, QTc = 480 ms

Axis: N/A.

Abnormalities on the ECG

- Complete (3rd degree) atrioventricular block (CAVB), later conducting to the ventricles with 2:1 block
- RBBB
- Prolonged PR interval in the two conducted beats, 250 ms.

ECG Test Answers
31, 32, 57.

ECG Synthesis
Complete atrioventricular block terminating with resumption of 2:1 AV conduction. Due to complete AV block, no QRS complexes can be seen in limb leads. We therefore do not know the frontal QRS axis. RBBB in itself is most commonly a benign finding, rarely, if ever, deteriorating to complete atrioventricular block. However, presence of additional conduction disturbances may mark an increased risk of advanced conduction block. In this case, a prolonged PR interval in the two conducted QRS complexes (last two in tracing) may be a marker of such disease. It is possible that left anterior or left posterior fascicular block existed as well; this is not known from the tracing.

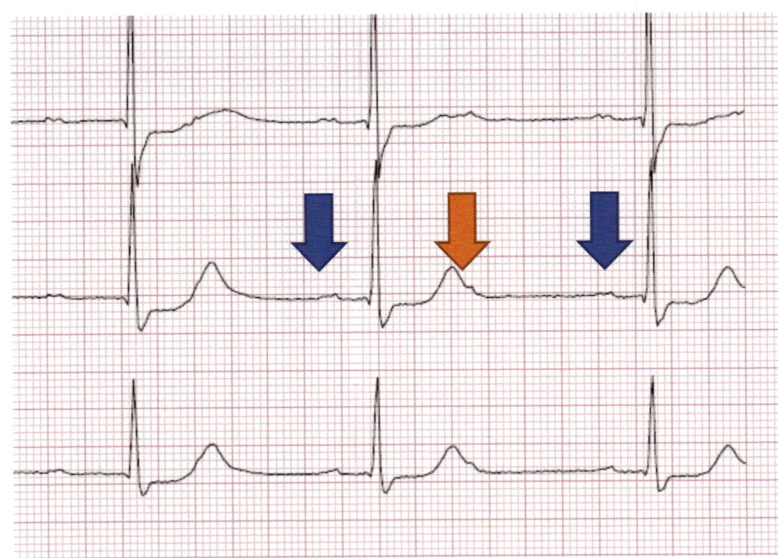

Enlargement of the second part of the ECG. Arrows mark 2:1 conduction; orange arrow marks non conducted p wave

A

B

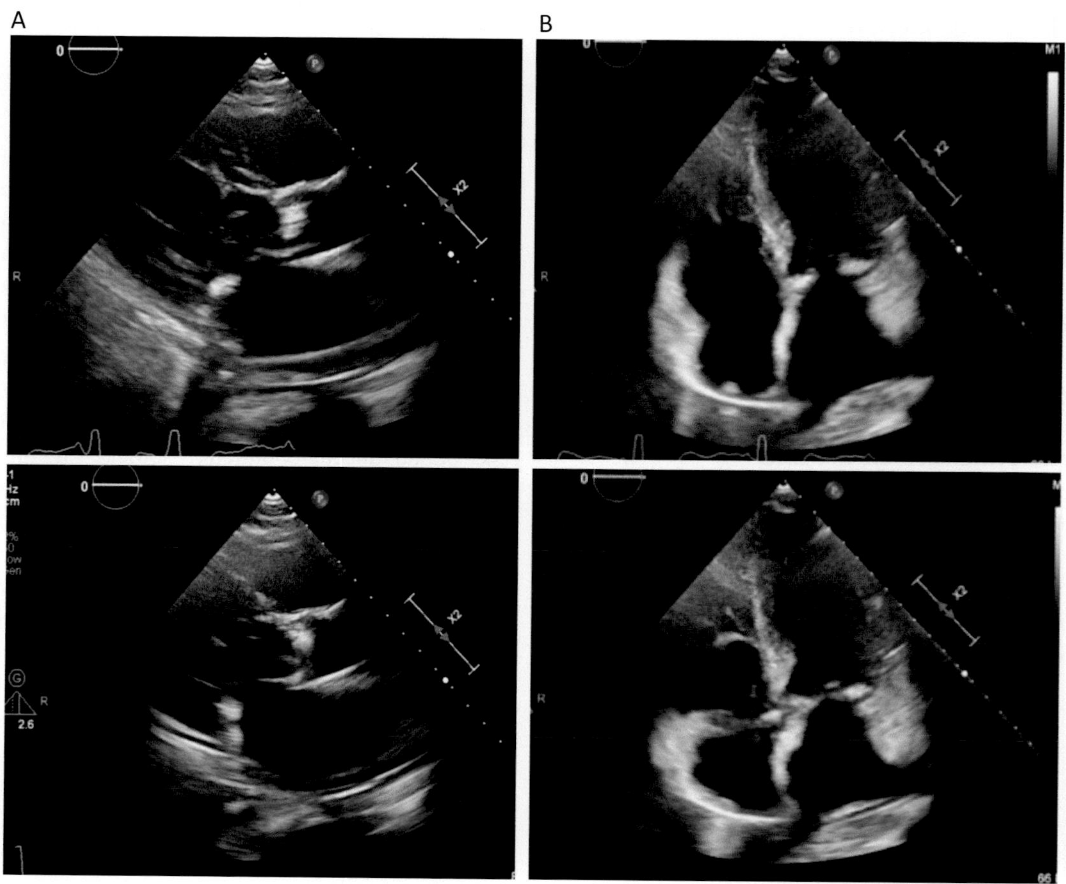

Parasternal long axis (A) and apical four chamber views (B) in systole and diastole show normal left ventricular size and function, and a mildly dilated left atrium. There is heavy calcification of the mitral annulus and the aortic valve

Echo interpretation

Parasternal long axis (A) and apical four chamber views (B) in systole and diastole show normal left ventricular size and function, and a mildly dilated left atrium. There is heavy calcification of the mitral annulus and aortic valve.

Echo Synthesis

The echocardiogram shows severe valvular calcification, probably due to age related degenerative valvular disease.

Cardiac Electrosonography Synthesis

This elderly patient has an echocardiogram showing heavy calcification, perhaps involving the cardiac electric conduction system. She presumably has prior signs of conduction disease, namely RBBB, possibly an additional hemiblock and a prolonged PR interval. This condition, if seen before the index event, should raise suspicion of impending atrioventricular block. The patient had emergent temporary pacemaker insertion in the emergency department, and later had a permanent pacemaker implanted.

6 Case 6

A 76 year old male with a medical history of hyperthyroidism and congestive heart failure, presented to the emergency department with 18 hours of weakness , shortness of breath and palpitations.

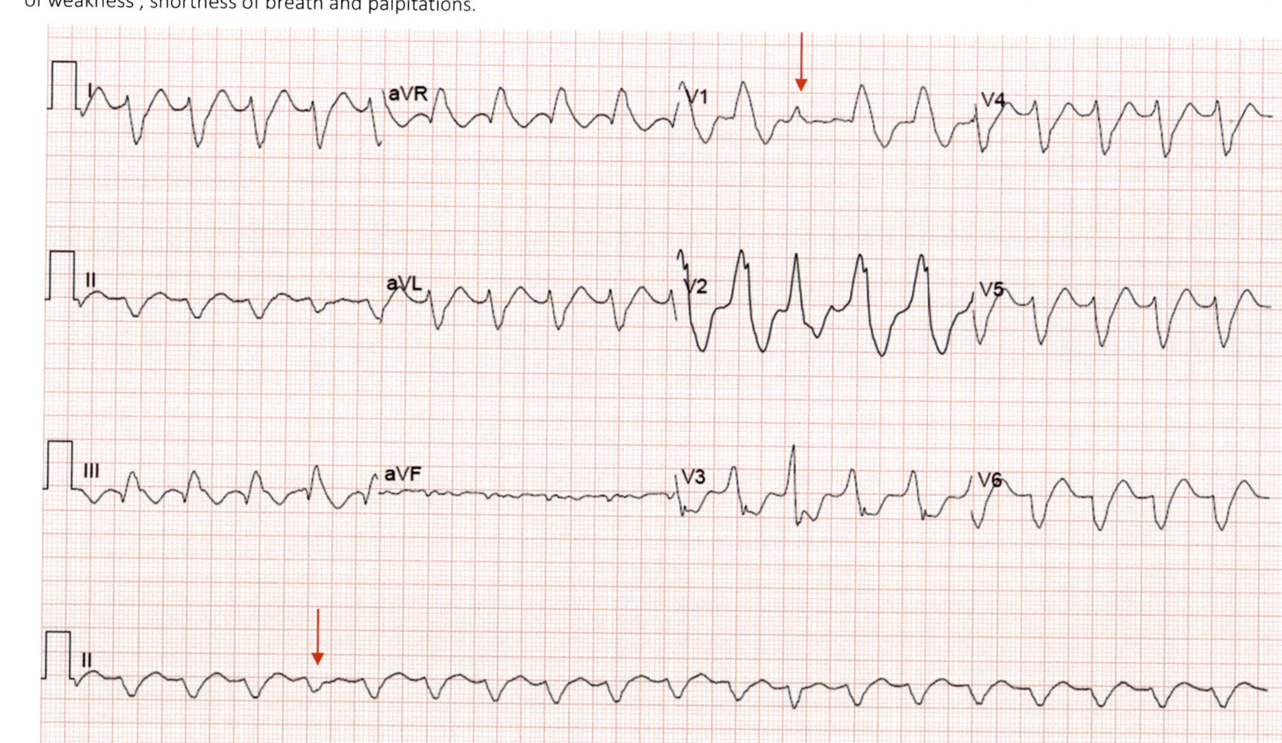

Additional Clinical History
Physical exam reveals a rapid, weak and regular pulse, no murmurs, elevated JVP with bilateral rales at lung bases
CXR shows pulmonary congestion

ECG interpretation

Rhythm: Wide complex tachycardia – ventricular tachycardia (VT).

Rate: 130 bpm

Intervals QRS = 170 ms

Axis: Northwest.

Abnormalities on the ECG:

- Wide complex tachycardia
- Abnormal axis.
- Fusion beats (2nd beat in leads V1,2,3 and 4th beat in the lead II rhythm strip)
- Time to first peak in II > 40 ms.

ECG Test Answers
24, 38.

ECG Synthesis

The differential diagnosis of wide complex tachycardia (WCT) includes monomorphic ventricular tachycardia (VT) or supraventricular tachycardia with aberrant conduction. Generally, in patients with a history of organic heart disease WCT is most likely to be of ventricular origin. Another important clue is the presence of AV dissociation which would support a diagnosis of VT. On the ECG of this patient there are fusion beats (arrows), resulting from VA dissociation and proving the diagnosis of VT. Fusion beats are defined as beats with a QRS of different, usually narrower morphology than the patient's baseline QRS. Other features supportive of the diagnosis of VT on this ECG are the abnormal northwest QRS axis, the very wide QRS complexes and positive QRS in aVR, and time to first peak in lead II greater than 40 ms.

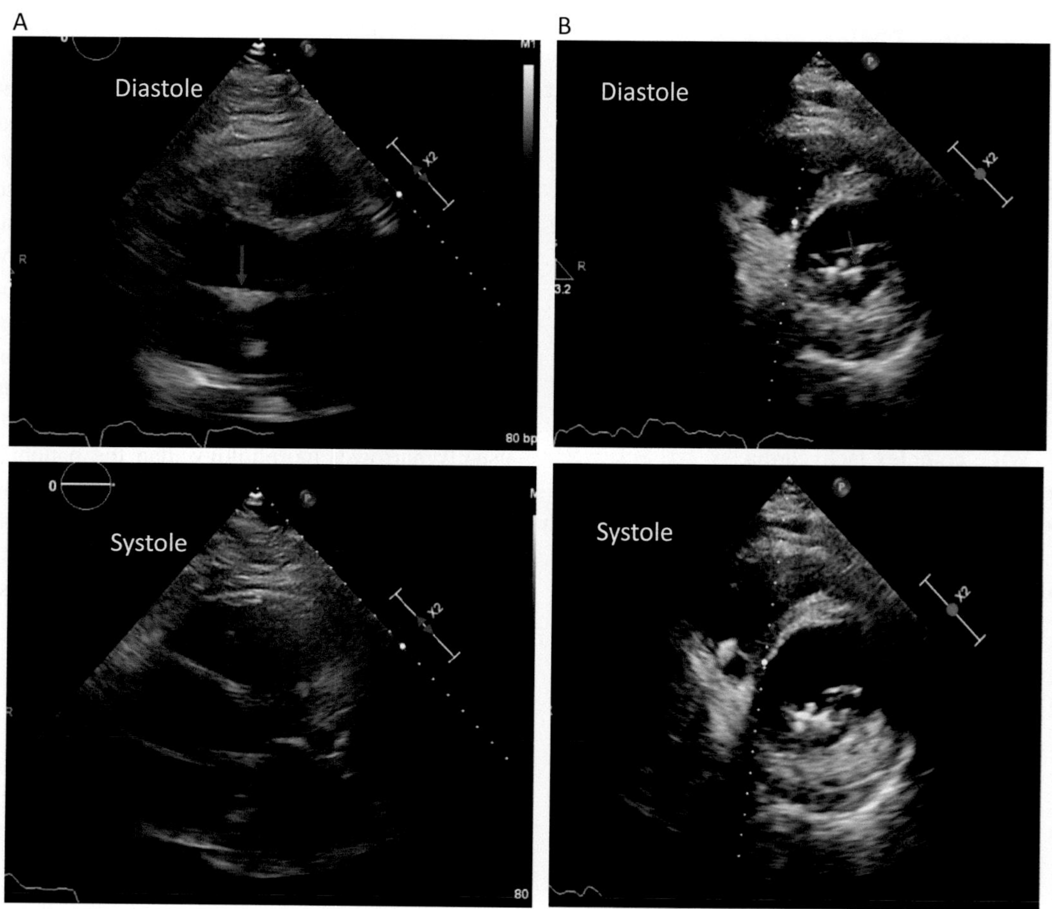

Parasternal long axis (A) and short axis views (B) are presented in systole and diastole. There are very small differences in area between systole and diastole indicative of severely reduced ventricular function

Echo Interpretation

Parasternal long axis (A) and short axis views (B) are presented in systole and diastole. There are very small differences in area between systole and diastole which indicates severely reduced left ventricular systolic function. A bright echodensity is seen on the mitral valve on both views (arrows). This finding appears to be a MitraClip device.

Echo Synthesis

The echocardiogram shows severely reduced left ventricular function. The patient has undergone previous percutaneous repair of his mitral valve presumably due to functional mitral regurgitation secondary to the cardiomyopathy.

Cardiac Electrosonography Synthesis

This patient presented with symptomatic wide complex tachycardia The history of congestive heart failure, the ECG features previously noted, and the severely reduced ventricular function demonstrated on echocardiogram establishes a diagnosis of ventricular tachycardia as a complication of his cardiomyopathy. It is probably scar related and brought about by a reentry mechanism. The patient was treated with amiodarone and eventually had an ablation of his ventricular tachycardia and implantation of an ICD.

7 Case 7

A 36 year old male presented with recurrent episodes of palpitations.

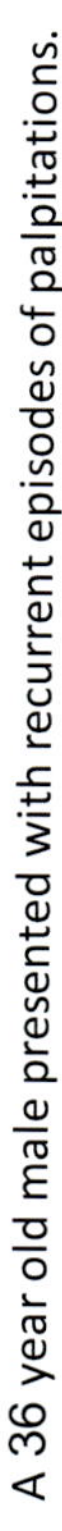

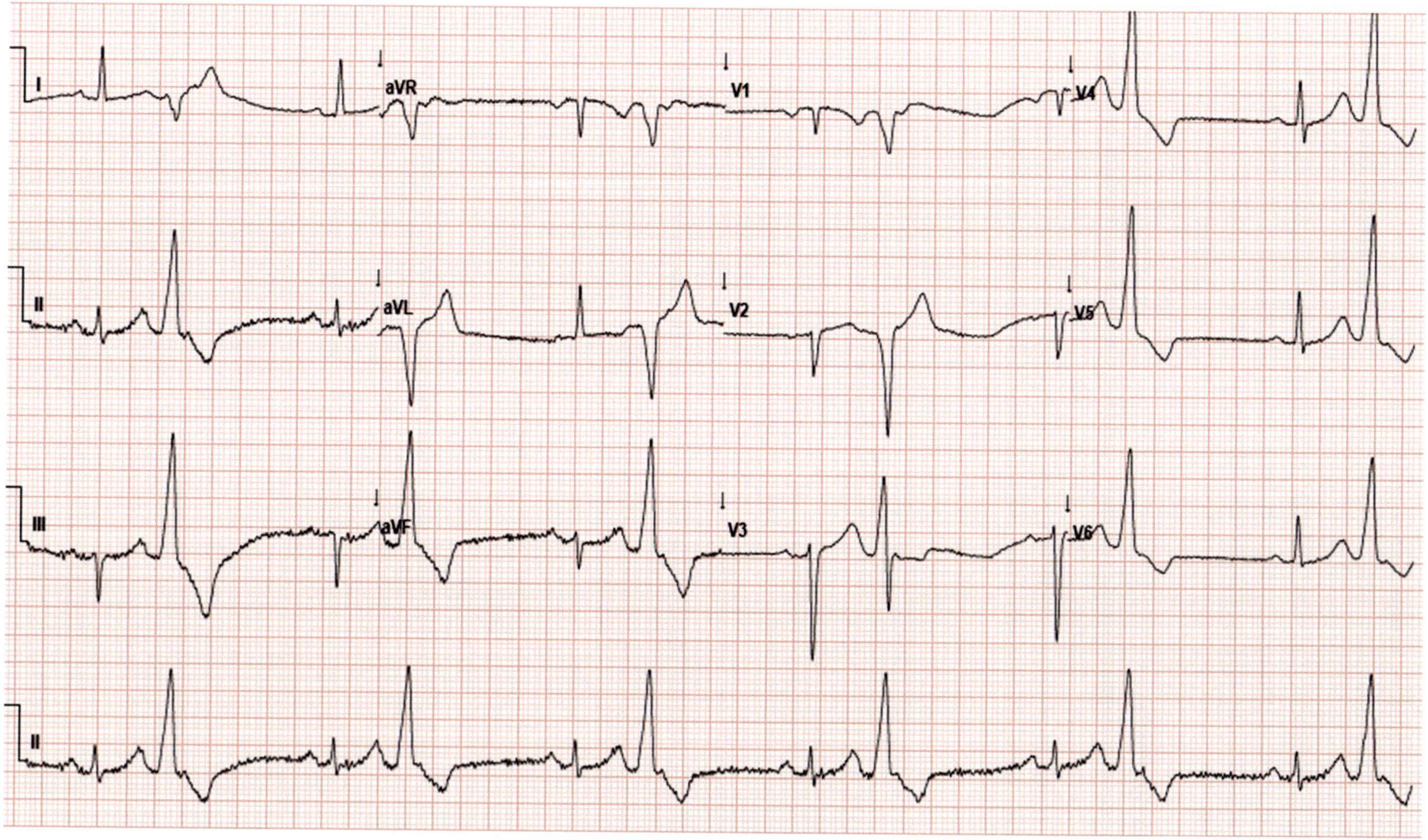

Physical exam revealed a regularly irregular rhythm.

ECG Interpretation

Rhythm: Sinus rhythm with frequent VPB's (ventricular bigeminy).

Rate: 71 bpm.

Intervals: QRS 98 ms, QTc 426 ms.

Axis: Normal.

Abnormalities on ECG

Frequent ventricular premature complexes in a bigeminal pattern.

ECG Test Answers

7, 22

ECG Synthesis

This patient presented with a bigeminal rhythm. The QRS complexes of the premature beats are not preceded by an obvious p wave, are relatively wide and have a different morphology from the native sinus beats. This makes them most likely of ventricular origin. These beats have an inferior axis (positive in leads II and III), an LBBB-like pattern in lead V1 (QS) and precordial transition at V3. This morphology is consistent with a right ventricular outflow tract origin, which is the most common origin of idiopathic PVC's. Echocardiography should be performed to ascertain whether the PVCS are idiopathic or associated with structural heart disease.

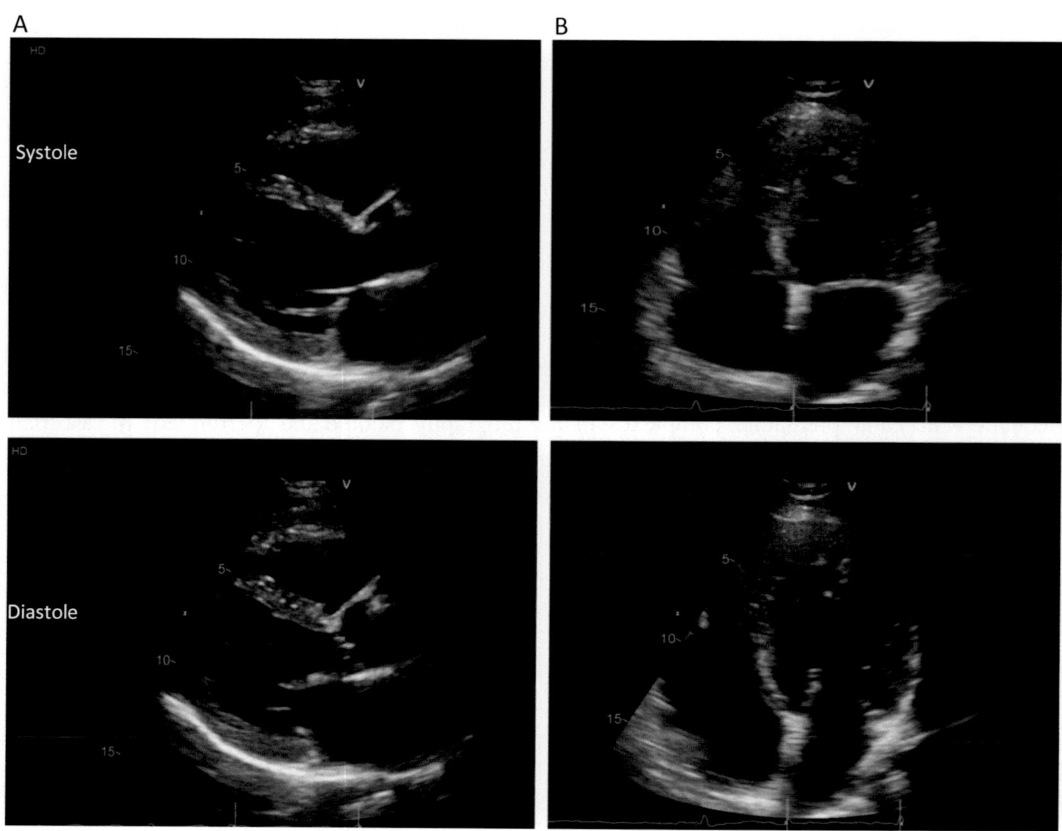

Parasternal long-axis (panel A) and apical four chamber (panel B) views demonstrated an enlarged left ventricle and left atrium. Note the small difference in left ventricular area in systole (mitral valve closed) and diastole (mitral valve open), indicating moderately reduced LV systolic function.

Echo Interpretation

Parasternal long-axis and apical four chamber views demonstrated an enlarged left ventricle and left atrium. Note the small difference in left ventricular area in systole (mitral valve closed) and diastole (mitral valve open), indicating moderately reduced LV systolic function.

Echo Synthesis

The echo shows LV dilatation with reduced function. The reduction in systolic function is global and not limited to specific regions, hence not suggestive of an ischemic etiology.

It is important to make sure the beat assessed for systolic function is a normal sinus beat, not a premature beat and not one that immediately follows a premature beat.

Cardiac Electrosonography Synthesis

This patient presented with ventricular bigeminy and reduced systolic function.

A large amount of premature beats may by itself cause reduction in systolic function, via a mechanism of 'tachycardia induced cardiomyopathy'. However, certain cardiomyopathies (e.g. arrhythmogenic right ventricular cardiomyopathy) may also be a cause of premature beats and it is difficult to determine in this case what the primary pathology is. The RVOT morphology of the premature beats supports a diagnosis of a primary arrhythmia causing secondary ventricular dysfunction.

8 Case 8

A 71 year old male with a a medical history of ischemic heart disease and congestive heart failure, presented to the emergency room with shortness of breath, palpitations and diaphoresis.

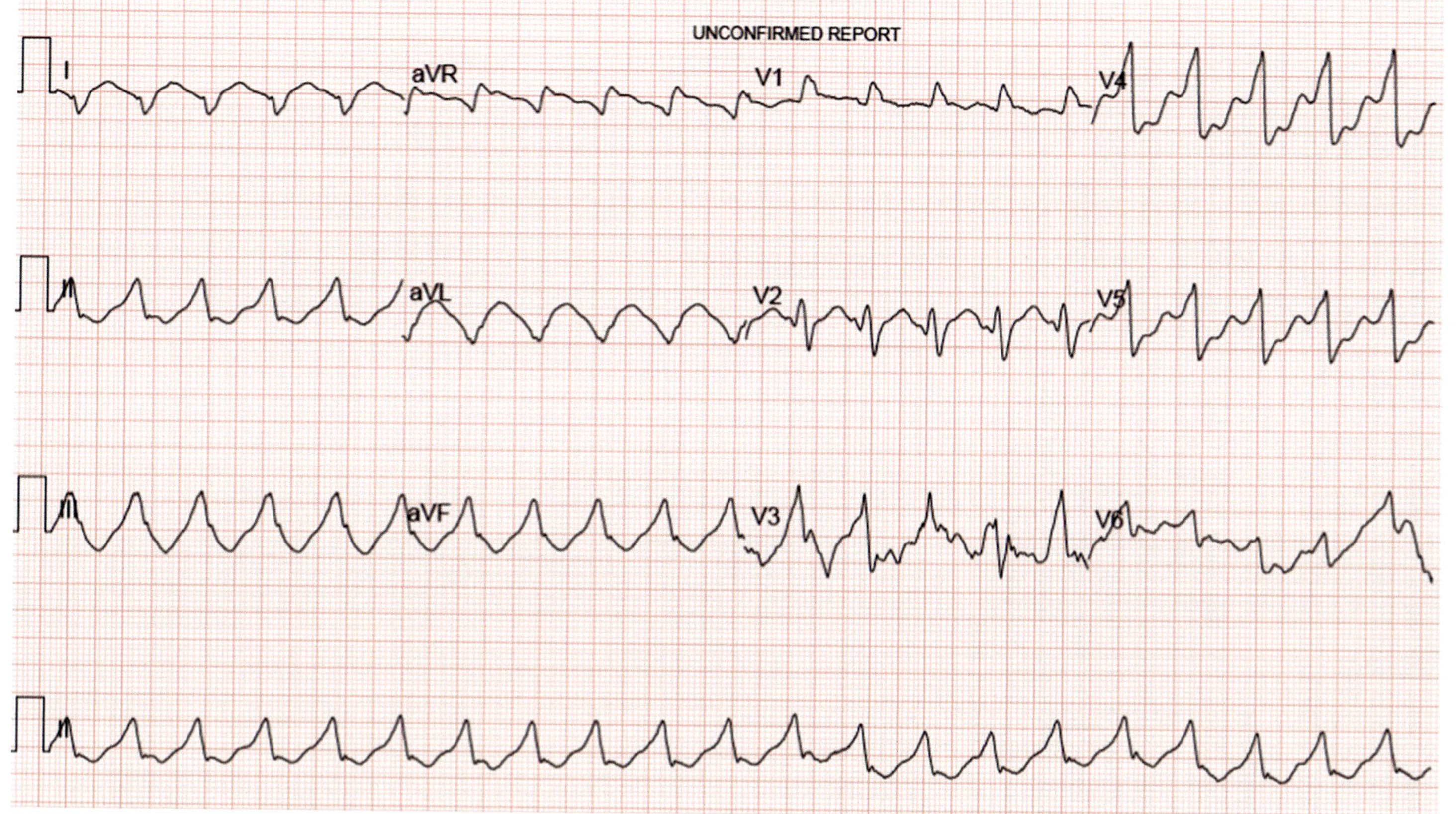

Additional Clinical Information:
Physical exam revealed rapid, regular and weak pulse. JVP was elevated with cannon a waves and there were bilateral rales on lung auscultation.

ECG Interpretation

Rhythm: Wide complex tachycardia

Rate: 145 BPM.

Intervals: QRS 200 ms (difficult to determine)

Axis: Right axis deviation.

Abnormalities on the ECG

- Wide complex tachycardia
- Time to first peak in leads II and aVR longer than 40 ms
- Initial QRS slope shallower than terminal part.

ECG Test Answers
24, 38

ECG Synthesis

This wide complex tachycardia is sustained monomorphic ventricular tachycardia. The patient is known for a history of ischemic heart disease and heart failure. The time to first peak in both leads II and aVR is longer than 40 ms, satisfying all three Basel Criteria (see tutorial). Right axis deviation, a very wide QRS complex and a shallow slope on the initial part of the QRS complex also support a diagnosis of VT. The initial part of the QRS complex has a shallow slope, sometimes called a 'pseudo-delta' wave, suggestive of possible epicardial origin of tachycardia. Emergent echo should be performed to assess left ventricular function and guide further management of the arrhythmia.

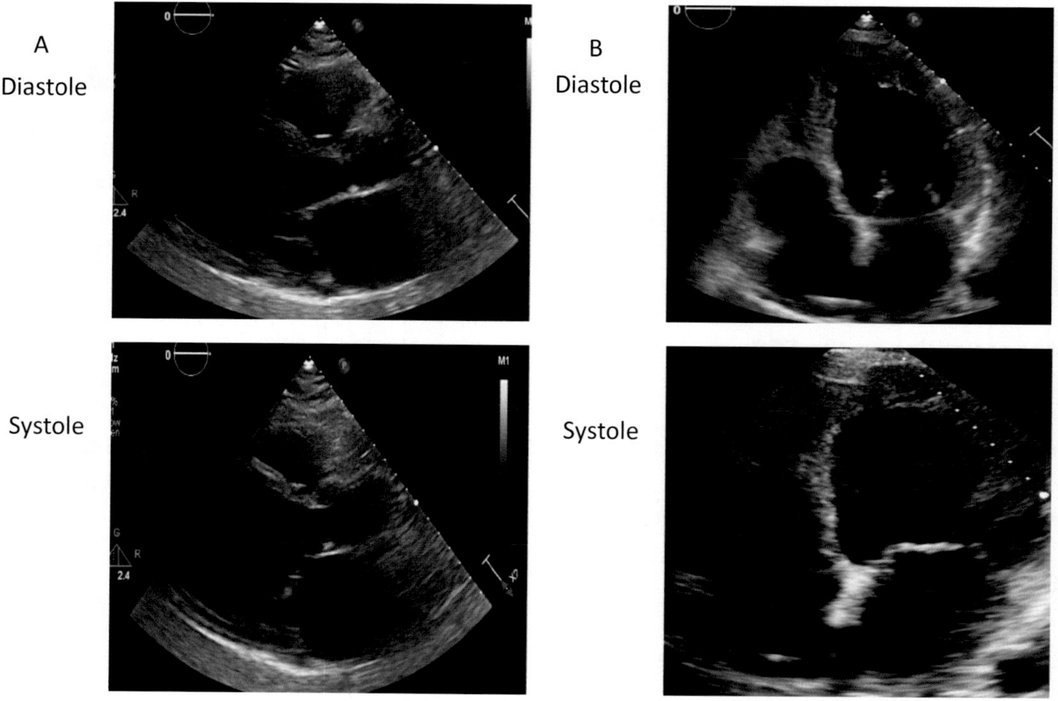

Parasternal long axis (A) and apical four chamber views (B) show a severely dilated left ventricle with severely reduced ejection fraction, estimated at 20–25%. This is evident by comparison of images in diastole (top, open mitral valve) and systole (bottom, closed mitral valve). The left atrium is enlarged

Echo Interpretation

Parasternal long axis (A) and apical four chamber views (B) show a severely dilated left ventricle with severely reduced ejection fraction, estimated at 20–25%. This is evident by comparison of images in diastole (top, open mitral valve) and systole (bottom, closed mitral valve). The left atrium is enlarged.

Echo Synthesis

The echocardiogram shows severely reduced left ventricular function with a dilated left atrium (LA). The dilated LA is presumably due to chronically elevated LA pressures secondary to the poor LV function. Once LV function is severely reduced it can be challenging by echocardiography to distinguish ischemic from non-ischemic cardiomyopathy. Clues to an ischemic etiology are multiple areas of thinned myocardium in coronary artery distributions and relatively preserved right ventricular function.

Cardiac Electrosonography Synthesis

The ECG was highly suggestive of VT, particularly given the clinical history. The echo finding of severely reduced LV function supports the diagnosis of VT. This patient is at high risk of sudden cardiac death due to his severely reduced left ventricular systolic function. The clinical event of sustained monomorphic ventricular tachycardia was terminated by emergent cardioversion. An ICD was implanted, as should be done in any patient with severely reduced left ventricular systolic function even before the VT episode (primary prevention). To prevent future episodes of ventricular tachycardia, this patient was successfully treated with amiodarone.

9 Case 9

A 74 year old female with weakness and palpitations.

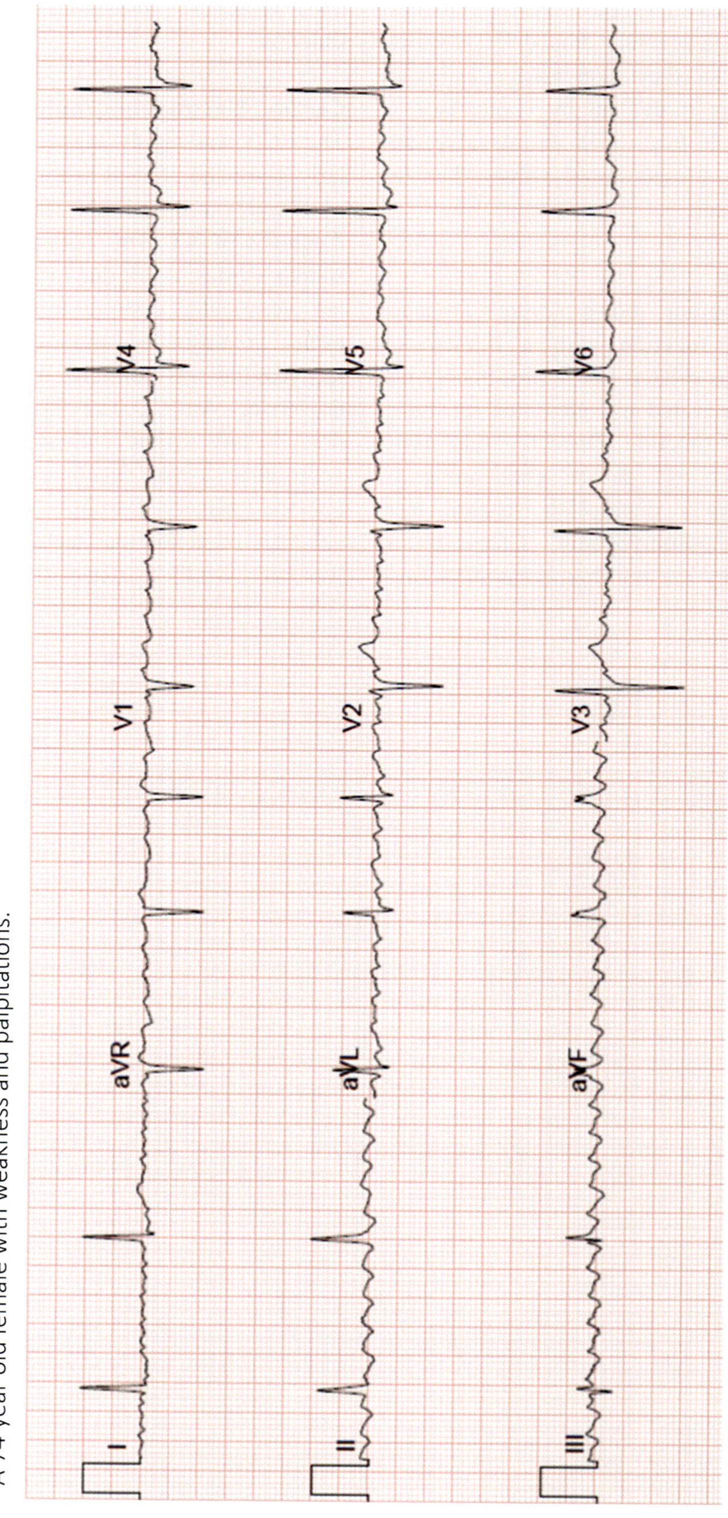

ECG Interpretation

Rhythm: Atrial flutter

Rate: 60 BPM.

Intervals: PR not measurable due to atrial flutter, QRS 98 ms

Axis: Normal.

Abnormalities on the ECG

- Sawtooth pattern
- Variable AV conduction

ECG Test Answers
17

ECG Synthesis
Sawtooth flutter waves at a rate of approximately 300 bpm which are negative in lead II and positive in V1 suggest a 'typical', cavotricuspid isthmus dependent atrial flutter. Note that variable AV block may cause irregular pulse. However this is usually 'regularly irregular', as opposed to atrial fibrillation where the rate is typically 'irregularly irregular'.

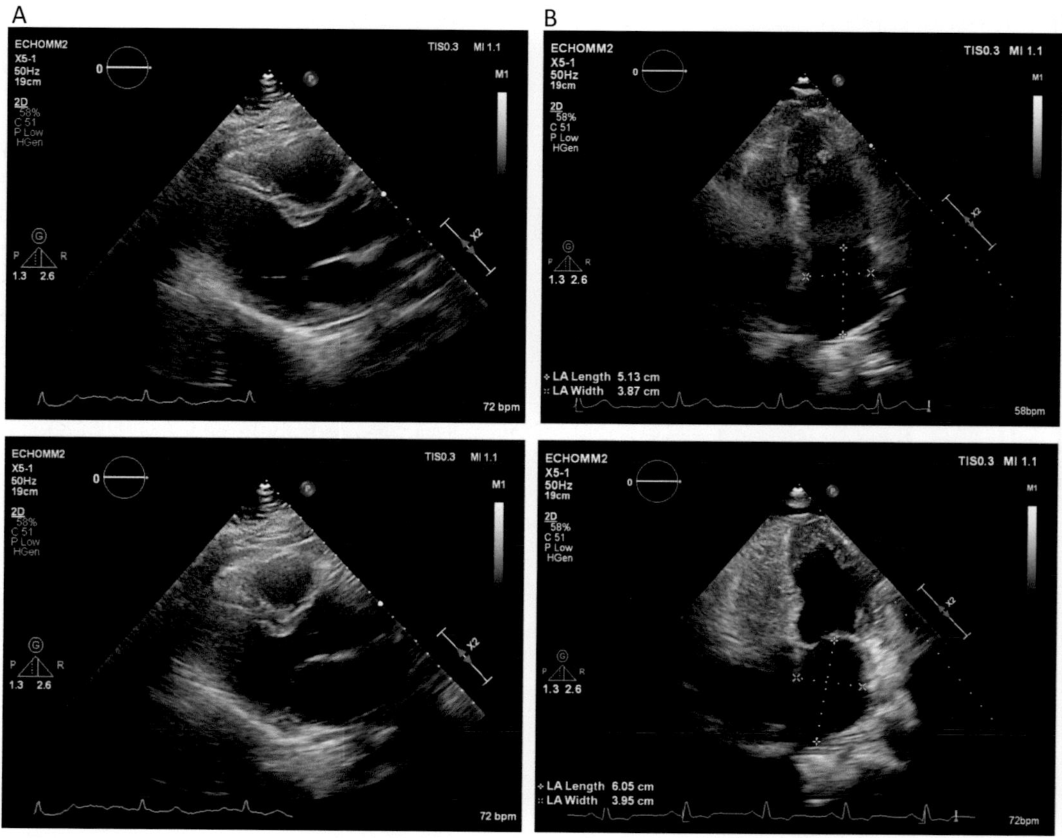

Parasternal long axis (A) and apical four chamber views (B) show mildly reduced systolic function and a dilated left atrium

Echo Interpretation

Parasternal long axis (A) and apical four chamber views (B) show mildly reduced systolic function and a dilated left atrium.

Echo Synthesis

The dilated atria may provide the substrate for typical atrial flutter.

Cardiac Electrosonography Synthesis

Atrial flutter probably explains this patient's weakness. The relatively slow atrioventricular conduction may be related to age or medications, and may cause chronotropic incompetence (inability to increase pulse rate to that required by the patient's activity). Additionally, lack of effective atrial contraction and AV synchrony may also contribute to this patient's symptoms of weakness. The mildly reduced function seen on echocardiography may be a result of, or a cause of the atrial arrhythmia and imaging should be repeated after treatment of the atrial flutter.

10 Case 10

A 46 year old male with no previous medical history presented with recurrent episodes of palpitations.

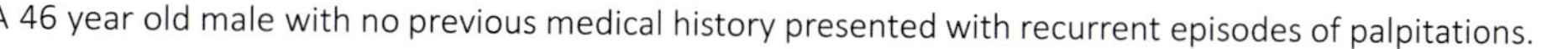

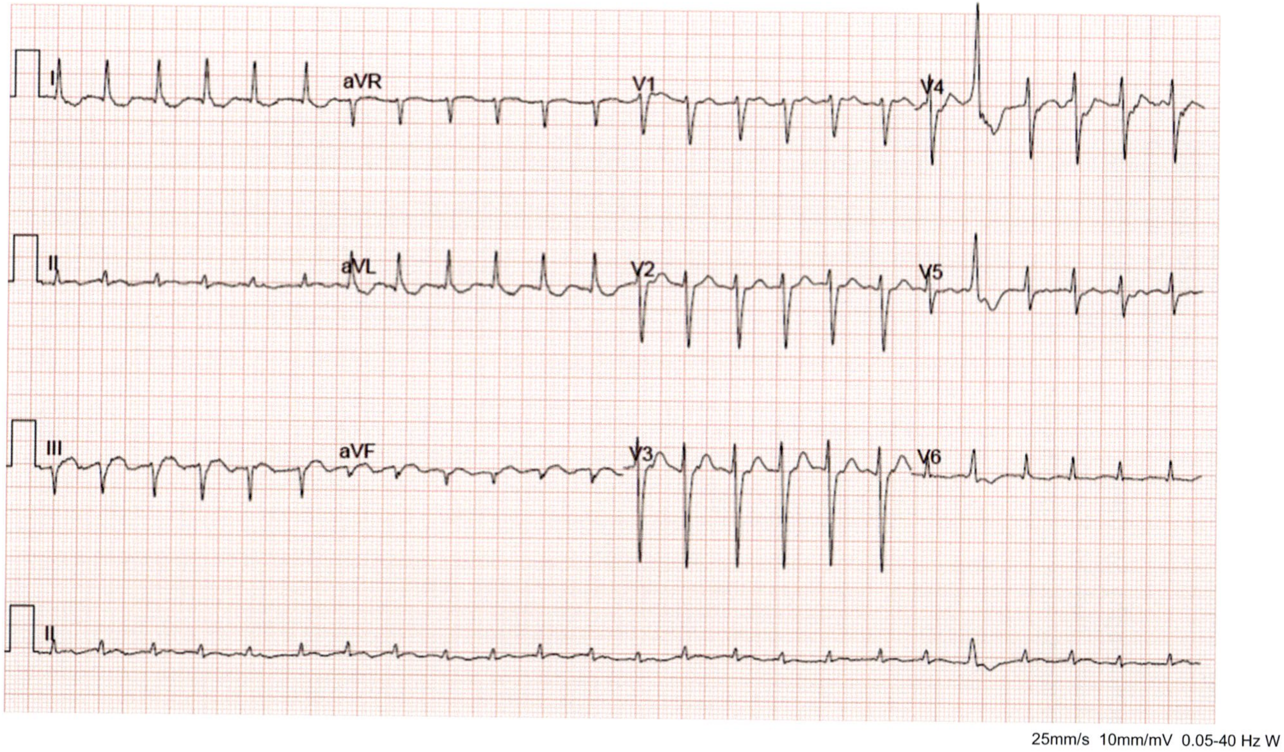

Additional Clinical History

The palpitations have sudden onset and offset. There is a sensation of neck pounding.

ECG Interpretation

Rhythm: Narrow complex tachycardia

Rate: 160 BPM.

Intervals: QRS 68

Axis: Normal.

Abnormalities on the ECG

- Narrow complex tachycardia
- Short RP interval

ECG Test Answers
16

ECG Synthesis

The history of sudden onset and offset palpitations with neck pounding and a narrow QRS complex is suggestive of paroxysmal supraventricular tachycardia (PSVT). The differential diagnosis of PSVT includes sinus tachycardia, atrial tachycardias and reentrant tachycardias. The absence of organized atrial activity before ventricular depolarization and the QRS complex suggests a reentrant mechanism such as atrioventricular nodal reentrant tachycardia (AVNRT) or an accessory pathway. Neck pounding is typical although not specific, for AVNRT, since the atria and ventricles contract almost simultaneously. This is also supported by a short RP interval. Echocardiography is important to rule out structural heart disease.

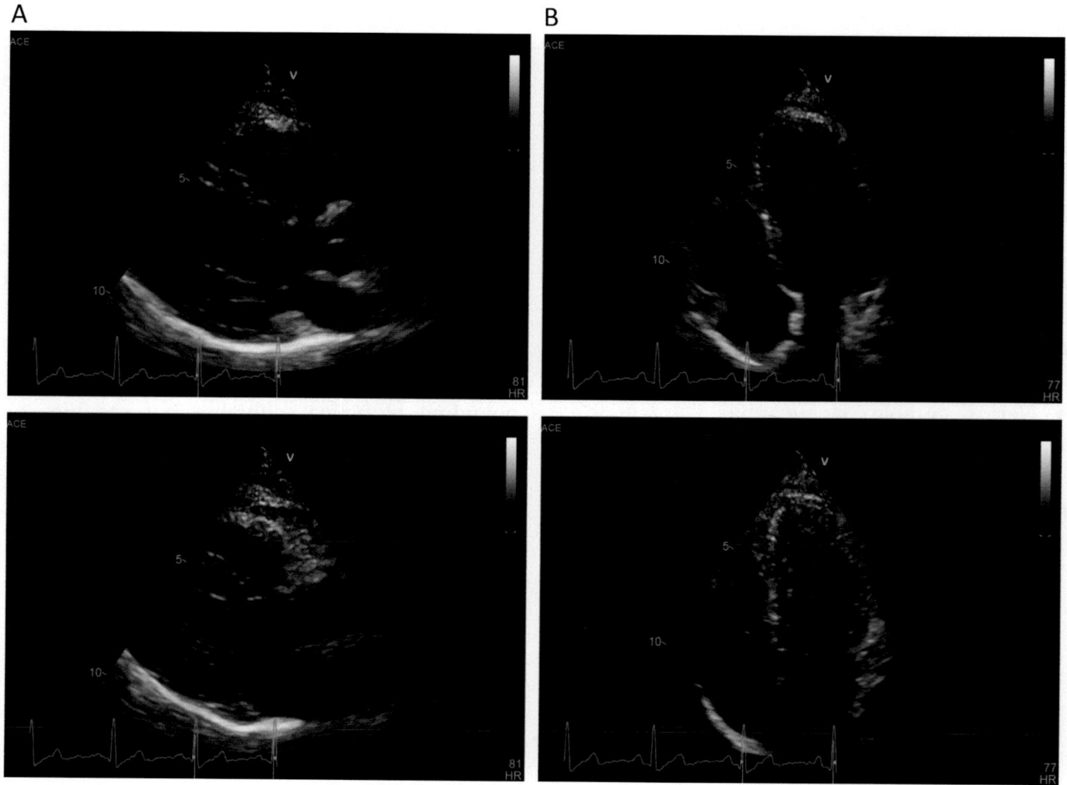

Parasternal long axis (A) and apical four chamber (B) views, comparing diastole (top image) and systole (bottom image), show normal left ventricular size and function

Echo Interpretation

Parasternal long axis (A) and apical four chamber (B) views, comparing diastole and systole, show normal left ventricular size and function.

Echo Synthesis

The echocardiogram is normal.

Cardiac Electrosonography Synthesis

In this otherwise young and healthy patient with a normal echocardiogram, the likely diagnosis is AVNRT. Orthodromic AVRT and atrial tachycardia are also possible however less likely. The patient received adenosine which terminated the tachycardia. Electrophysiologic study confirmed the diagnosis of AVNRT. The slow pathway was successfully ablated and there were no recurrences.

11 Case 11

A 59 year old female presents with long episodes of palpitations and lightheadedness.

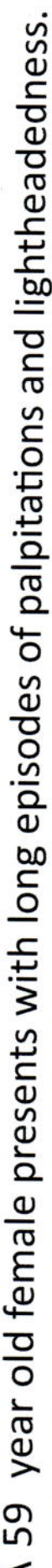

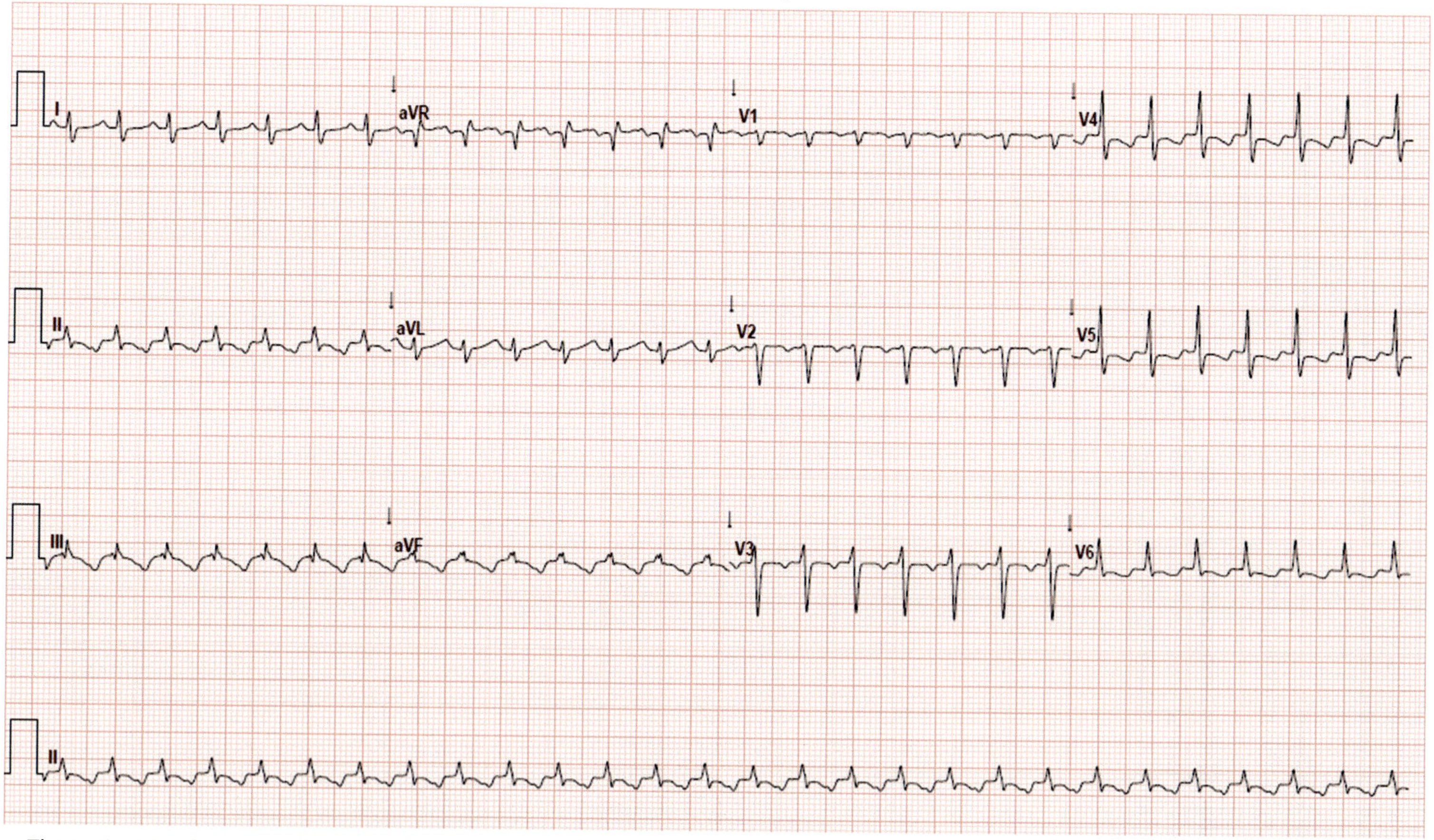

The patient is a heavy smoker with a known history of COPD.

ECG Interpretation

Rhythm: Narrow complex tachycardia

Rate: 166 BPM.

Intervals: QRS 100 ms, QTc 460 ms

Axis: normal.

Abnormalities on ECG

Narrow complex tachycardia.
Very long RP interval (RP > PR).

Test Answers
14, 77

ECG Synthesis

Narrow complex tachycardia with a very long RP interval suggests atrial tachycardia. This is perhaps supported by the episodes being prolonged. However, the differential diagnosis includes atypical atrioventricular nodal reentry tachycardia (AVNRT) or atrioventricular reentry tachycardia (AVRT) with a lateral accessory pathway. In this ECG, the A:V ratio appears to be 1:1. However, the caregiver should carefully look for p waves hidden within the QRS complexes, in which case an atypical atrial flutter with 2:1 conduction may exist. Vagal maneuvers or administration of adenosine should answer this question. The patient is a known smoker with a history of COPD. This is the probable explanation for the low voltage in limb leads, except for lead I. The formal diagnosis of low voltage in limb leads requires the QRS complex to be less than 5 mV in **all** limb leads. Echo imaging is necessary to rule cardiac pathology, in particular evidence of right heart strain given the history of smoking and COPD.

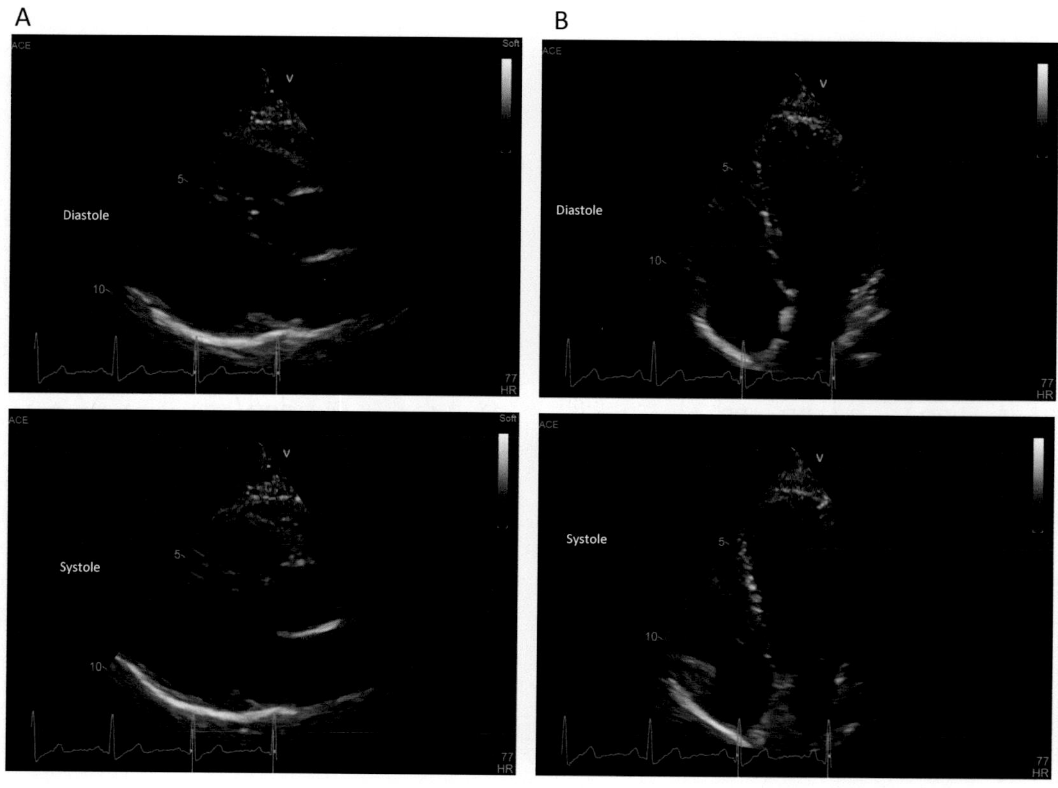

Parasternal long axis (panel A) and apical four chamber (panel B) views reveal normal left ventricular function

Echo Interpretation

The patient's echo is unremarkable. Comparison of echo images in diastole and in systole, in two different views, shows normal left ventricular systolic function. The estimated left ventricular ejection fraction was 55%. The apical 4 chamber view (B) does not show signs of cor pulmonale despite the patient's history of pulmonary disease.

Echo Synthesis

Normal echocardiogram.

Cardiac Electrosonography Synthesis

This patient had symptomatic atrial tachycardia. Atrial tachycardia, as opposed to AVNRT or AVRT, is commonly associated with some cardiac pathology. Although the echo was normal, in this case a possible contributor is the patient's severe lung disease. Patients with COPD sometimes present with multifocal atrial tachycardia, defined as an atrial tachycardia with at least three different P wave morphologies. This is not the case here. This patient had her COPD treatment optimized. She was counseled on smoking cessation, and was treated with antiarrhythmic medications.

12 Case 12

A 24 year old male with no previous medical history presented with episodes of palpitations.

ECG Interpretation

Rhythm: Normal sinus rhythm

Rate: 63 BPM.

Intervals: PR 96 ms, QRS 126 ms QTc 393 ms

Axis: normal.

Abnormalities on ECG
Short PR interval.
   "Delta" wave.

Test Answers
7, 33

ECG Synthesis
The ECG shows sinus rhythm with a short PR interval and a gentle upslope (delta wave) at the initiation of the QRS complex most obvious in leads 1, L, V4–V6. The combination of these two findings on baseline ECG represents preexcitation due to Wolff-Parkinson-White syndrome (WPW). This patient has an accessory pathway conducting antegradely (from atria to ventricles) when in normal sinus rhythm; this causes shortening of the PR interval and early depolarization of the ventricles, leading to the characteristic delta wave. It is important to note that these features of WPW are not always evident on baseline ECG, a condition referred to as "concealed" WPW. The accessory pathway predisposes him to episodes of rapid supraventricular tachycardia through a reentrant circuit. Rarely, WPW is associated with other structural heart disease and echocardiography is necessary to rule out this possibility.

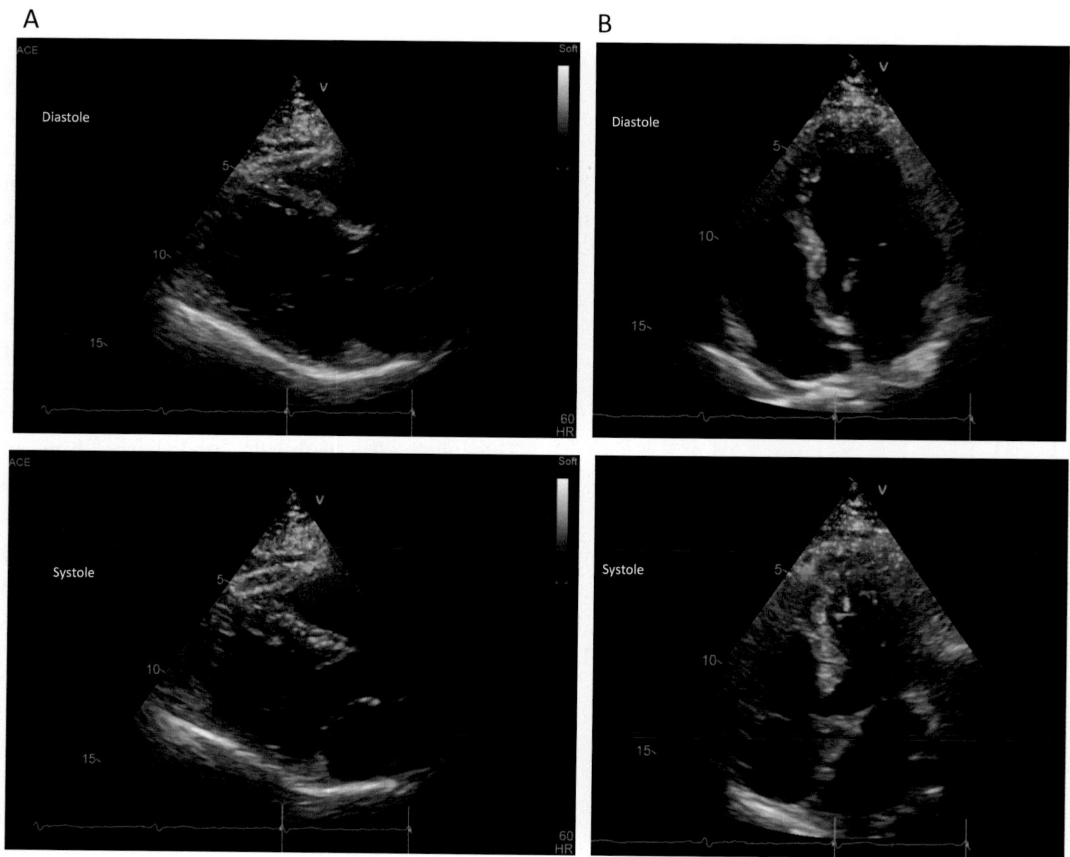

Parasternal long axis (A) and apical 4 chamber (B) views in diastole and systole show normal left ventricular systolic function

Echo Interpretation

Parasternal long axis (A) and apical 4 chamber (B) views in diastole and systole show normal left ventricular systolic function. There are no signs of Ebstein's anomaly, a congenital anomaly of the tricuspid valve predisposing to WPW syndrome. However the vast majority of patients with WPW syndrome do not have Ebstein's anomaly.

Echo Synthesis

Normal echocardiogram.

Cardiac Electrosonography Synthesis

This patient presents with palpitations and a WPW pattern on ECG. He likely has episodes of tachyarrhythmia, therefore may be diagnosed with WPW syndrome.

The most common tachyarrhythmia in patients with WPW is orthodromic AVRT. This is a symptomatic, not life- threatening condition. However, uncommonly a patient with WPW may have an episode of atrial fibrillation. If this very rapid, chaotic atrial rhythm should conduct to the ventricles via an accessory pathway, a rapid wide complex tachycardia may result that may deteriorate to polymorphic ventricular tachycardia and VF. Therefore, WPW is considered a possible cause of sudden cardiac death. Mapping and ablation of this patient's accessory pathway cured his symptoms and abolished the risk of fatal arrhythmias.

13 Case 13

Clinical History

Clinical History
A 44-year-old female presented to the emergency department with sudden onset of shortness of breath with palpitations.

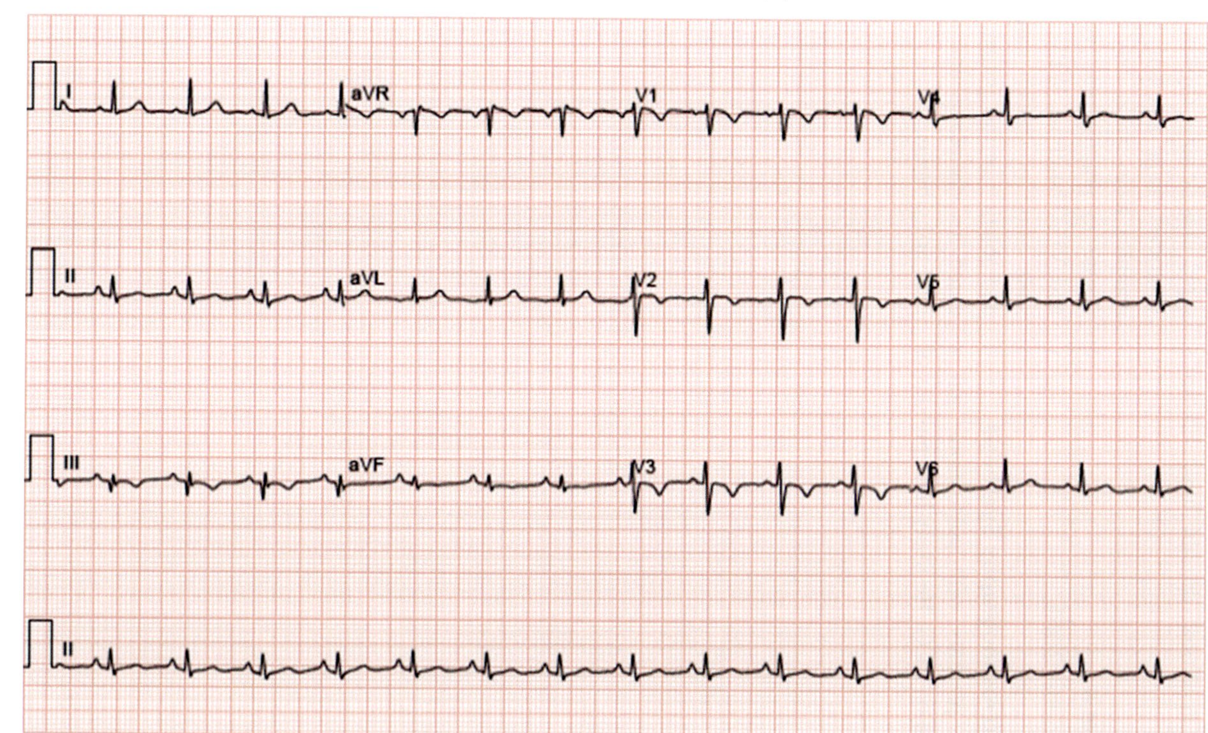

Additional Clinical History
Her past medical history was significant for lower limb venous insufficiency. She was hospitalized with COVID-19 two months before her current admission. She was taking oral contraceptives and was not a smoker. Her father had venous thromboembolism. Blood pressure was 132/71 mmHg, heart rate of 122 bpm, temperature of 36.4 degrees, and oxygen saturation was 95% in room air. She was tachypneic with a respiratory rate of 36 breaths per minute. Heart examination was significant for fast and regular heart sounds with a 2/6 systolic murmur intensified with inhalation. Lung auscultation was clear, examination of her lower limbs did not show signs of deep vein thrombosis, and she had elevated jugular venous pressure

Additional information
Lab work revealed significant leukocytosis, d-dimer of 14,000 ng/mL, hsTnT of 1427 ng/L.

ECG Interpretation

Rhyth: Sinus

Rate: 100 bpm.

Intervals: PR = 180 ms, QRS = 100 ms, QRS = 380 ms, RR = 670 ms, QTC Baz = 464 – normal intervals.

Axis: Normal.

Abnormalities on the ECG

- Sinus Tachycardia
- T-wave inversion V1-V3
- Right atrial abnormality
- Q wave in lead III.

ECG Test Answers

5, 10, 51

ECG Synthesis

The ECG demonstrated T-wave inversion in leads V1-V3 and right atrial abnormality due to right sided strain. Transthoracic echocardiography demonstrate decreased LV systolic function with a severely dilated right ventricle with evidence of pressure and volume overload. Since the patient's biomarkers (hsTnI) were positive, he is considered an intermediate high risk pulmonary embolism and was treated with catheter directed therapy with a bolus of 3 mg of tPA and a continuous infusion of 1 mg per hour.

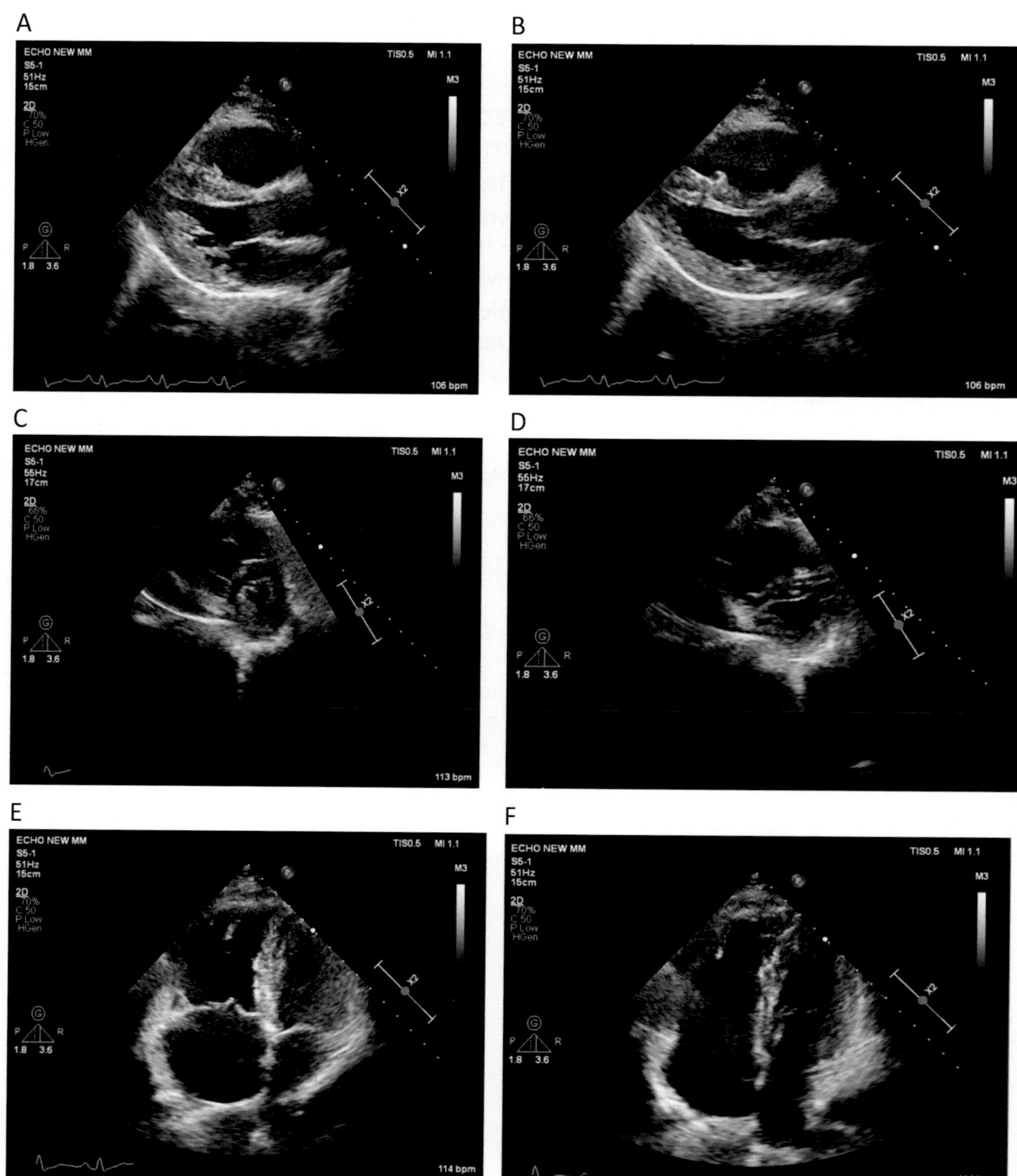

Transthoracic parasternal long axis imaging in systole (A) and diastole (B). Transthoracic parasternal short axis imaging in systole (C) and diastole (D). Apical 4-chambers imaging in systole (E) and diastole (F)

Echo Interpretation

Transthoracic parasternal long axis imaging in systole (A) and diastole (B) demonstrates decreased LV systolic function. Parasternal short axis imaging in systole (C) and diastole (D) showed severe dilatation of all segments of the right ventricle with septal flattening in systole and diastole suggesting volume and pressure overload. Apical 4-chamber imaging in systole (E) and diastole (F) shows reduced LV systolic function, and reconfirms the dilatation and decreased systolic function of the right ventricle.

Echo Synthesis

Echo images demonstrate reduced LV systolic function and a severely dilated right ventricle, with evidence of pressure and volume overload.

Cardiac Electrosonography Synthesis

This patient, presenting with sudden onset shortness of breath and palpitations, has signs of right sided strain on ECG and echocardiography.

The differential diagnosis includes pulmonary embolism. Ischemia is also a possibility. The presence of pressure overload on the right ventricle suggests pulmonary embolism. CT eventually confirmed the diagnosis of pulmonary embolism.

Clinical History

Clinical History

A 79-year-old female presented to the emergency department with syncope witnessed at home after a short walk in the park.

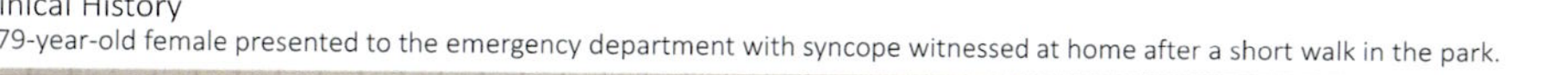

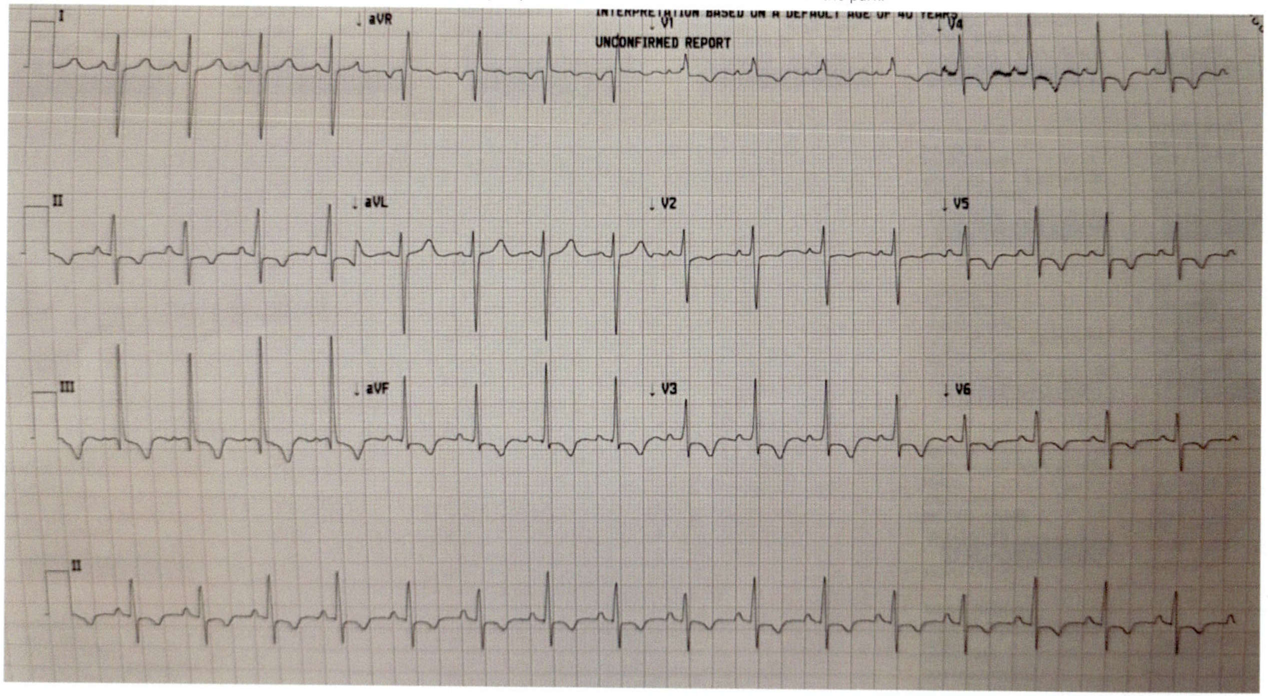

Additional Clinical History

The emergency medical team arrived at the scene and found the patient conscious, but they could not obtain a measurable systolic blood pressure. On arrival to the emergency department, the patient's condition deteriorated. She became bradycardic and hypotensive and eventually progressed to asystolic cardiac arrest.
Cardiopulmonary resuscitation (CPR), including advanced medical therapy with adrenaline, calcium gluconate, and sodium bicarbonate, was initiated followed by return of spontaneous circulation (ROSC).

ECG Interpretation

Rhythm: Sinus

Rate: 100 bpm.

Intervals: PR = 170 ms, QRS = 105 ms, QT = 370 ms, RR = 670 ms, QTC Baz = 452 – normal intervals.

Axis: Right axis deviation.

Abnormalities on the ECG

- Right axis deviation
- Diffuse T-wave inversion
- ST depression in leads II, aVF, V3-6.
- S1Q3T3 sign

ECG Test Answers

10, 38, 51, 77.

ECG Synthesis

The ECG demonstrated diffuse T-wave inversion with ST depression in leads II, aVF and V3-6. The combination known as 'S1Q3T3' is a well known sign of pulmonary embolism. It is not very sensitive (if it does not exist, PE is not ruled out) but in an appropriate clinical setting it should raise the suspicion of PE. The significance of diffuse T wave depression in this ECG is not clear but is probably a marker of severity. Ischemia may also be considered.

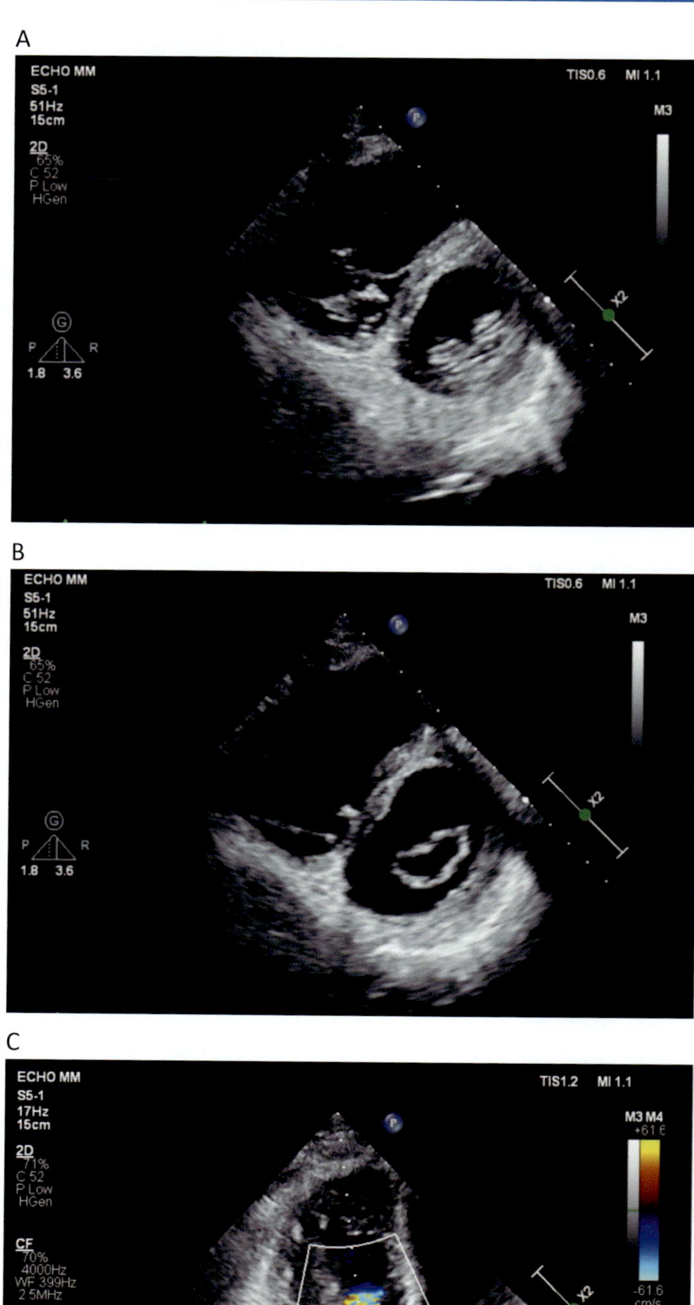

Transthoracic parasternal short axis imaging in systole (A) and diastole (B). Apical 4- chambers imaging in systole (C)

Echo Interpretation

Transthoracic parasternal short axis imaging in systole (A) and diastole (B) showed severe dilatation of all segments of the right ventricle with septal flattening in systole and diastole suggesting volume and pressure overload. Apical 4-chamber imaging in systole (C) shows reduced LV systolic function, confirming the dilatation and decreased systolic function of the right ventricle and severe tricuspid regurgitation.

Echo Synthesis

Bedside echo images demonstrate reduced LV systolic function with a severely dilated right ventricle. There is evidence of pressure and volume overload and tricuspid regurgitation.

Cardiac Electrosonography Synthesis

This patient presented with shock, the ECG showed sinus tachycardia and signs of right sided strain on the ECG.

The differential diagnosis includes ischemia and pulmonary embolism. The presence of pressure overload on the right ventricle is also evident by acute severe tricuspid regurgitation. The pulmonary embolism response team was activated for consideration of immediate reperfusion strategy.

References

Albleihed L, Al-Salameh T. Wide complex tachycardias. Emerg Med Clin North Am. 2022;40(4):733–53.

Brugada J, et al. 2019 ESC Guidelines for the management of patients with supraventricular tachycardia. Eur Heart J. 2020;41(5):655–720.

Brugada J, et al. 2019 ESC Guidelines for the management of patients with supraventricular tachycardia. Eur Heart J. 2020;41(5):655–720.

Pulmonary Embolism, Springer, 2022, p. 269–287.

Goudis CA, et al. Electrocardiographic abnormalities and cardiac arrhythmias in chronic obstructive pulmonary disease. Int J Cardiol. 2015;15(199):264–73.

Kahle AK, et al. Management of ventricular tachycardia in patients with ischemic cardiomyopathy: contemporary armamentarium. Europace. 2022;24(4):538–51.

Lerman BB, et al. Idiopathic right ventricular outflow tract tachycardia: a clinical approach. Pacing Clin Electrophysiol. 1996;19(12 Pt 1):2120–37.

Nelson WP. Diagnostic and prognostic implications of surface recordings from patients with atrioventricular block. Card Electrophysiol Clin. 2016;8(1):25–35.

Orzan F, et al. Associated cardiac lesions in patients with radiation-induced complete heart block. Int J Cardiol 1993 PMID 8314649

Pollak A, Falk RH. Pacemaker therapy in patients with atrial fibrillation. Am Heart J. 1993;125:824–30.

Rahamim E, et al. Illustrative Cases of Multimodality Imaging in the Diagnosis and Management of Pulmonary Embolism. In: Herzog E, editor., et al., Pulmonary Embolism. Springer; 2022. p. 269–87.

Eldad Rahamim et al. Illustrative Cases of Multimodality Imaging in the Diagnosis and Management of Pulmonary Embolism, In: Eyal Herzog Editor,

Rohde JM, et al. Inpatient management of acute atrial fibrillation and atrial flutter in non-pregnant hospitalized patients. Michigan Medicine University of Michigan 2021.

Sawhney NS, et al. Diagnosis and management of typical atrial flutter. Cardiol Clin. 2009;27(1):55–67.

Clinical Cases of Electrosonography in Patients with Neurological Symptoms

David Leibowitz, Muhamed Saric,
Sophia Dongas, Megan Job, Yair Elitzur,
and Eyal Herzog

Abstract

In this chapter the authors provide representative cases of patients presenting to health care system with clinical complaints of neurologic symptoms. Acute neurologic events may have a cardiac source and the use of cardiac electrosonography in the evaluation of these challenging patients is demonstrated in a variety of clinical scenarios.

Keywords

ECG · Echocardiography · Cerebrovascular accident · Embolism · Congestive heart failure · Atrial fibrillation · Myxoma

D. Leibowitz (✉) · Y. Elitzur · E. Herzog
The Heart Institute Department of Cardiology
Hadassah Medical Center, Hebrew University
of Jerusalem, Jerusalem, Israel
e-mail: oleibo@hadassah.org.il

M. Saric · S. Dongas · M. Job
Leon H. Charney Division of Cardiology, New York
University School of Medicine, 560 First Avenue,
New York, NY, USA

A 62-year-old woman with a history of hypertension and mitral valve replacement with a bioprothesis presented to the emergency department with new-onset left-sided weakness.

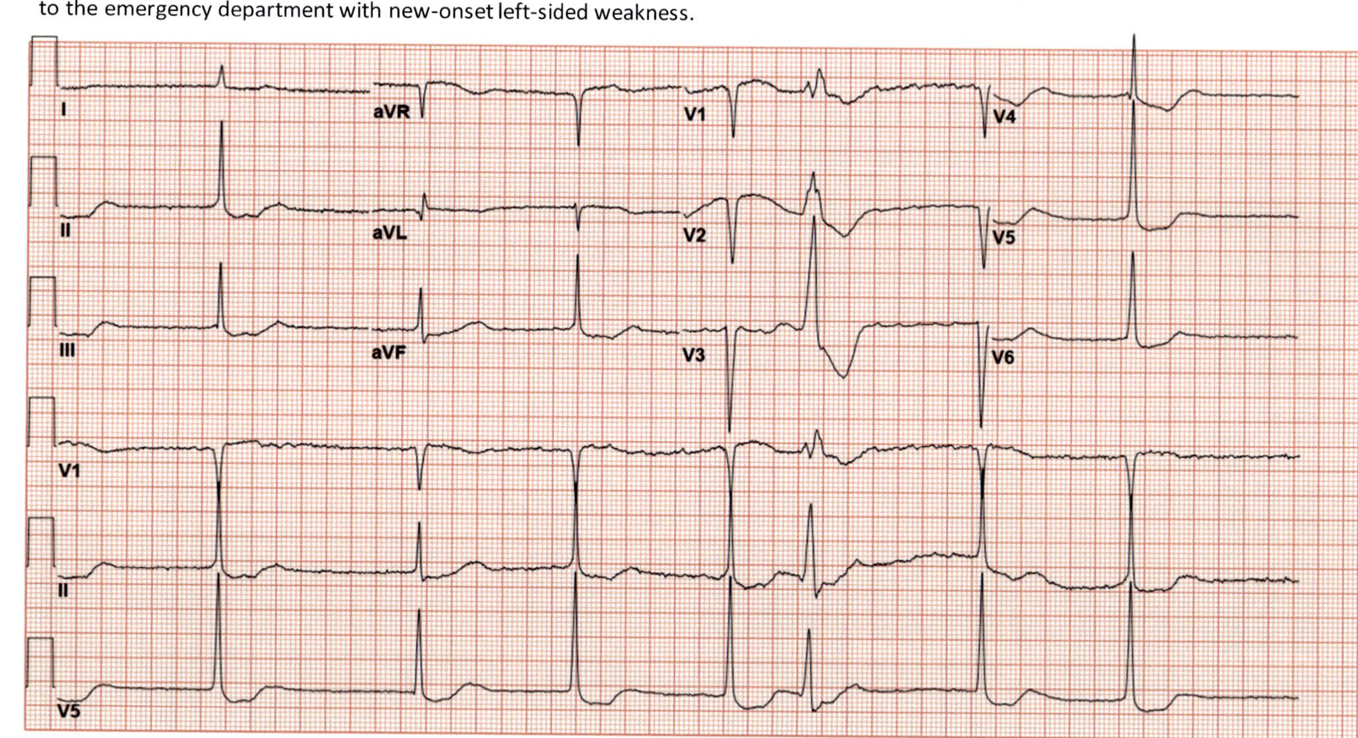

Additional Clinical History

In addition to neurologic findings, her physical exam was remarkable for irregular pulse and bradycardia.

Additional Information

Urgent computed tomography (CT) of the brain revealed no intracranial hemorrhage. Brain MRI revealed multiple strokes in multiple vascular territories of various age

ECG Interpretation

Rhythm: Atrial fibrillation with a premature ventricular complex.
Rate: 50 bpm.
Intervals: PR not measurable due to Afib, QRS 92 ms; QTc = 453 ms.
Axis: Normal.

ECG Abnormalities

- Anteroseptal infarct, age undetermined.
- Minimal voltage criteria for LVH, may be normal variant diffuse ST abnormalities.

ECG Test Answers
18, 22, 40, 68, 77.

ECG Synthesis
The ECG demonstrated atrial fibrillation with slow ventricular response (bradycardia at 50 bpm), a finding probably related to the history of hypertension and mitral valve disease. The premature ventricular complex is a non-specific finding which is common in many types of cardiac pathology but may occur in a normal left ventricle as well. In addition, there are signs of left ventricular hypertrophy with repolarization abnormalities and a possible old anteroseptal infarct.

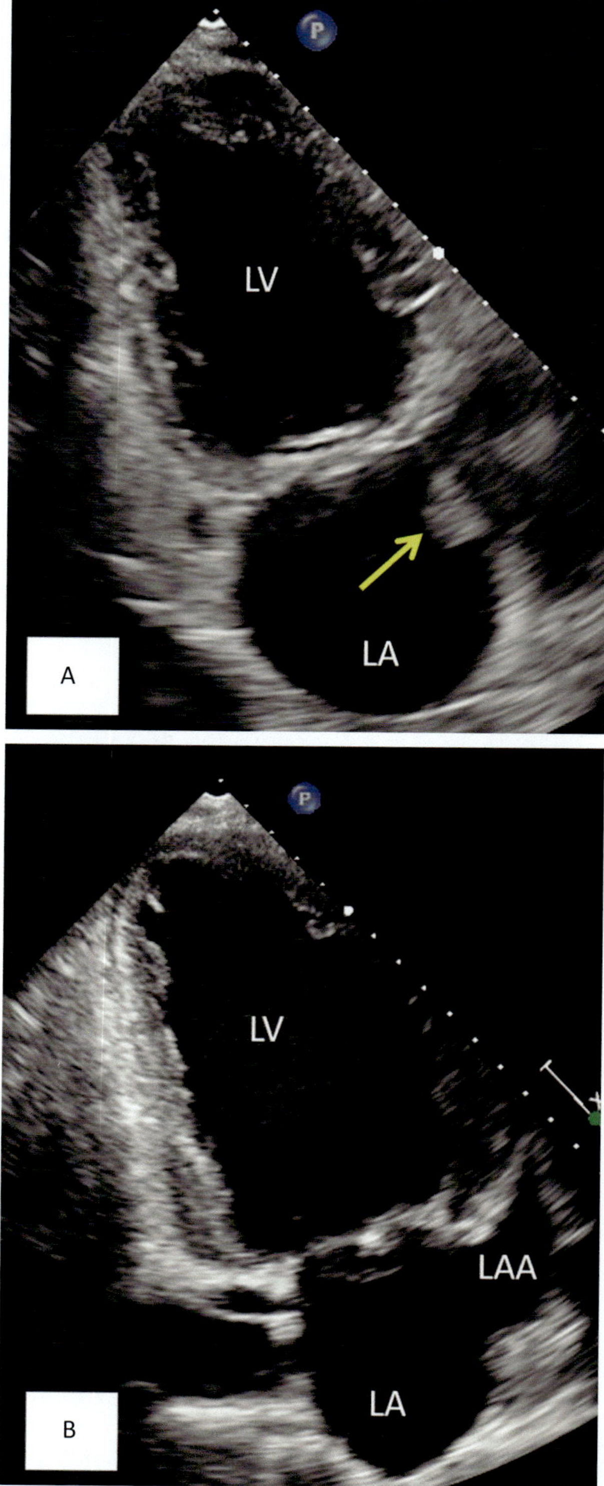

Panel A reveals a large thrombus (arrow) emanating from the left atrial appendage seen on apical 2 chamber view. For comparison, Panel B demonstrates a normal appearance of the left atrial appendage in this view

Echo Interpretation

The echo revealed a dilated left atrium with a large echodensity in the region of the left atrial appendage in the apical 2-chamber view. The prosthetic mitral valve had normal function.

Echo Synthesis

The large mass in the left atrial appendage (LAA) in the setting of atrial fibrillation and brain MRI suggestive of cardioembolic strokes is most consistent with a thrombus.

Cardiac Electrosonography Synthesis

The finding of atrial fibrillation on EKG in a patient presenting with an acute stroke should always raise the possibility of a thromboembolic origin. Brain MRI findings of multiple strokes in multiple vascular territories of various age further support the embolic cause. This suspicion was confirmed by echocardiography. It should be noted that the sensitivity of transthoracic echo for LAA thrombus is low and the diagnosis generally requires transesophageal echo. In nonvalvular atrial fibrillation, the vast majority of thrombi (> 90%) are located in the left atrial appendage.

2 Case 2

A 29-year-old man with a history of bicuspid aortic valve presented to the emergency department with fever, weakness, left upper quadrant abdominal pain and lower extremity edema.

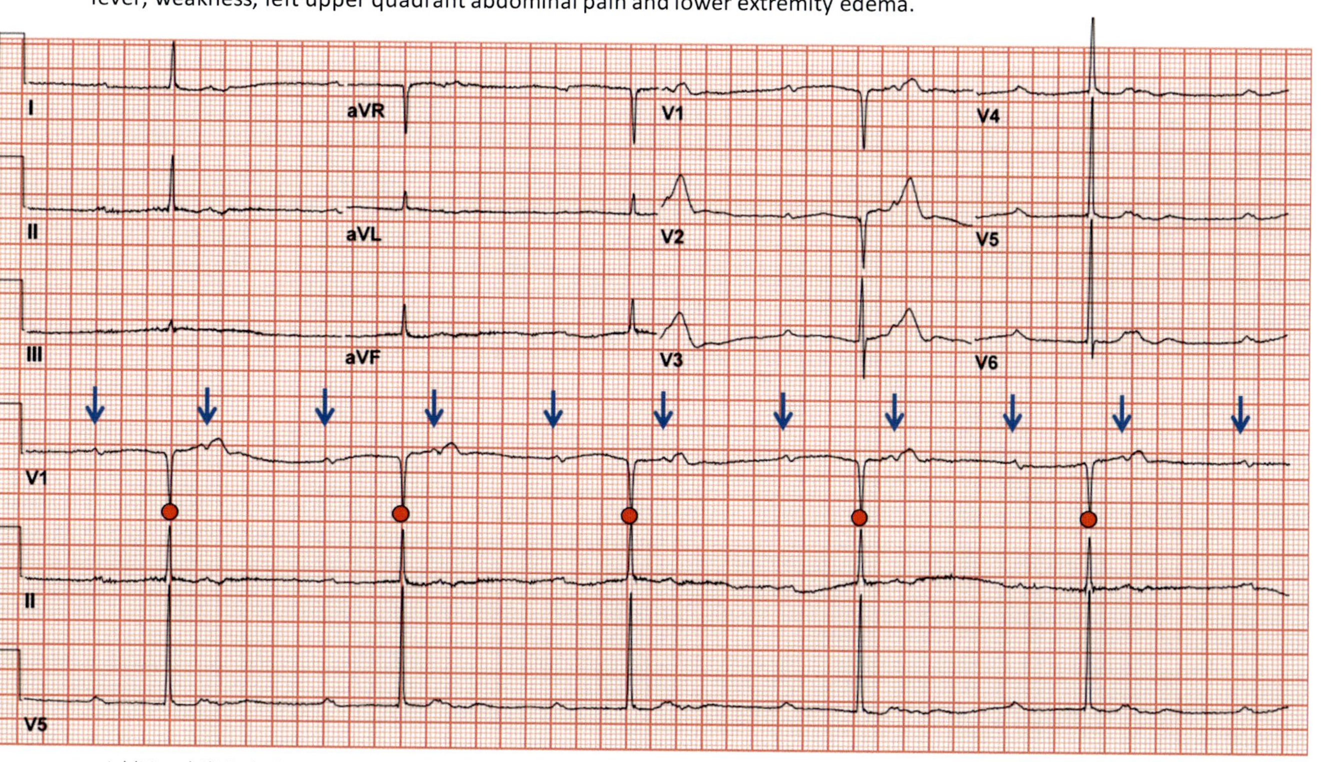

Additional Clinical History

On presentation, four out of four blood cultures promptly grew methicillin sensitive *Staphylococcus aureus*. Laboratory findings demonstrated elevated white blood count, thrombocytopenia and elevated levels of C-reactive protein.

Additional Information

Computed tomography (CT) of the abdomen demonstrated hepatosplenomegaly and multiple splenic and bilateral renal infarcts

ECG Interpretation

Rhythm: Sinus rhythm with complete AV block and a nodal escape rhythm.
Rate: Atrial rate 60 bpm; ventricular rate at 33 bpm.
Intervals: PR not measurable due to AV dissociation, QRS 80 ms; QTc = 374 ms.
Axis: Normal.

ECG Abnormalities

- Complete heart block.
- AV dissociation with an atrial rate of 60 bpm (blue arrows) and ventricular rate at 33 bpm (red dots) Narrow-complex junctional escape rhythm.
- Left ventricular hypertrophy.

ECG Test Answers

7, 32, 34, 40.

ECG Synthesis

The EKG demonstrated complete (3rd degree) atrioventricular block (AVB) with AV dissociation; atria are in sinus rhythm and there is junctional narrow-complex escape rhythm with a slow ventricular rate at 33 bpm. The causes of AVB include degenerative disease of the conduction system, medications which depress conduction such as beta blockers, and ischemic heart disease. AVB in a young patient in the setting of fever and valvular disease suggests the possibility of aortic valve endocarditis with abscess formation and echocardiography should be emergently performed.

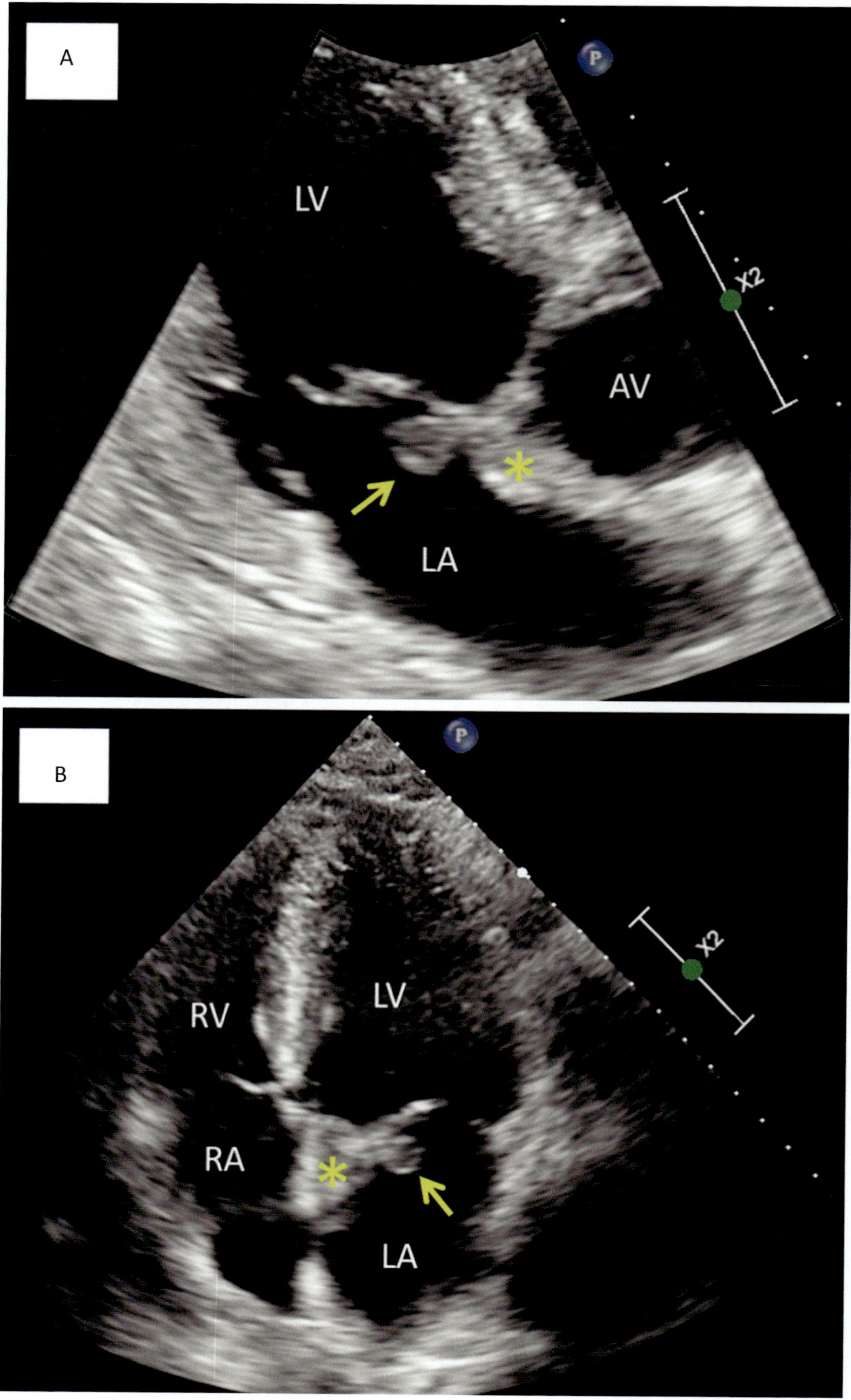

TTE imaging demonstrated a large mobile echodensity adjacent to the aortic valve (asterisk) with extension into the intervalvular fibrosa (arrow) in the parasternal long axis view (panel A) and apical 4-chamber view (Panel B). AV, aortic valve; LA, left atrium; LV, left ventricle; RA, right atrium; RV, right ventricle

Echo Interpretation

TTE imaging demonstrated a large, mobile shaggy echodensity adjacent to the aortic valve with extension into the intervalvular fibrosa (arrow) in the parasternal long axis view and apical 4-chamber view. The native aortic valve was bicuspid with a raphe between the right and non coronary cusps.

Echo Synthesis

Echodensities on echo imaging may represent vegetation, thrombus or primary/secondary tumor. The finding of an echodensity adjacent to a bicuspid aortic valve in a patient with Staphylococcus in multiple blood cultures is highly suggestive of vegetation. The extension into the intervalvular fibrosa is highly suggestive of an abscess.

Cardiac Electrosonography Synthesis

The finding of complete AVB on EKG in a patient presenting with embolic events and aortic valve vegetation should always raise the possibility of an aortic valve abscess. This diagnosis is crucial as it is an indication for prompt referral for cardiac surgery. Although in this case the diagnosis was made on transthoracic echocardiography (TTE) it is not generally a sensitive test for this complication and transesophageal echo is recommended to establish the diagnosis. TEE in this case confirmed the findings on TTE and the patient was referred for emergent surgery.

A 47 year old male with a history of smoking presented to the ED with acute diplopia and difficulty speaking which resolved spontaneously after 20 minutes.

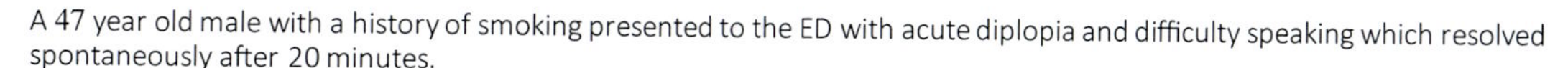

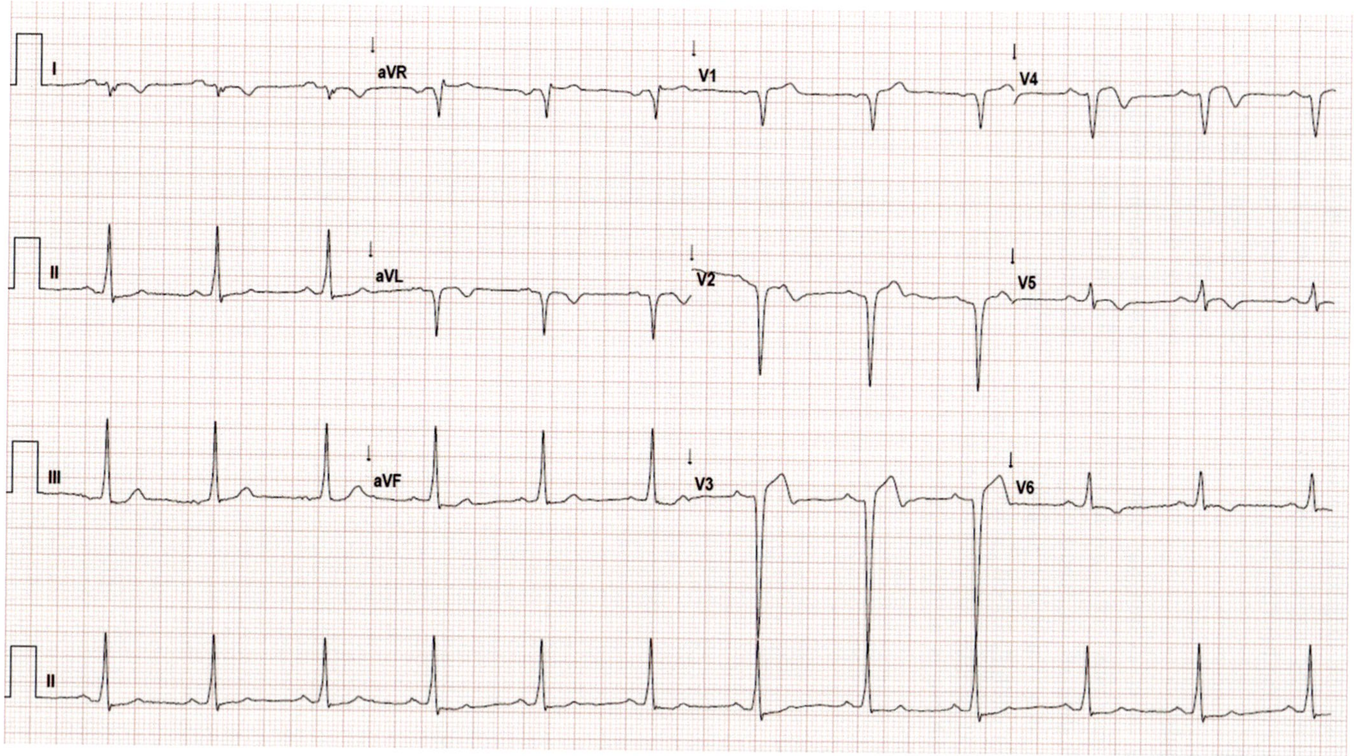

Additional Clinical History

Two months prior to presentation the patient had an acute anterior wall infarction with emergent PCI of the LAD. Echo at that time showed significantly decreased LV function without evidence of LV thrombus.

Additional information

CT angiography did not reveal vascular pathology of the head and neck. MRI diffusion was consistent with a small cerebral infarction.

ECG Interpretation

Rhythm: Sinus
Rate: 70 bpm.
Intervals: PR 170 ms, QRS 70 ms, QTc 390 ms
Axis: normal (+95)

Abnormalities on the ECG

- Q waves in 1,aVL, V1 to V4
- T wave inversion (including biphasic T) in 1, aVL, V2 to V6

ECG Test Answers

7, 66, 68.

ECG Synthesis

This patient has ECG evidence of an extensive anterior wall MI involving the anteroseptum as well as the lateral wall, as evident by q wave distribution and lack of r waves. Lateral wall involvement is demonstrated in leads 1 and aVL more than V5 and V6, where an inverted T wave is the sign of the infarction. The presence of Q waves and t wave inversions suggests an old infarction. This ECG raises the possibility of a complication of extensive anterior wall MI such as left ventricular thrombus as an etiology of the clinical neurologic complaints.

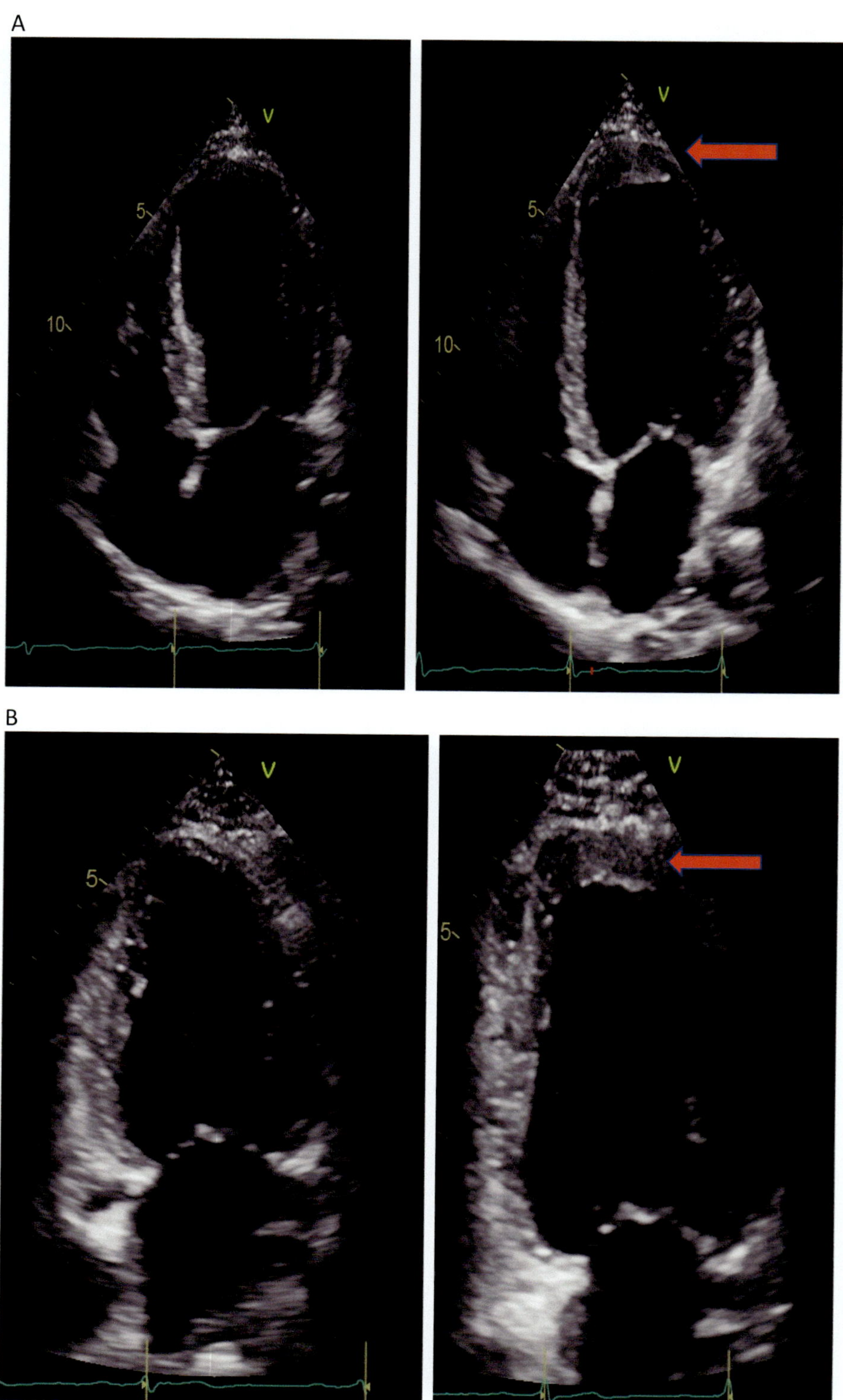

Apical four chamber (A) and apical two chamber (B) views with images from the initial echo performed 2 months earlier on the left and images from the current admission on the right. The arrows indicate a new echodensity on the current study in the area of the akinetic LV apex

Echo Interpretation

Apical four chamber (A) and apical two chamber (B) views with images from the initial echo performed 2 months earlier on the left and images from the current admission on the right. The arrows indicate a new echodensity on the current study in the area of the akinetic LV apex.

Echo Synthesis

The differential diagnosis of an intracardiac echodensity on echo includes thrombus, primary or secondary malignancy or infective material/vegetation. Factors such as clinical history, the echocardiographic appearance and importantly the location of the finding are helpful to determine the etiology. In this case, the clinical history of recent anterior wall infarction and the location of the echodensity in the infarcted area was highly suggestive of intracardiac thrombus.

Cardiac Electrosonography Synthesis

In this patient, electrosonography revealed evidence on ECG of a old extensive anterior wall myocardial infarction. The recent clinical history of anterior wall MI and the ECG findings in a young patient with a new cerebrovascular event raised the clinical suspicion of cardioembolic stroke due to left ventricular thrombus. The finding on emergency echo of a new echodensity in the area of the akinetic LV apex confirmed this clinical suspicion and the patient was started on anticoagulation therapy with resolution of the echocardiographic finding.

A 43 year old female with no past medical history presented to the ED with parasthesias and weakness in her left upper extremity which resolved after 30 minutes.

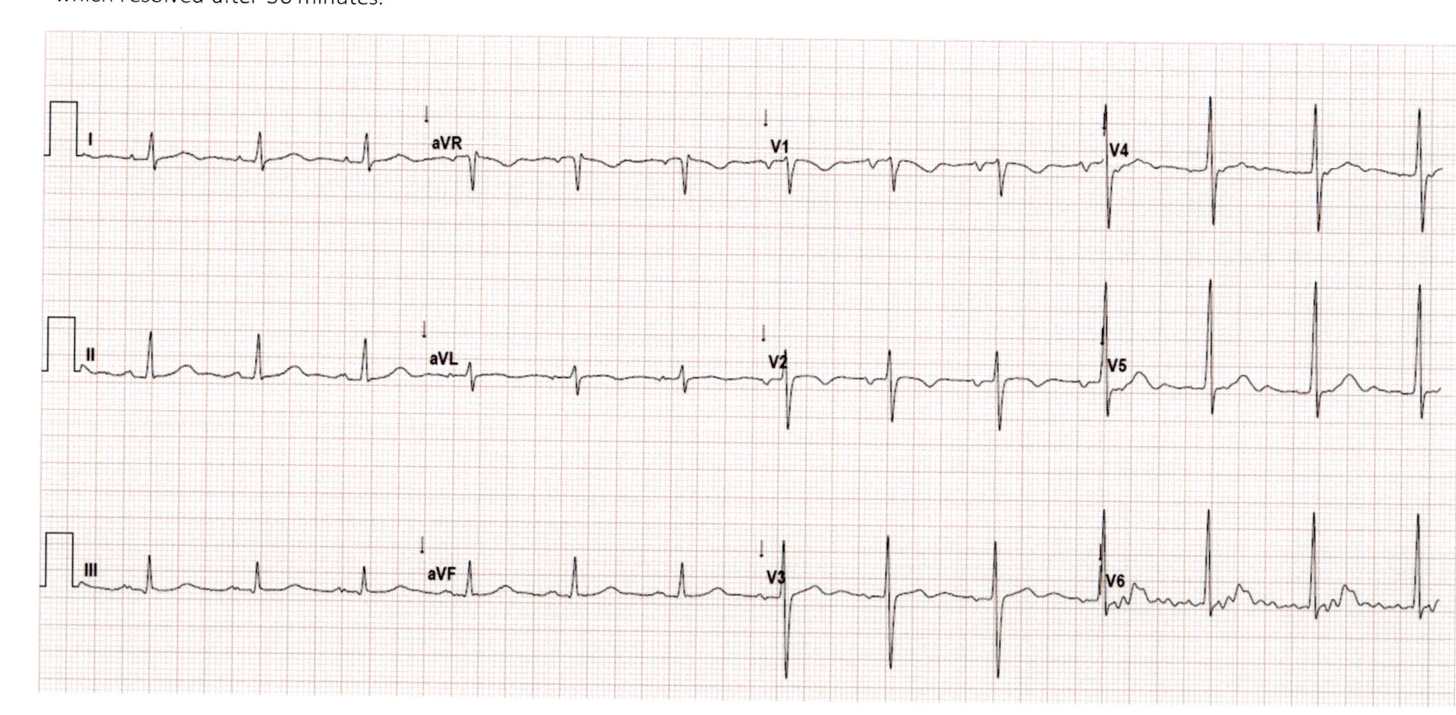

Additional Clinical History

On physical exam an additional heart sound early in diastole was noted with a short diastolic murmur.

Additional information

CT angiography did not reveal vascular pathology of the head and neck. MRI diffusion was consistent with two small cerebral infarctions in distinct vascular territories.

ECG Interpretation

Rhythm: Sinus.
Rate: 77 bpm.
Intervals: PR 148 ms, QRS 100 ms, QTC 431 ms.
Axis: Normal.

Abnormalities on the ECG

Possible LA enlargement (negative p wave in V1 deeper than 1 mm and wider than 40 ms).

ECG Test Answers

6, 7

ECG Synthesis

In this patient the ECG shows possible left atrial abnormality. It is only evident in lead V1 and not in lead II.

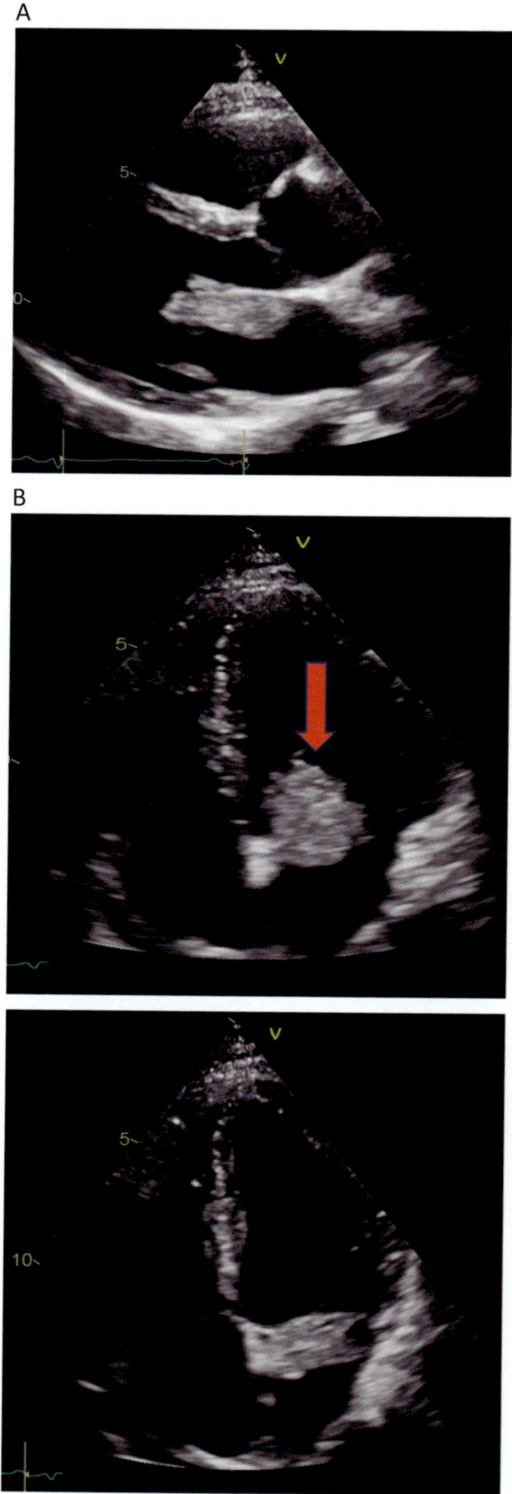

Parasternal long axis (panel A) and apical 4 chamber views (panel B) clearly depict a large echodensity in the left atrium with diastolic prolapse into the left ventricle (top image, arrow) which appears to originate from the left atrial aspect of the interatrial septum

Echo Interpretation

Parasternal long axis and apical 4 chamber views clearly depict a large echodensity in the left atrium with diastolic prolapse into the left ventricle (arrow) which appears to originate from the left atrial aspect of the interatrial septum.

Echo Synthesis

The differential diagnosis of an intracardiac echodensity on echo includes thrombus, primary or secondary malignancy or infective material/ vegetation. The location of the highly mobile echodensity on the interatrial septum is typical for cardiac myxoma. This region is not susceptible to formation of thrombus or vegetation and so these diagnoses would be highly unlikely to explain the finding.

Cardiac Electrosonography Synthesis

In this patient, ECG findings of possible left atrial enlargement in the absence of other obvious cardiac disease on the ECG, suggested pathology involving the left atrium. This was confirmed on emergent echo with findings consistent with a large myxoma in the left atrium presumably responsible for the multiple embolic events seen on MRI imaging. The finding on cardiac exam is consistent with a "tumor plop" caused by diastolic obstruction of the mitral annulus by the left atrial mass. The patient was referred to cardiothoracic surgery for excision of the myxoma.

A 67 year old male with a history atrial fibrillation and chronic ischemic heart disease presented with one hour of difficulty speaking and right arm weakness

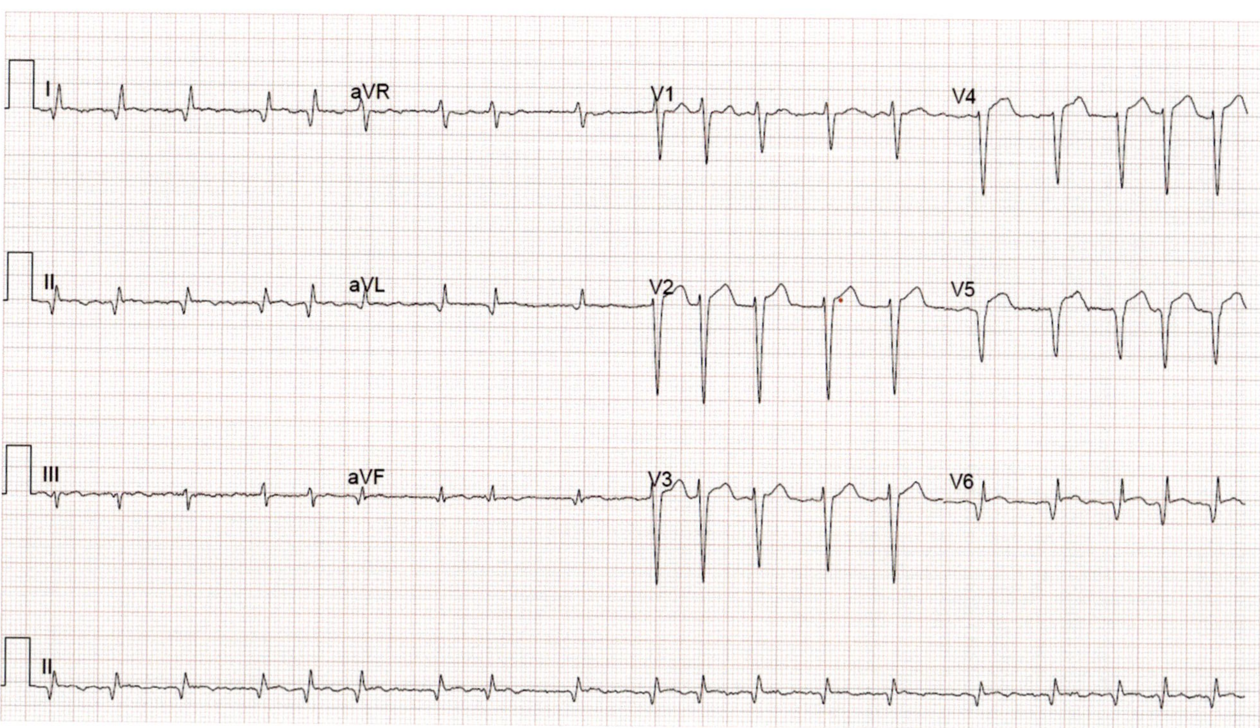

Additional Clinical History

Two months prior to presentation the patient had an episode of gastrointestinal bleeding and anticoagulation was stopped.

Additional information

Pulse was irregular with a blood pressure of 150/110 mmHg. MRI diffusion was consistent with cerebral infarction.

ECG Interpretation

Rhythm: Atrial fibrillation.
Rate: 110 bpm.
Intervals: QRS = 110 ms, QTc = 400 ms.
Axis: Normal.

Abnormalities on the ECG

- Old extensive anterior wall MI
- Poor R wave progression (r wave in V3 < 3 mm)
- Q wave in 1,2, aVL, V5, V6
- Atrial fibrillation

ECG Test Answers
18, 66, 68, 70, 79.

ECG Synthesis
In the context of a search for possible sources of emboli, the ECG in this patient raises two possible sources:

- Atrial fibrillation giving rise to a left atrial thrombus.
- Prior extensive anterior wall myocardial infarction, suggesting the possibility of a left ventricular mural thrombus.

The extent of infarction in this case requires some discussion. There is clear evidence of lateral wall involvement, manifest in the ECG as pathologic Q waves (deeper than 2 mm and wider than 40 ms, greater in voltage than 0.25 of the R wave) in V6. Pathologic Q waves are obviously found in V5, as well as L1 and aVL. Poor R wave progression (r wave smaller than 3 mm in V3) is suggestive of anteroseptal involvement. These findings define the infarction as 'extensive'. However, there is also a Q wave in limb lead II. This wave, although not large, fulfills in itself the criteria for 'pathologic Q wave'. Nevertheless, there is no consistent Q wave in leads III or aVF; the Q wave in not to be found in two contiguous leads. We therefore do not regard it as a definite sign of inferior wall infarction.

Echocardiography is needed to clarify the extent of infarction, the extent of damage to left ventricular systolic function, and the presence of a ventricular or atrial clot as a source of emboli. This patient will require anticoagulant treatment regardless of the findings on echo, since he has atrial fibrillation and is at high risk of embolus (has a high CHADSVASC score). Nevertheless, the finding or ruling out of thrombus will have implications on the possibility to treat the arrhythmia by anti arrhythmic drugs, cardioversion or ablation.

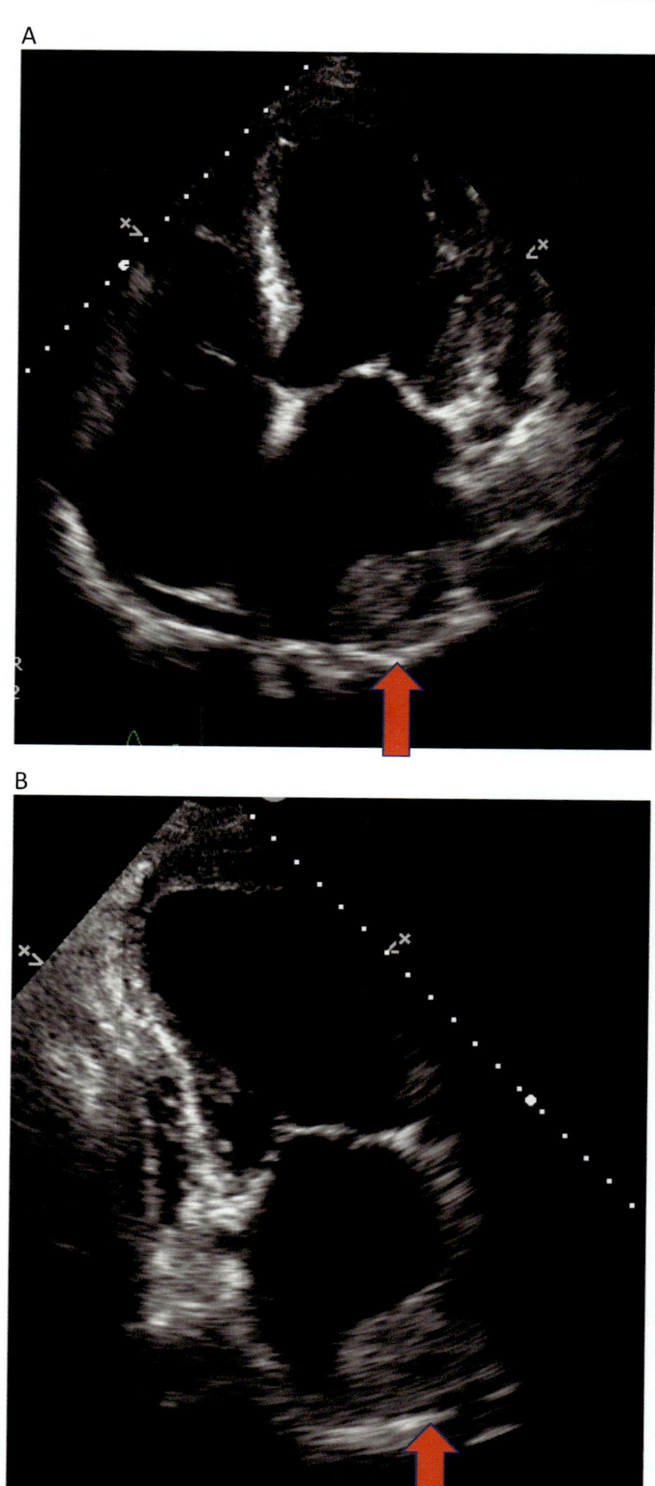

Apical four chamber (A) and apical two chamber (B) views of the echocardiogram performed which demonstrate a large echodensity in the base of the left atrium. The arrows highlight this echodensity, which shows a broad attachment to the left atrial free wall

Echo Interpretation

Apical four chamber (A) and apical two chamber (B) views demonstrate a large echodensity in the body of the left atrium with a broad attachment to the left atrial free wall.

Echo Synthesis

The differential diagnosis of an intracardiac echodensity on echo includes thrombus, primary or secondary malignancy or infective material/vegetation. Factors such as clinical history, the echocardiographic appearance and importantly the location of the finding are helpful to determine the etiology. In this case, the clinical history of atrial fibrillation with recent stoppage of anticoagulant therapy and the location of the echodensity in the left atrium were most consistent with a diagnosis of left atrial thrombus.

Cardiac Electrosonography Synthesis

In this hypertensive patient the differential diagnosis of the neurologic event included hypertensive crisis as well as ischemic or cardioembolic stroke with major implications for treatment. Using "electrosonography", the ECG revealed evidence of atrial fibrillation with an old extensive anterior wall myocardial infarction, raising the possibility of either a left ventricular or left atrial thrombus. Although the sensitivity of transthoracic echocardiography for left atrial thrombus is low, in our patient the finding of an echodensity in left atrium in a patient with atrial fibrillation and no anticoagulant therapy established the likely diagnosis of cardioembolic stroke and the patient was started on anticoagulation therapy with resolution of the echocardiographic finding.

References

Camaj A, et al. Left ventricular thrombus following acute myocardial infarction. J Am Coll Cardiol. 2022;79:1010–22.

Griborio-Guzman AG, et al. Cardiac myxoma: clinical presentation, diagnosis and management. Heart. 2022;108:827–33.

Saric M, Armour AC, Arnaout MS, Chaudhry FA, Grimm RA, Kronzon I, Landeck BF, Maganti K, Michelena HI, Tolstrup K. Guidelines for the use of echocardiography in the evaluation of a cardiac source of embolism. J Am Soc Echocardiogr. 2016;29(1):1–42.

Suwa et al. Atrial fibrillation and stroke: importance of left atrium as assessed by echocardiography. J Echocardiography. 2022;20:69–76.

Clinical Cases of Electrosonography in Adult Congenital Heart Disease

Dan G. Halpern, Adam J. Small, Yair Elitzur, Eyal Herzog, and David Leibowitz

Abstract

The revolutionary survival of patients with congenital heart disease (CHD) into adulthood demands familiarity with the most common congenital heart lesions. This chapter provides examples of adult CHD cases and caveats based on history, physical exam, ECG and transthoracic echocardiography that would improve mastery in identification and management of CHD cases.

Keywords

ECG · Echocardiography · Electrosonography · Congenital heart disease · Adult congenital heart disease · Shunts · Cyanosis · Endocardial cushion defects · Tetralogy of Fallot · Atrial septal defect · Ventricular septal defect · Pulmonary hypertension · Eisenmenger syndrome · Ebstein anomaly

D. G. Halpern (✉) · A. J. Small
Adult Congenital Heart Disease, NYU Grossman School of Medicine, NYU Langone Health, New York, USA
e-mail: Dan.Halpern@nyulangone.org

Y. Elitzur · E. Herzog · D. Leibowitz
The Heart Institute, Department of Cardiology, Hadassah Medical Center, Hebrew University of Jerusalem, Jerusalem, Israel

1 Case 1

A 30 year-old woman was noted to have an abnormal EKG during preoperative evaluation prior to gynecological surgery

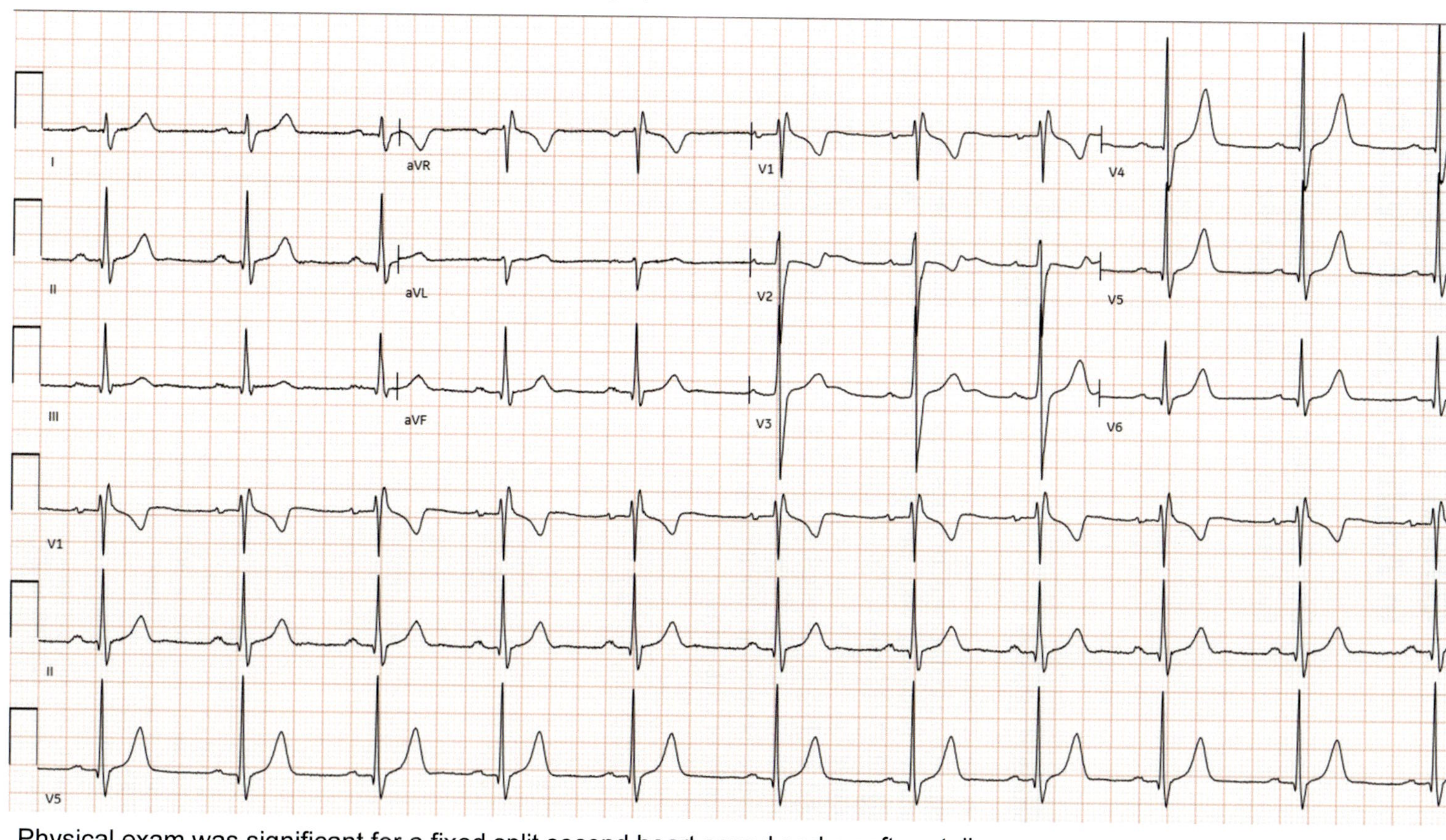

Physical exam was significant for a fixed split second heart sound and a soft systolic murmur

- ECG interpretation
  - Sinus rhythm
  - 63 bpm
  - PR 188 ms, QRS 114 ms, QTc 382 ms

- Abnormalities on the ECG
  - Incomplete right bundle branch block
  - Right axis deviation

- ECG test answers
  - 7, 38, 58

- ECG synthesis
  - This ECG shows right axis deviation. Causes include normal variation, syndromes causing acute or chronic right ventricular overload, and conduction defect (left posterior fascicular block). The finding of incomplete right bundle branch block supports a diagnosis of right ventricular overload in this patient and echocardiography was performed prior to the planned procedure.

A

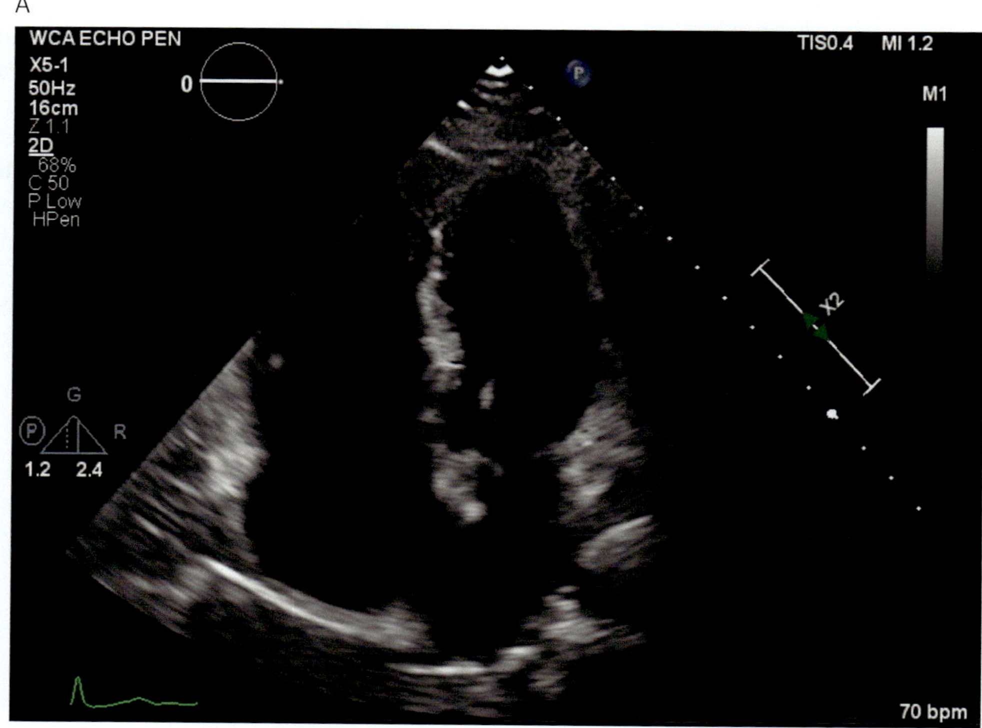

B

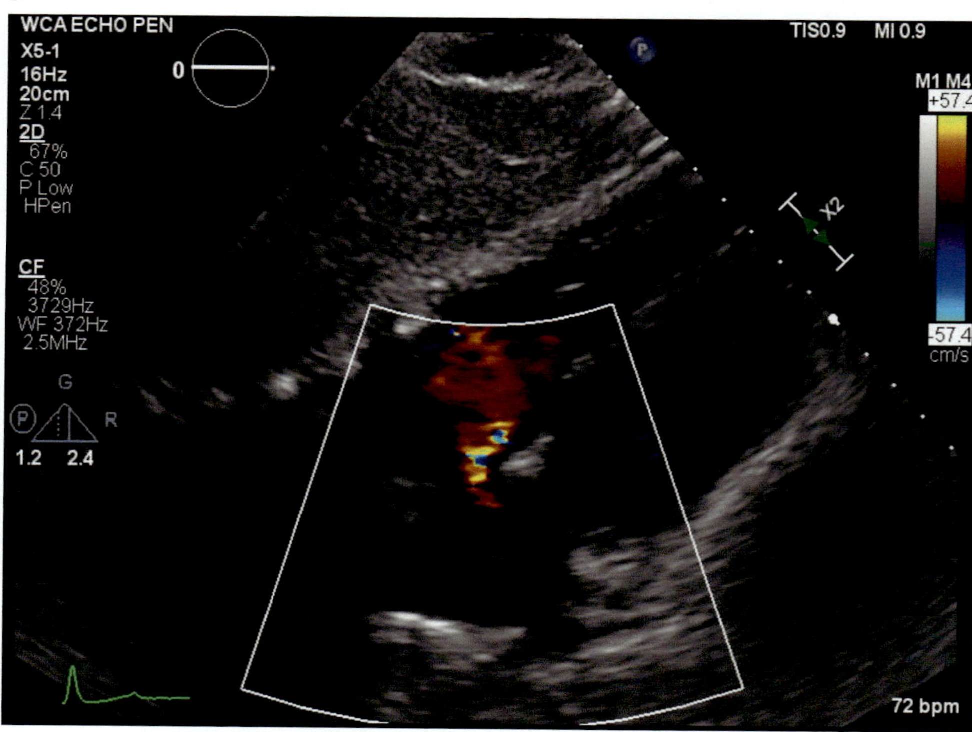

Panel A shows an apical 4 chamber view with an enlarged right atrium and right ventricle. Panel B is a subcostal view showing a color Doppler jet from the left atrium through the intertrial septum into the right atrium

Echo Interpretation

Generally in the apical 4 chamber view, the width of the right ventricle (RV) should be about 2/3rds of the width of the left ventricle. In the apical 4 chamber image presented in panel A the RV diameter is clearly wider than that of the LV, consistent with RV enlargement. The echo dropout seen in the middle of the interatrial septum is common and should not be considered diagnostic of atrial septal defect without corroborating color Doppler evidence of an atrial septal defect. The finding of atrial septal defect is confirmed by the subcostal image seen in panel B, which demonstrates a color flow jet traversing the interatrial septum.

Echo Synthesis

The findings of RV dilatation along with color Doppler flow through the inter-atrial septum is consistent with an ostium secundum atrial septal defect with a hemodynamically significant left to right shunt.

Cardiac Electrosonography Synthesis

The right axis on routine preoperative ECG suggested the possibility of RV overload, a finding confirmed by the echo which established secundum ASD, the most common type of ASD, as the diagnosis. The finding of incomplete RBBB is consistent with this diagnosis as well. Ostium primum ASD generally presents with left axis deviation on ECG. Given the presence of right sided enlargement suggestive of hemodynamically significant shunt, this ASD should be closed either percutaneously or surgically after ruling out significant pulmonary hypertension.

2 Case 2

A 19 year old male presented with an acute stroke and a resting O2 saturation of 85% on room air.

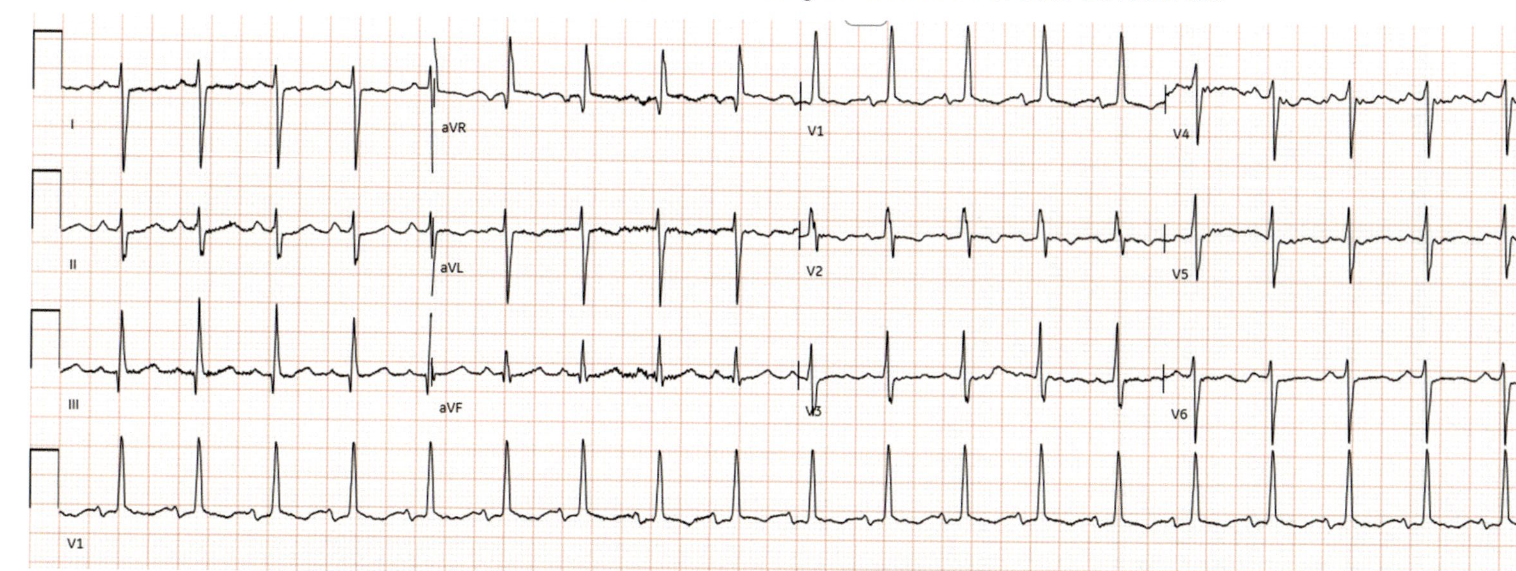

Physical exam was significant for central cyanosis, clubbed fingernails and on heart auscultation an accentuated second heart sound without murmurs.

ECG interpretation

Rhythm: Sinus tachycardia.

Rate: 115 bpm.

Intervals: PR 146 ms, QRS 78 ms, QTc 334 ms.

Axis: Right axis.

Abnormalities on the ECG

Sinus tachycardia.

Right axis deviation.

Right ventricular hypertrophy with repolarization changes.

Non specific ST-T changes.

ECG Test Answers

5, 10, 38, 41, 81

ECG Synthesis

This ECG shows sinus tachycardia with right axis deviation (RAD) and right ventricular hypertrophy (RVH). RVH is diagnosed when there is RAD as well as R/S ratio > 1 or the R > 7 mm in lead V1. Increased R/S ratio may also be seen in posterior infarcts, right bundle branch blocks, lead misplacement and Wolf-Parkinson- White syndrome. The presence of a right bundle branch block or right atrial dilatation may be supportive of right sided heart involvement. Conditions where RVH pattern is diagnosed include cor pulmonale, pulmonary hypertension, congenital heart disease, pulmonary embolism, valvular diseases affecting the right heart (e.g. mitral/pulmonary/tricuspid valve disease) and other pulmonary diseases (e.g. chronic obstructive pulmonary disease, sarcoidosis, obstructive sleep apnea).

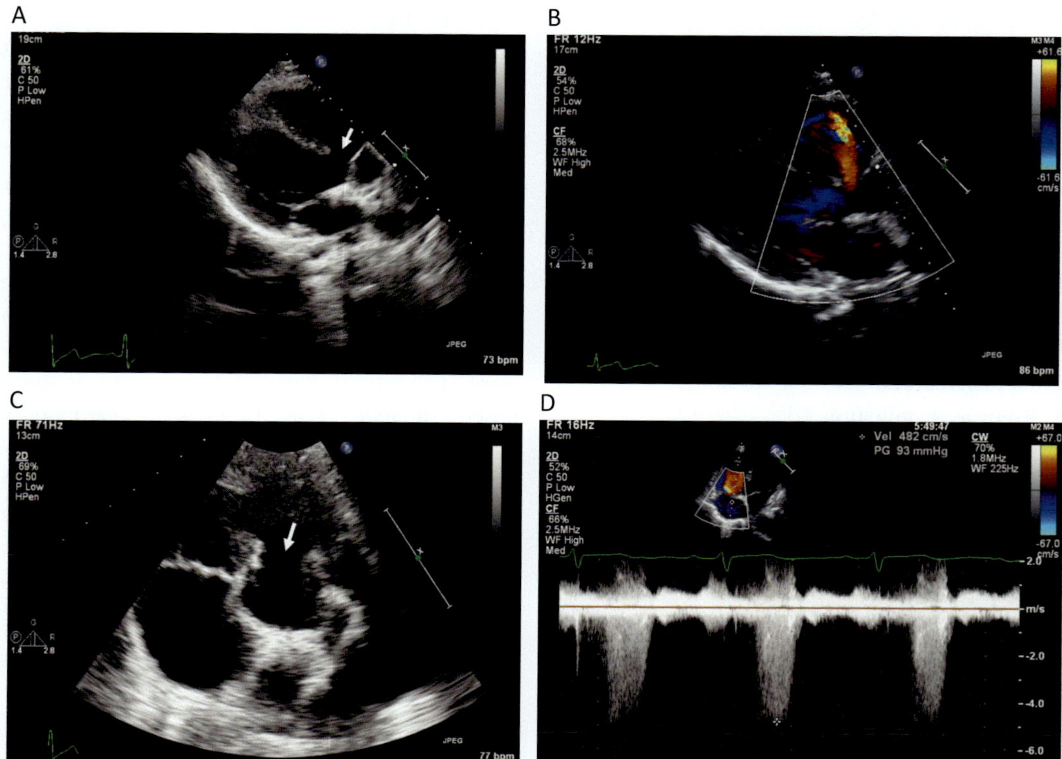

Panel A shows a parasternal long axis view with a large ventricular septal defect (VSD) below the aortic valve (arrow). Panel B shows the same image with color Doppler demonstrating predominately right to left shunt though the VSD. Panel C is a parasternal short-axis view showing the missing septum from the membranous area (10 o'clock) extending toward the outlet area (2 o'clock) (arrow). Panel D shows an elevated tricuspid regurgitation jet (4.8 m/s) consistent with severe pulmonary hypertension

Echo Interpretation

There is a large ventricular septal defect (VSD) with bidirectional flow—predominantly right to left (since right-to-left shunt results in cyanosis). It extends from the membranous septum (10 o'clock on the short axis view) extending to the outlet septum (2 o'clock; outlet VSD is also referred to as doubly committed or supra-cristal). There was also evidence of right atrial enlargement and a hypertrophied and enlarged right ventricle with evidence of pulmonary hypertension.

Echo Synthesis

The echo revealed a large membranous-outlet VSD with predominantly right to left shunting and evidence of pulmonary hypertension in a cyanotic patient. Prior to the development of pulmonary hypertension, VSDs through left-to-right shunting cause left sided heart enlargement. Ultimately, with the development of fixed pulmonary vascular disease, the shunt reverses causing cyanosis, and the right ventricle enlarges and hypertrophies. This syndrome is referred to as Eisenmenger syndrome. The clinical implications of VSDs could be judged by the velocities across them—small restrictive have elevated systolic velocities and less likely to develop pulmonary hypertension, whereas large non-restrictive ones (such as in this case) have low velocities and are prone to develop pulmonary vascular disease. Of note, the tricuspid regurgitation jet may be contaminated by the VSD jet and can be misleading when estimating right ventricular systolic pressure.

Cardiac Electrosonography Synthesis

The ECG demonstrates right ventricular hypertrophy and the echo confirms right ventricular enlargement and hypertrophy as well as pulmonary hypertension in the setting of a large VSD. The clinical scenario is consistent with Eisenmenger syndrome with a large unrestrictive VSD resulting in cyanosis and susceptibility to right to left shunt embolic complications such as stroke. The patient underwent cardiac catheterization that confirmed elevated pulmonary vascular resistance and was placed on advanced pulmonary hypertension therapies and anticoagulation.

3 Case 3

A 49 year-old woman reports being a "blue baby" and having heart surgery in infancy. She presents for a year of progressive dyspnea on exertion.

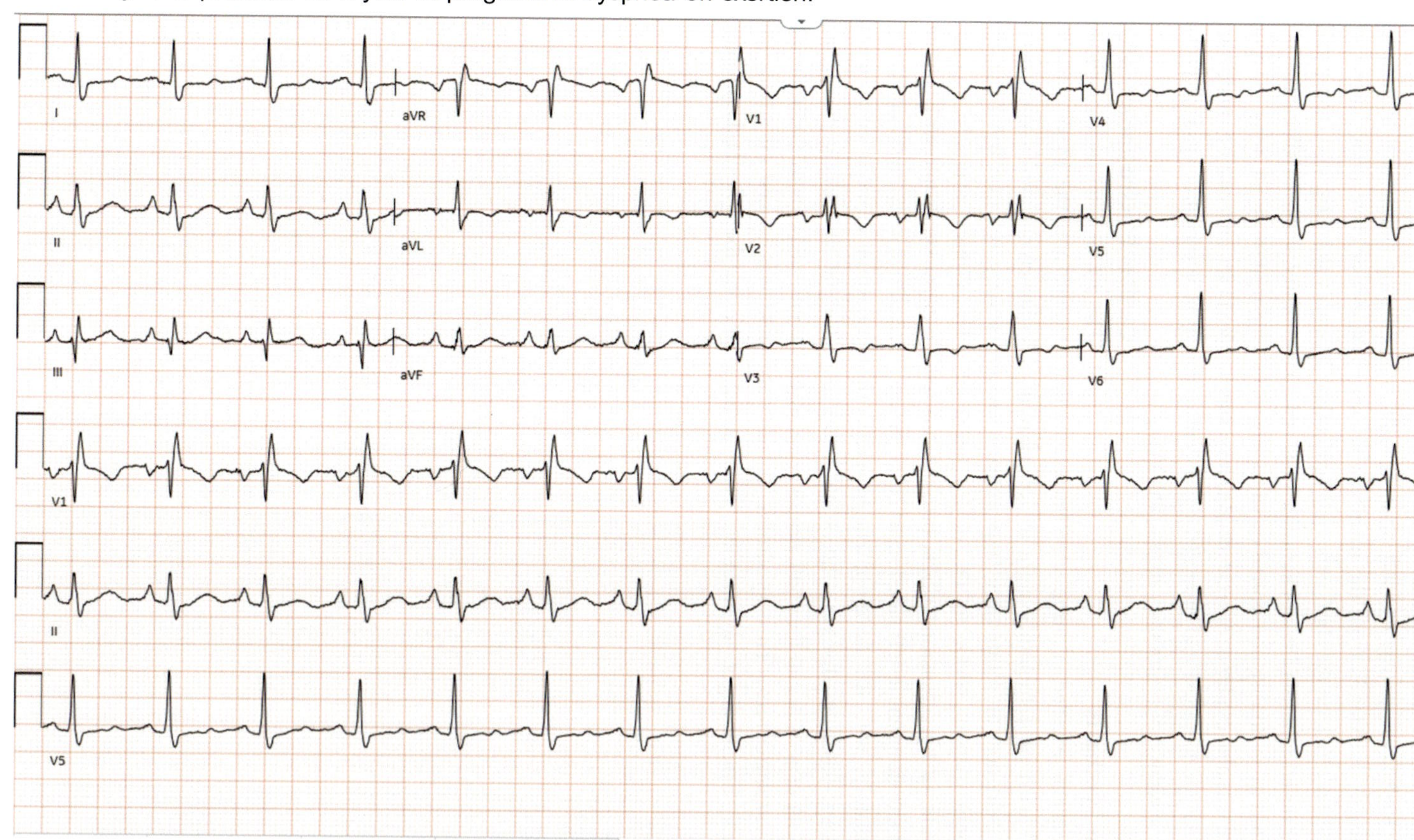

On physical exam she has a widely split S2, a I/VI systolic ejection murmur and a I/IV diastolic murmur

ECG Interpretation

Rhythm: Sinus.

Rate: 88 bpm.

Intervals: PR 172 ms, QRS 112 ms, QTc 484 ms.

Axis: Normal.

Abnormalities on the ECG
Incomplete right bundle branch block.
Right atrial enlargement.

ECG Test Answers
5, 7, 58, 82

ECG Synthesis
This ECG shows right atrial enlargement and right bundle-branch block, which may signal right-sided volume overload, for example due to tricuspid regurgitation, pulmonary regurgitation, or congenital heart disease such as inter-atrial communication. Incomplete—or complete—right bundle branch block is commonly seen in tetralogy of Fallot.

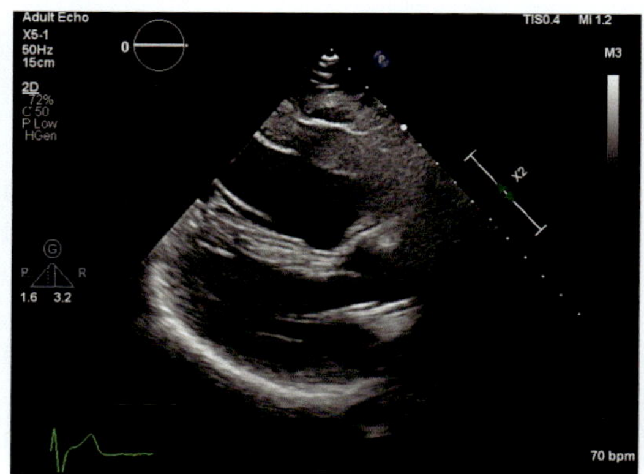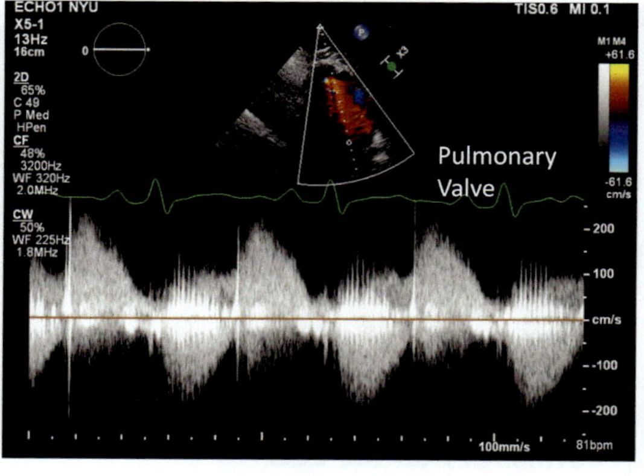

The left panel, a parasternal long-axis view, demonstrates right ventricular dilation and hypertrophy. The right panel a continuous wave Doppler tracing over the pulmonic valve in parasternal short axis view, demonstrates severe pulmonary regurgitation

Echo Interpretation

In the parasternal long-axis view, the width of the right ventricular outflow tract (RVOT), the width of the aortic root, and the anterior–posterior dimension of the left atrium should all be roughly the same. The thickness of the right ventricular free wall should be less than 5 mm. Here the right ventricular outflow tract is markedly dilated and there is right ventricular hypertrophy.

Pulmonary valve continuous wave Doppler demonstrates severe pulmonary regurgitation. The diastolic Doppler signal is dense, there is fast deceleration of diastolic flow, and there is no pressure gradient between the pulmonary artery and the right ventricle at end-diastole. This is consistent with severe pulmonary valve regurgitation.

Echo Synthesis

Severe pulmonary regurgitation causes chronic volume overload of the right ventricle. As seen here, right ventricular dilation is commonly seen.

Concomitant right ventricular hypertrophy is common in tetralogy of Fallot.

Cardiac Electrosonography Synthesis

Tetralogy of Fallot is the most common cyanotic congenital heart disease (note history of being a "blue baby"). Tetralogy of Fallot includes right ventricular outflow obstruction, ventricular septal defect, over-riding aorta, and right ventricular hypertrophy. Initial repair includes establishment of unobstructed pulmonary blood flow and closure of the ventricular septal defect. In adulthood, the primary hemodynamic abnormality after initial repair is often pulmonary regurgitation. This patient has right atrial abnormality and incomplete right bundle branch block on ECG, suggestive of right-sided heart disease. The echocardiogram demonstrates hemodynamically significant pulmonary regurgitation with resultant right ventricular volume overload. Given the degree of right ventricular enlargement and the symptoms, pulmonary valve replacement is warranted.

4 Case 4

A 50 year old male without previous medical history presented with multiple embolic events.

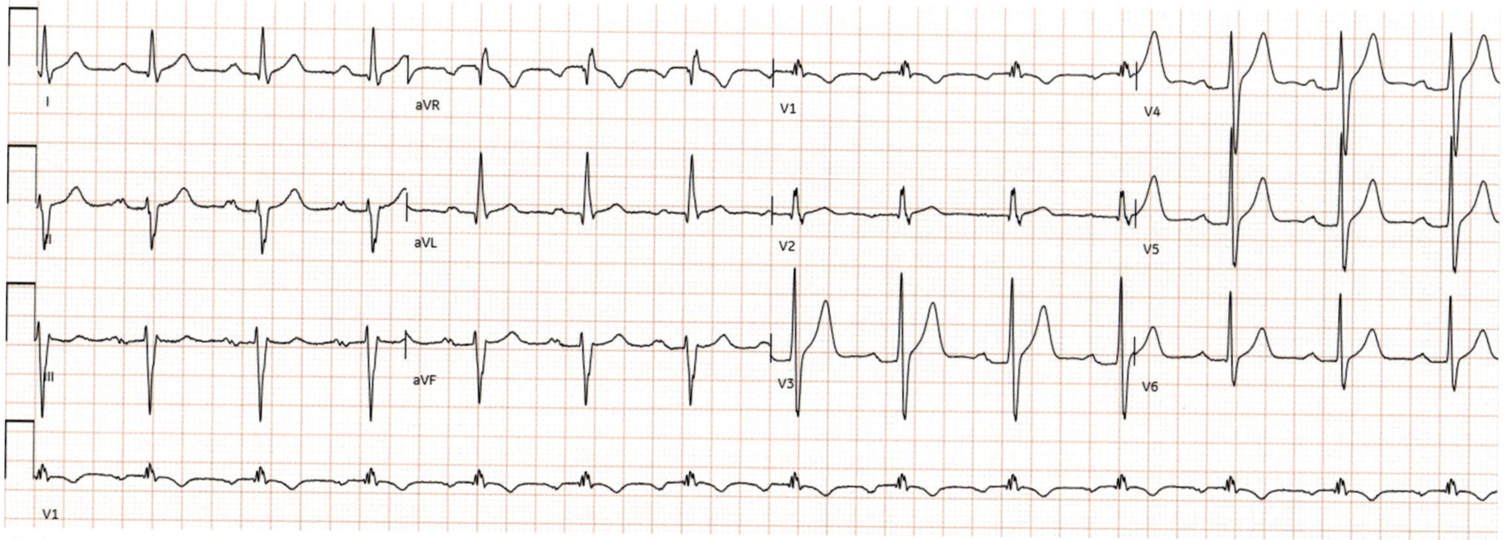

On physical exam he has a normal S1, widely fixed split S2 and an apical III/VI systolic ejection murmur.

ECG interpretation

Rhythm: Sinus.

Rate: 83 bpm.

PR 225 ms, QRS 120 ms, QTc 423 ms.

Axis: Left.

Abnormalities on the ECG

First degree atrioventricular (AV) block.
Left axis deviation.
Complete right bundle branch block.

ECG Test Answers

7, 28, 57, 59

ECG Synthesis

ECG shows first degree AV block, left axis deviation and right bundle branch block. In an older individual this pattern would be seen with tri-fascicular block, a degenerative conduction abnormality, yet in younger patients a congenital heart defect may be suspected. Left axis deviation is seen in endocardial cushion defects because of a posteriorly displaced AV node and elongated bundles. A complete RBBB should raise suspicion of right ventricular volume or pressure overload.

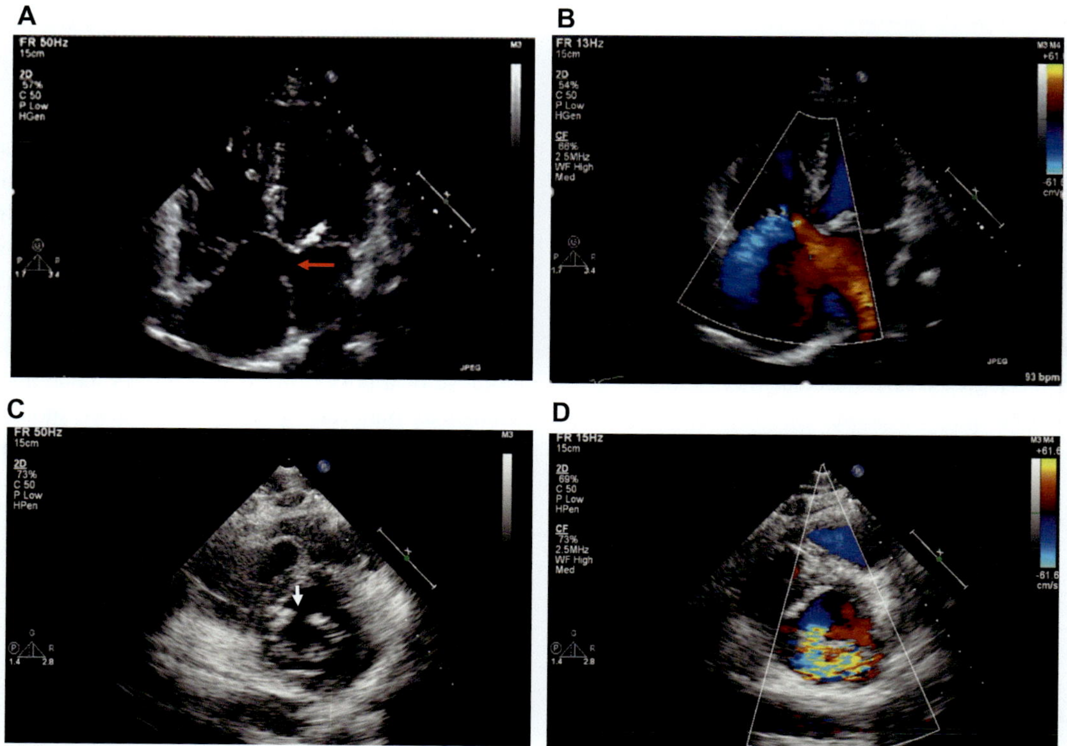

Panels A shows an apical 4 chamber view with right ventricular enlargement, a large atrial septal defect (arrow) and a thickened anterior mitral leaflet. Both AV valves are situated on the same level. Panel B depicts the left to right shunt through the atrial septal defect. Panel C shows a parasternal short-axis view depicting the mitral valve. The arrow shows a cleft within the anterior mitral leaflet. Panel D adds color and shows significant mitral regurgitation through the cleft mitral valve.

Echo Interpretation

An atrial septal defect (ASD) located at the basal-anterior portion of the atrial septum in the endocardial cushion portion of the heart would be a primum ASD. A left-to-right shunt is seen through the ASD is seen with the expected right sided heart enlargement. The anterior mitral leaflet is thickened and a cleft with mitral regurgitation is diagnosed and both AV valves are located at the same level (normally the tricuspid valve is more apically positioned). Primum ASD with cleft mitral valve or partial AV canal defect is the diagnosis.

Echo Synthesis

The endocardial cushion defects range from complete absence of atrial and septal endocardial cushion walls resulting in complete AV canal to partial defects that may include a primum ASD and/or an inlet VSD. These defects commonly have a cleft mitral valve which represents a halted development of the anterior mitral leaflet from embryonic mural and the superior bridging leaflets. Since the mitral valve developed defectively, in this condition it is commonly referred to the left AV valve. These defects also have a gooseneck deformity of the left ventricular outflow tract with possible obstruction as well as both AV valves are located at the same annular level. Endocardial cushion defects are commonly seen in Down's syndrome patients.

Cardiac Electrosonography Synthesis

The combination of an ASD and left axis deviation on ECG with mitral regurgitation raises suspicion of an endocardial cushion defect or partial AV canal defect. ASD with a right sided deviation on ECG is associated with other types of ASDs, most notably with secundum ASD. The patient was surgically operated on with patch closure of the primum ASD and repair of the cleft mitral valve.

A 30 year-old man presented with a month of progressive dyspnea on exertion. He was born in Ecuador and moved within the last year.

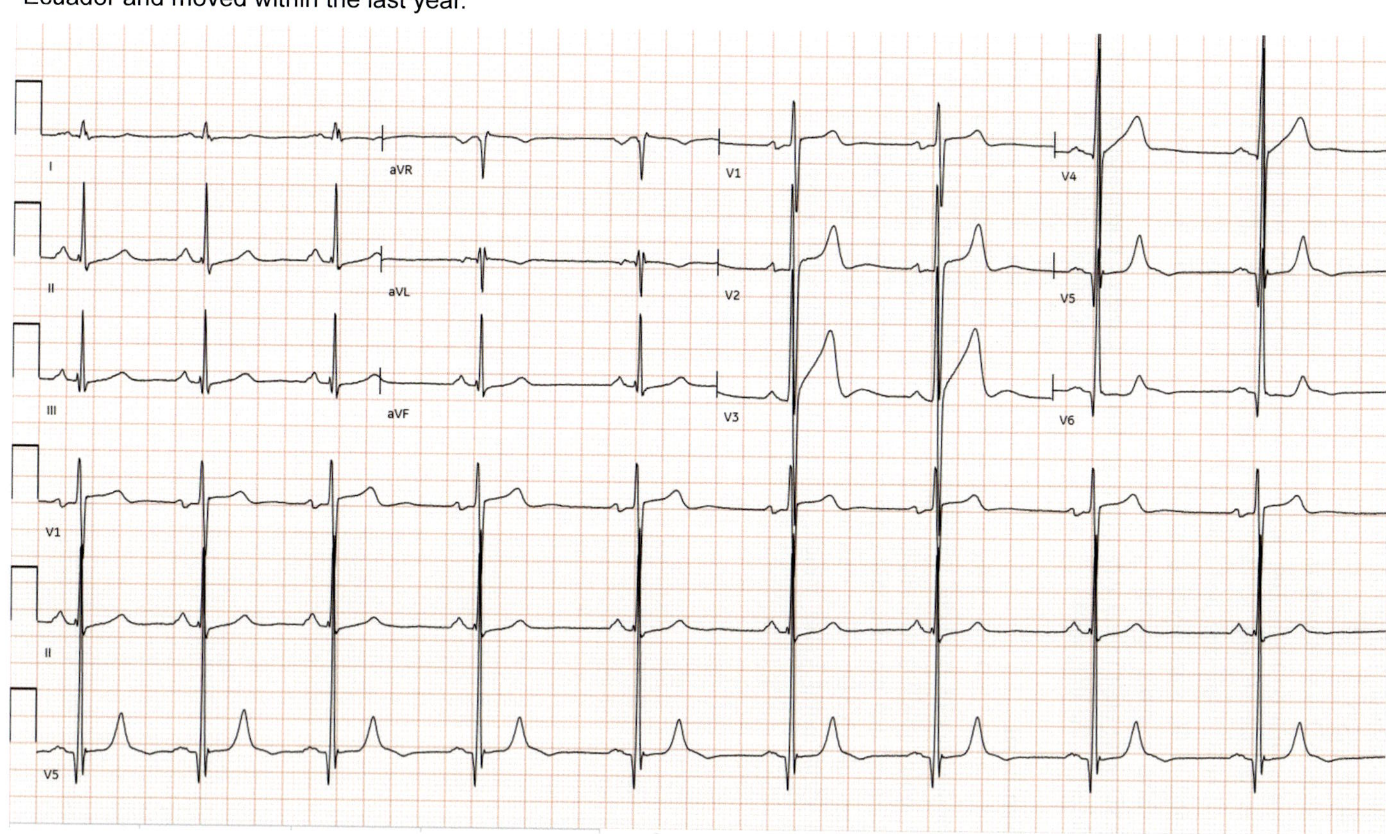

On exam his oxyhemoglobin saturation is 96%. He has a continuous, "machinery-like" murmur at the left upper sternal border.

ECG Interpretation

Rhythm: Sinus bradycardia with sinus arrhythmia.

Rate: 55 bpm.

Intervals: PR 166 ms, QRS 92 ms, QTc 419 ms

Axis: Normal.

Abnormalities on the ECG
Left ventricular hypertrophy.

ECG Test Answers
9, 40

ECG Synthesis
Ths ECG shows high QRS voltage in the precordial leads consistent with left ventricular hypertrophy. This may signal either eccentric or concentric left ventricular hypertrophy. In this patient, eccentric hypertrophy (left ventricular enlargement) results from chronic left-sided volume overload from the patent ductus arteriosus.

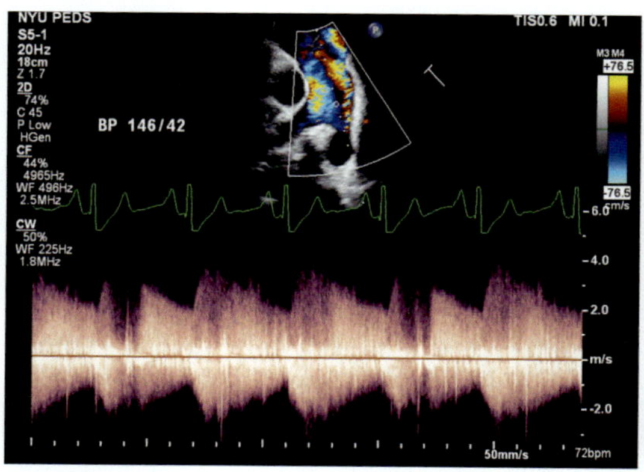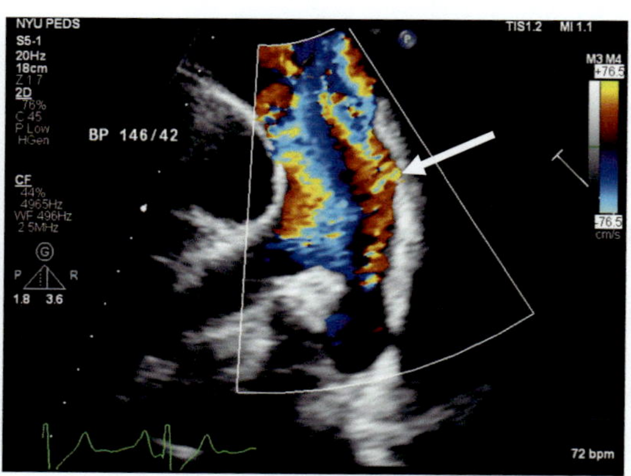

Both images were taken from the parasternal short axis view of the pulmonary artery. The left panel, a continuous wave Doppler tracing, demonstrates a continuous shunt into the pulmonary artery. The right panel, a color Doppler still image, demonstrates a flow signal into the proximal left pulmonary artery (arrow).

Echo Interpretation

In the parasternal short axis view at the level of the pulmonary artery bifurcation, a patent ductus arteriosus is seen. There is continuous flow into the proximal left pulmonary artery (from the aorta) seen on spectral Doppler interrogation. In the right panel, color Doppler interrogation demonstrates flow from the patent ductus arteriosus into the pulmonary artery (white arrow).

Echo Synthesis

Patent ductus arteriosus, a connection between the aortic arch and the pulmonary artery, causes a continuous left-to-right shunt as shown in this case.

Cardiac Electrosonography Synthesis

Patent ductus arteriosus, in the absence of elevated pulmonary vascular resistance, causes a left-to-right shunt and left ventricular volume overload. Pulmonary over-circulation and LV volume overload may lead to congestive heart failure. EKG in a large PDA may demonstrate left ventricular hypertrophy, a reflection of the chamber dilation caused by the volume load. Color Doppler demonstrates flow through the ductus into the pulmonary artery; spectral Doppler demonstrates a continuous left-to-right shunt with higher velocity in systole. In this patient, symptoms and left-sided chamber dilation warrant repair, which can be done either surgically or by transcatheter technique.

6 Case 6

22 year old male present with increasing dyspnea on exertion

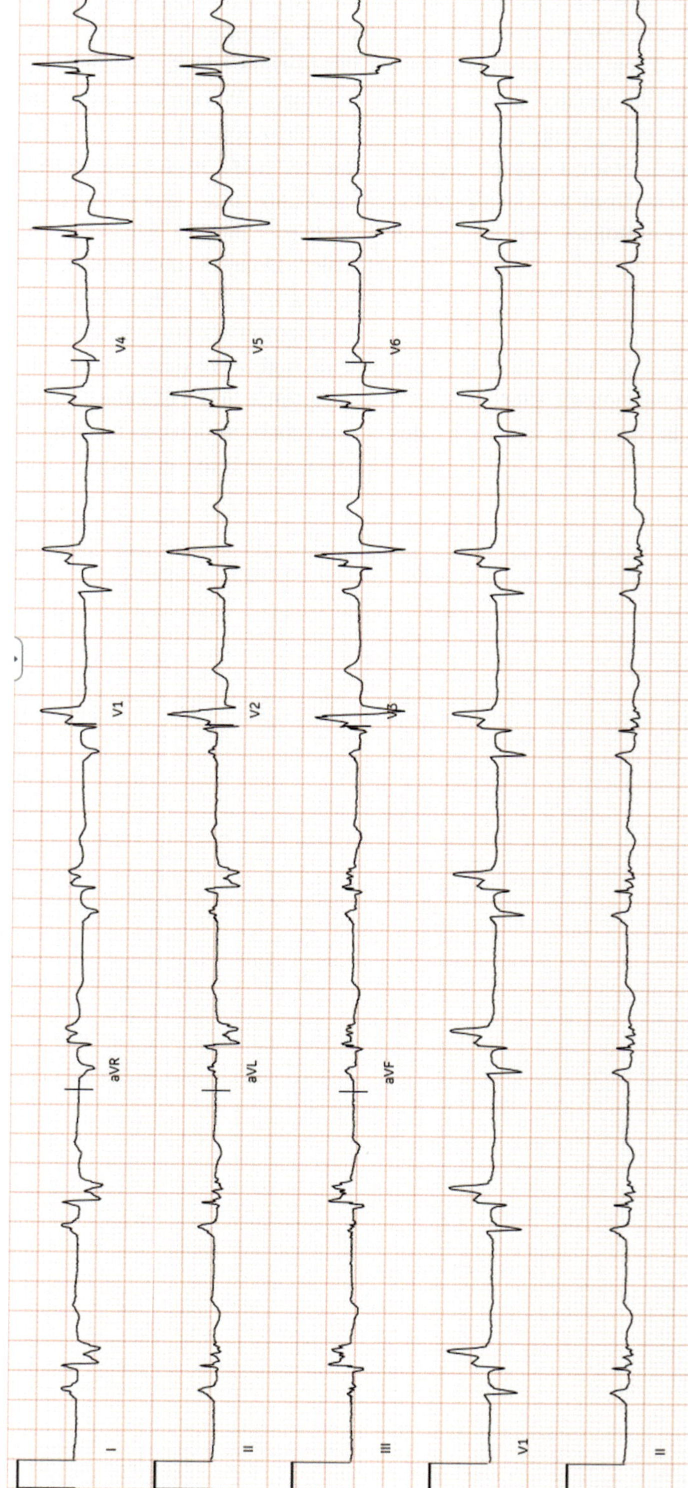

On physical exam there is a loud and split S1 (making a "sail sound"), a split S2 as well as a loud holosystolic murmur loudest at the left sternal border.

ECG interpretation

Rhythm: Sinus bradycardia.

Rate: 55 bpm.

Intervals: PR 220 ms, QRS 240 ms, QTc 498 ms

Axis: Borderline right.

Abnormalities on the ECG
Dilated right atrium.
First degree AV block.
Complete right bundle branch block.

Right ventricular hypertrophy.
Prolonged QT interval.

ECG test answers
5, 9, 28, 51, 57, 82

ECG synthesis
ECG shows a severely enlarged right atrium with large p waves often referred to as "Himalayan P waves" and features of a dilated right ventricle (i.e. complete RBBB and RVH). The degree of "fractionations" of the RBBB generally coincides with the degree of right ventricular enlargement and dysfunction.

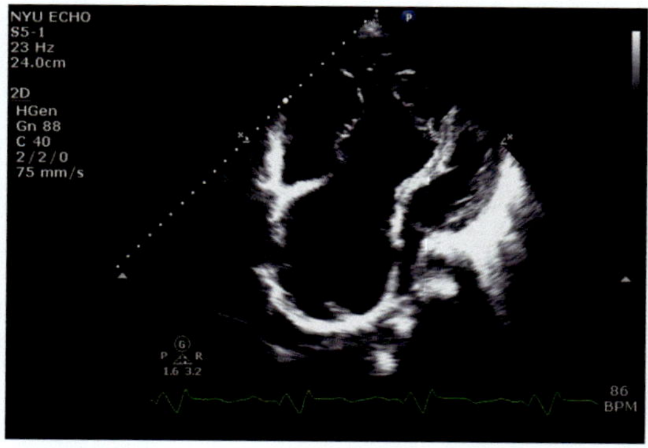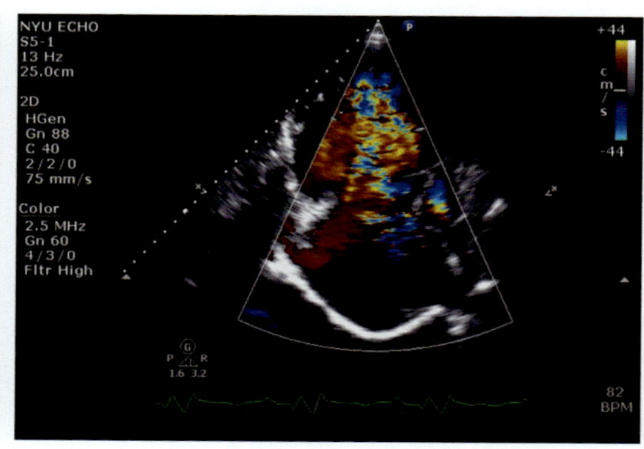

Both images were taken are from the apical 4 chamber view. The left panel shows a massive right atrium (including an "atrialized" portion of the right ventricle) as well as an apically displaced tricuspid valve (the anterior tricuspid leaflet appears enlarged and the septal tricuspid leaflet appears diminutive). The right panel, a color Doppler still image, demonstrates the torrential tricuspid regurgitation due to severe malcoaptation of the deformed tricuspid valve

Echo Interpretation

The echo shows apical displacement of the tricuspid valve, an enlarged anterior tricuspid leaflet and diminutive septal and posterior tricuspid leaflets with severe tricuspid regurgitation. The right atrium and ventricle are severely enlarged (the area between the leaflets and the true tricuspid annulus is referred to as "atrialized" portion of right ventricle) with reduced function. The left ventricle exhibits normal function. No obvious atrial septal defect or patent foramen ovale seen. The finding of apical displacement of the tricuspid valve provides the diagnosis of Ebstein Anomaly (EA) of the tricuspid valve.

Echo Synthesis

EA is the result of failure of the tricuspid leaflets to embryonically delaminate or "peel off" the myocardium appearing as an apically displaced tricuspid valve. The anterior tricuspid leaflet appears as an enlarged sail and the other leaflets are diminutive. Echocardiography confirms the diagnosis with an apical displacement of the tricuspid valve annulus more then 0.8 cm/m^2 compared to the mitral valve annulus. Echocardiographic findings of EA are predominantly associated with tricuspid regurgitation; however other associated features include right ventricular myopathy, inter-atrial communications (80%), pulmonary valve stenosis and left ventricular non-compaction.

Cardiac Electrosonography Synthesis

ECG in EA shows giant P waves ("Himalayan P waves") and complete RBBB; the width and fractionations of the RBBB are associated with the degree of RV size and dysfunction. It is important to rule out accessory pathways (i.e. Wolff-Parkinson-White) as they can be multiple and common (25%). This patient underwent a successful surgical cone procedure in which the large anterior tricuspid leaflet was manipulated and sutured to the true tricuspid valve annulus to allow valve competency together with right atrial size reduction by plication.

References

Gatzoulis MA et al. Diagnosis and management of adult congenital heart disease. Chapter 52. Eisenmenger syndrome. 3rd ed. Elsevier; 2018. pp 528.

Gatzoulis MA et al. Diagnosis and management of adult congenital heart disease, 3rd ed. Chapter 43. Ebstein Anomaly. Elsevier; 2018: p. 442.

Harrigan RA, Jones K. ABC of clinical electrocardiography. Conditions affecting the right side of the heart. BMJ. 2002;324(7347):1201–4. Review.

Huehnergarth KV, Gurvitz M, Stout KK, Otto CM. Repaired tetralogy of Fallot in the adult: monitoring and management. Heart 2008;1663–9 94.

Schneider DJ, Moore JW. Patent ductus arteriosus. Circulation. 2006;114:1873–82.

Webb G, Gatzoulis MA. Atrial septal defects in the adult: recent progress and overview. Circulation. 2006;114:1645–53.

Webb G, Gatzoulis MA. Atrial septal defects in the adult: recent progress and overview. Circulation. 2006;114:1645–53.

Clinical Cases of Chest Sonography

Adam Rothman, Alexander Davidovich,
Janet Shapiro, Eyal Herzog, David Leibowitz,
and Yair Elitzur

Abstract

Our tutorial described the basic principles of chest sonography, and provided a review of pulmonary anatomy, ultrasound probe positioning, and a discussion of the most common ultrasound findings (both normal and pathologic). In this chapter, we work through a series of case-based scenarios designed to practice combining patient history and symptom presentation, ECG, and chest sonography interpretation with the overall aim of correctly identifying various pulmonary diagnoses and helping direct appropriate management plans.

Keywords

ECG · Ultrasound · Chest electrosonography · Shortness of breath · Cough · Lung sliding · A-lines · B-lines · Lung point · Pleural effusion · Pulmonary edema

A. Rothman (✉)
Mount Sinai West, Institute for Critical Care
Medicine, Icahn School of Medicine at Mount Sinai,
New York, USA
e-mail: Adam.Rothman@mountsinai.org

A. Davidovich · J. Shapiro
Mount Sinai Morningside, Institute for Critical Care
Medicine, Icahn School of Medicine at Mount Sinai,
New York, USA

E. Herzog · D. Leibowitz · Y. Elitzur
The Heart Institute, Department of Cardiology,
Hadassah Medical Center, Hebrew University
of Jerusalem, Jerusalem, Israel

1 Case 1

A 32-year-old-woman with no prior medical history presented with progressive shortness of breath, chest pain, and episodes of hemoptysis.

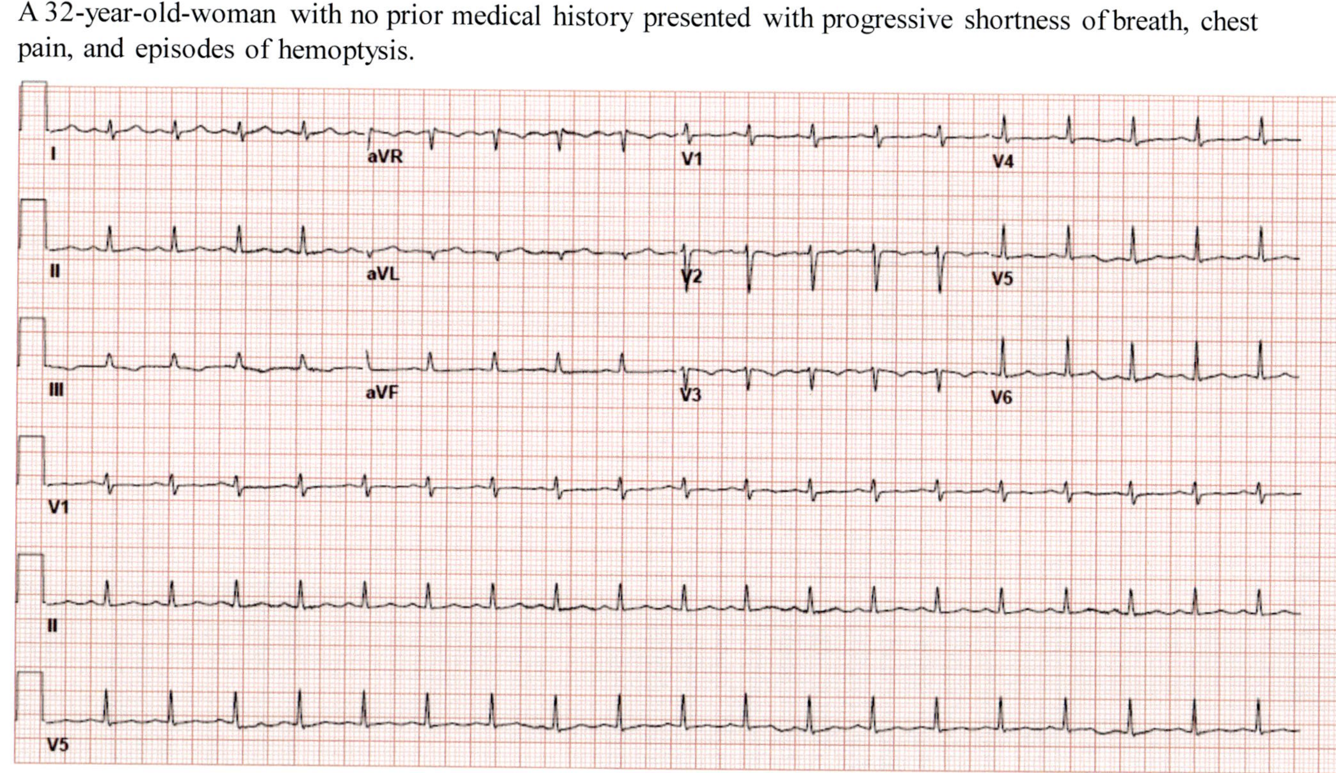

Additional Clinical History
She reported subjective feeling of fever and chills and received treatment with antibiotics as an outpatient for a bacterial pneumonia 1 month prior.

Additional Information
CXR showed mild hazy reticular changes with a large right pleural effusion and associated atelectasis or pneumonia.

ECG Interpretation

Rhythm: Sinus

Rate: 117 bpm

Intervals: PR 170 ms, QRS = 70 ms QTc = 364 ms

Axis: Normal

Abnormalities on the ECG

- Sinus tachycardia
- R/S ratio in V1 > 1, intrinsicoid deflection in V1 shorter than 50 ms, T wave inversion in V2 (but also in V3).

ECG Test Answers
10, 40, 81

ECG Synthesis
The ECG shows sinus tachycardia which is non specific and to be expected under the clinical circumstances. Some signs may be consistent with right ventricular hypertrophy, however these are also not specific. In the setting of shortness of breath, sinus tachycardia and ECG signs of possible right ventricular strain, pulmonary embolus must be considered in the differential diagnosis, among other possibilities. Echocardiography and chest sonography are essential for further rapid point of care workup.

A

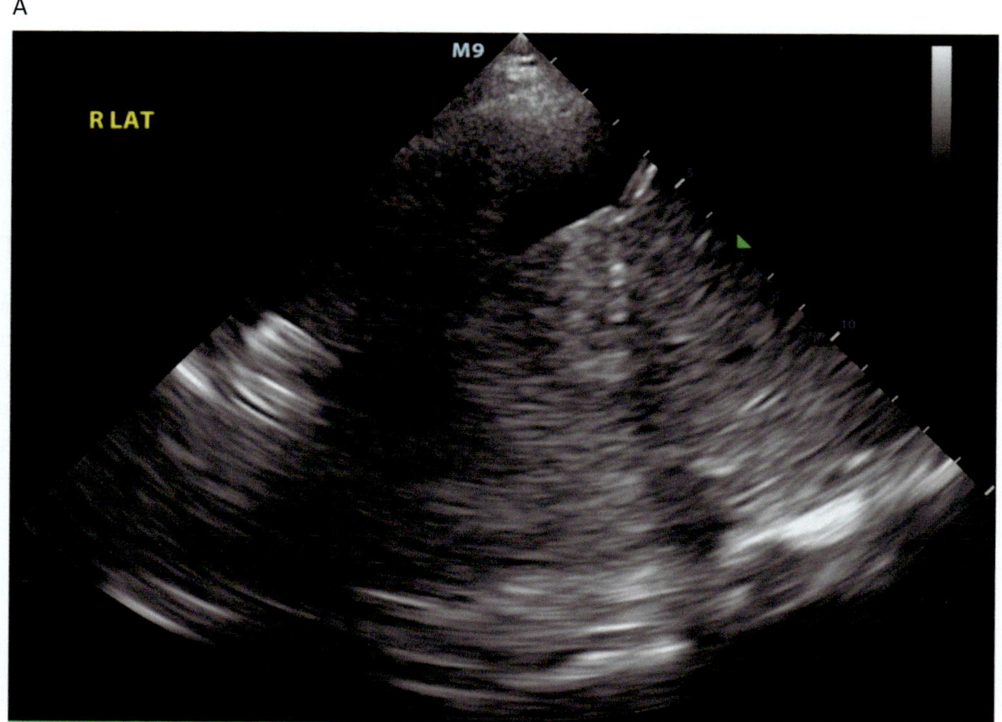

B

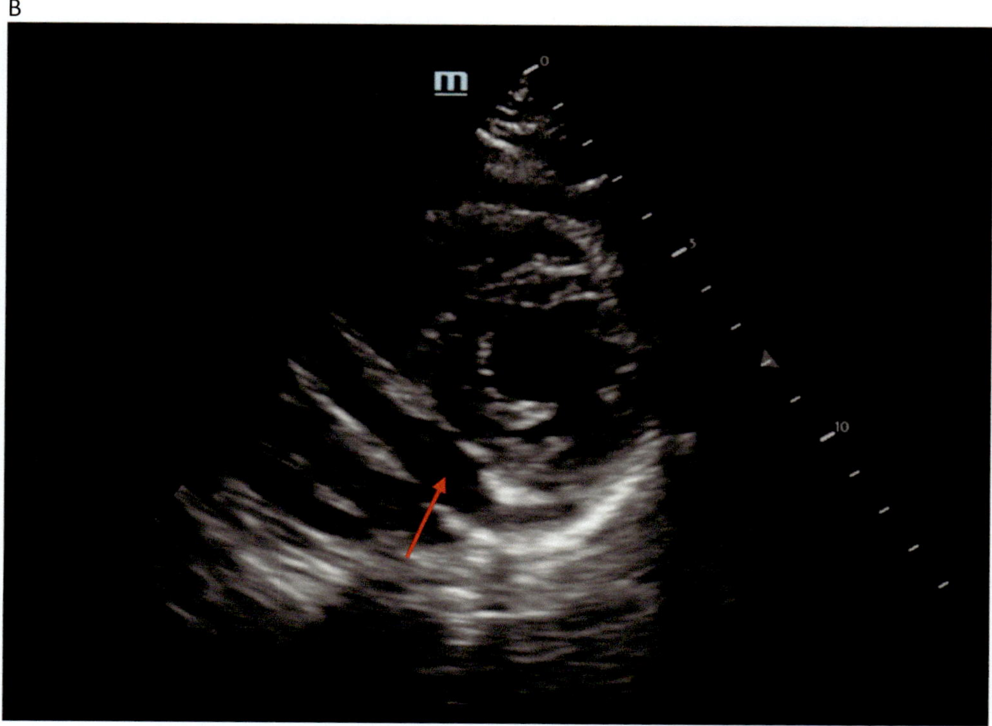

Panel A is a chest ultrasound showing a simple-appearing pleural effusion with an associated large consolidation ("hepatization") in the lower lung field (abutting the diaphragm). Panel B is a parasternal short-axis echocardiographic view showing a pericardial effusion (arrow)

Ultrasound Interpretation

Panel A is a chest ultrasound showing a simple-appearing pleural effusion with an associated large consolidation ("hepatization") in the lower lung field (abutting the diaphragm). Panel B is a parasternal short-axis echocardiographic view showing a pericardial effusion (arrow).

Ultrasound Synthesis

The pleural effusion associated with a large lung consolidation is most indicative of either an atelectatic or infectious disease process. In view of the pericardial effusion, additional etiologies, including autoimmune and neoplastic disease processes, should be considered.

Chest Electrosonography Synthesis

The ECG findings of tachycardia and signs of right heart strain is consistent with the chest ultrasound finding of a lung consolidation and pleural effusion. The echo finding of a pericardial effusion suggests that the pathological process involves this space as well. The patient ultimately underwent thoracentesis and eventually, pericardiocentesis, with subsequent cytology from the thoracentesis positive for a metastatic lung adenocarcinoma.

2 Case 2

An 83-year-old man with history of chronic obstructive pulmonary disease, diabetes mellitus, hypertension, deep vein thrombosis and normal pressure hydrocephalus presents with productive cough, fatigue, fevers, and hypoxia.

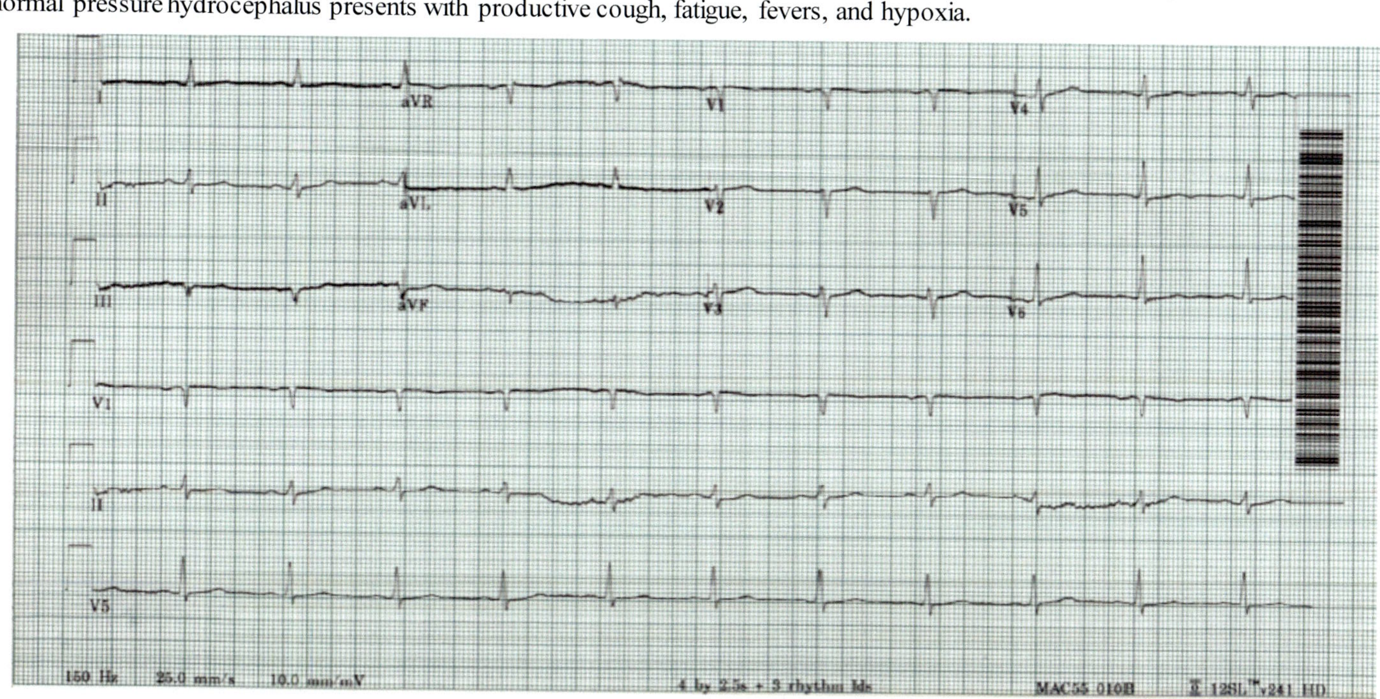

Additional Clinical History

The patient has underlying dementia and is bedbound at baseline. On exam, the patient has diminished breath sounds throughout the right hemithorax.

Additional Information

Chest X-ray shows near complete opacification of the right hemithorax, with possible trace left pleural effusion. Non-contrast CT Chest shows a large right pleural effusion with extensive collapse/atelectasis of portions of the right lung

ECG Interpretation

Rhythm: Sinus

Rate: 70 bpm

Intervals: QRS = 100 ms QTc = 420 ms PR = 190 ms.

Axis: Normal

Abnormalities on the ECG

None. This ECG is borderline for low voltage QRS, as R + S in limb leads is 5 mm. It is also borderline for poor R wave progression. However the formal criteria require R + S in limb leads to be **less** than 5 mm, and R/S transition to be in V5,6 to make these diagnoses. Both of these may be a sign of chronic lung disease.

ECG Test Answers

7

ECG Synthesis

The ECG does not clearly point to any pathology, however may suggest a possibility of lung disease, which is well known in this patient's medical history.

A

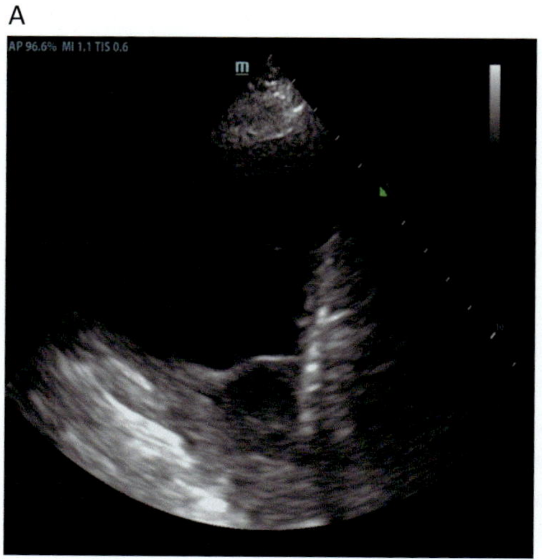

B

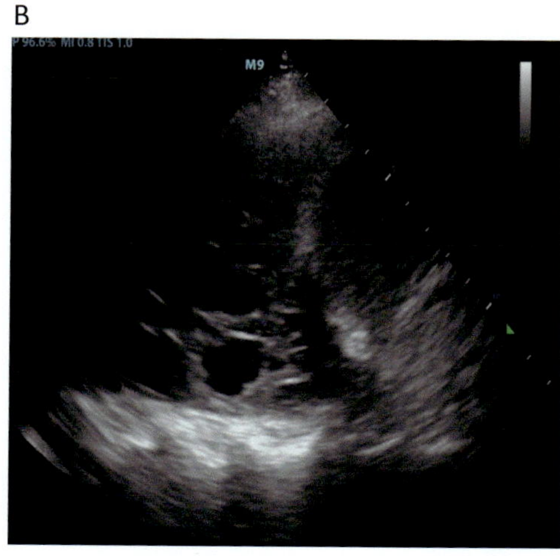

C

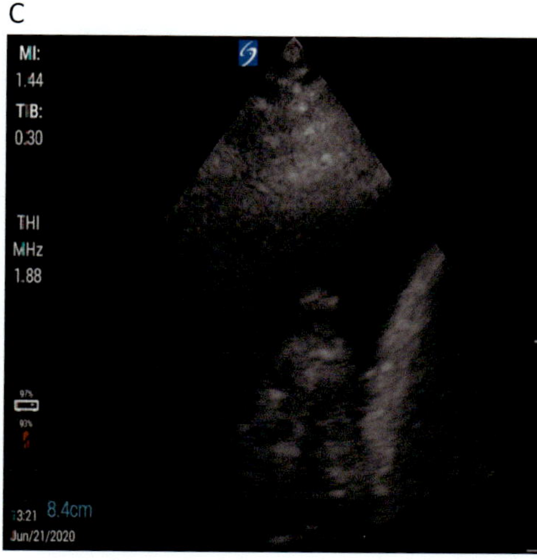

Panel A depicts a large, complex effusion with septations and the plankton sign (debris within the fluid) Panel B shows significant loculated fluid collections within the larger effusion Panel C demonstrates an area of lung consolidation within the large effusion

Ultrasound Interpretation

Panel A depicts a large, complex effusion with septations and the plankton sign (debris within the fluid).

Panel B shows significant loculated fluid collections within the larger effusion.

Panel C demonstrates an area of lung consolidation within the large effusion.

Ultrasound Synthesis

Given the complex appearance of the effusion, associated with a lung consolidation and new cough, fevers, and hypoxia, this is most concerning for an infected pleural space (empyema).

Chest Electrosonography Synthesis

The patient was started on broad-spectrum antibiotics, and then underwent right-sided small-bore (pigtail) chest tube placement. Pleural fluid studies were notable for a pH 7.10, glucose less than 5, and white blood cell count of 2800 (neutrophil-predominant). These results supported the diagnosis of empyema suspected on chest ultrasound imaging.

3 Case 3

A 37-year-old woman with a past medical history of alcoholic cirrhosis, presented with hematemesis. She underwent endoscopy with banding of an esophageal varix. Her hospital course was then complicated by worsening shortness of breath and hypoxia.

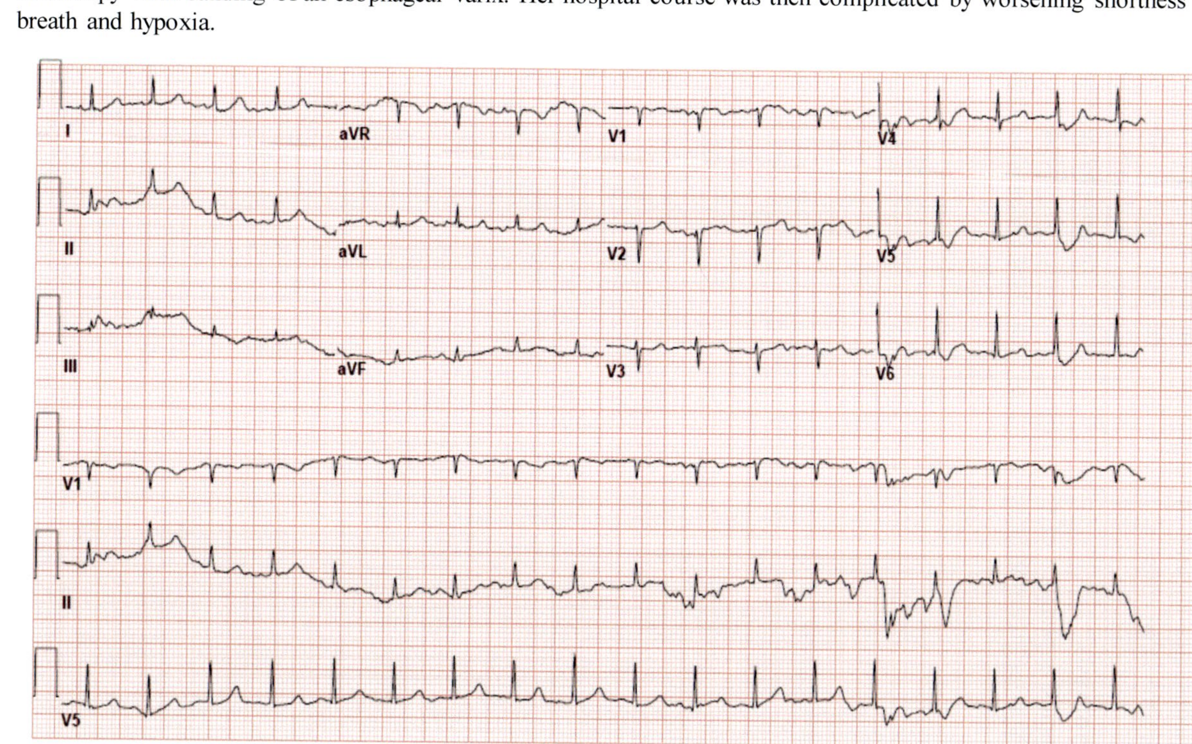

Additional Clinical History

On exam, the patient had scleral icterus and mild abdominal distention, with absent breath sounds throughout the right hemithorax.

Additional History

Chest X-ray showed near complete opacification of the right hemithorax, with mass effect and mediastinal shift to the left.

ECG Interpretation

Rhythm: Sinus tachycardia.

Rate: 110 bpm.

Intervals: PR = 160 ms,   QRS = 70 ms
QTc = 404 ms.

Axis: Normal.

Abnormalities on the ECG
Sinus tachycardia.

ECG Test Answers
10

ECG Synthesis
The rhythm in this ECG is difficult to interpret as there is a lot of artifact and the p waves appear very small, however it does appear to be sinus tachycardia. In this case the ECG shows an atrial tachyarrhythmia, possibly atrial flutter. This is a non-specific finding and additional cardiothoracic imaging is warranted to further evaluate the complaints.

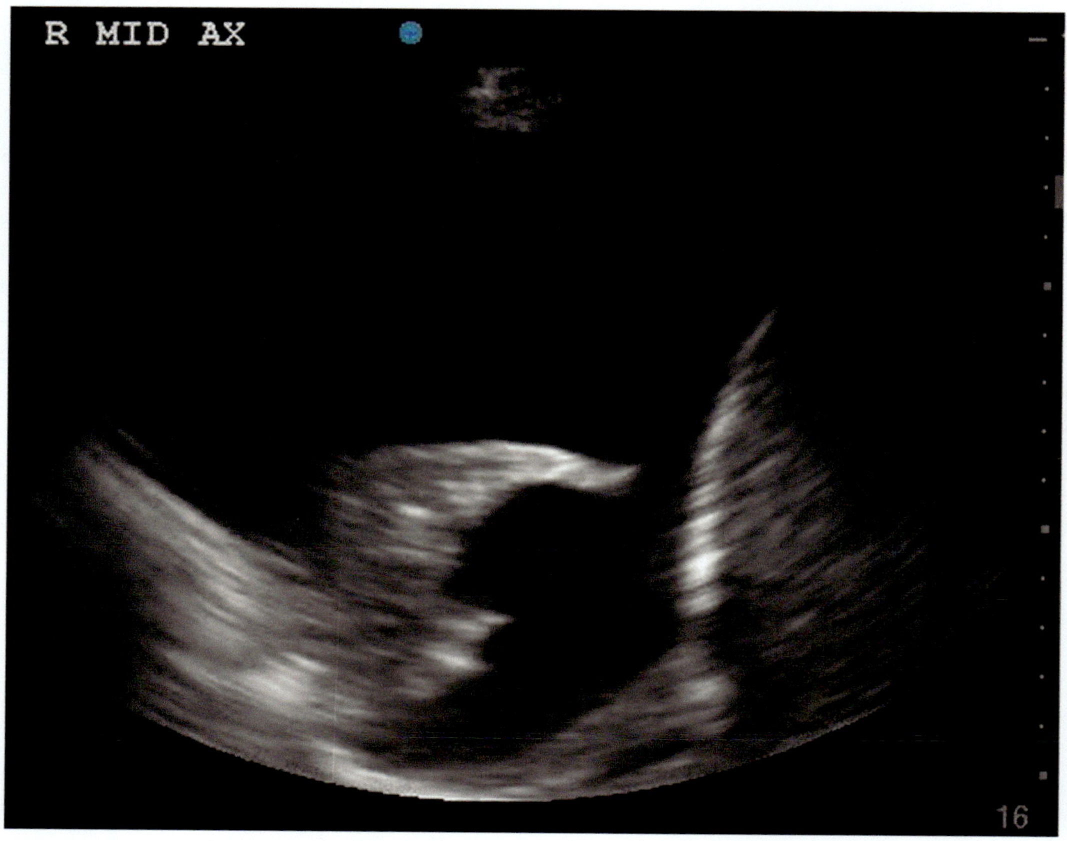

There is a large, simple-appearing effusion with a collapsed area of the lung appearing to float within the surrounding fluid ("jellyfish sign")

Ultrasound Interpretation

There is a large, simple-appearing effusion with a collapsed area of the lung appearing to float within the surrounding fluid ("jellyfish sign").

Ultrasound Synthesis

Given the large right-sided effusion, and known decompensated alcoholic cirrhosis, these findings are most suggestive of a hepatic hydrothorax.

Chest Electrosonography Synthesis

The patient underwent diagnostic and therapeutic thoracentesis, with pleural fluid studies consistent with a transudative effusion. Following the procedure, the patient had improvement in her respiratory status.

A 67-year-old woman with past medical history of hypertension, diabetes, and congestive heart failure, presented with several weeks of worsening shortness of breath and cough.

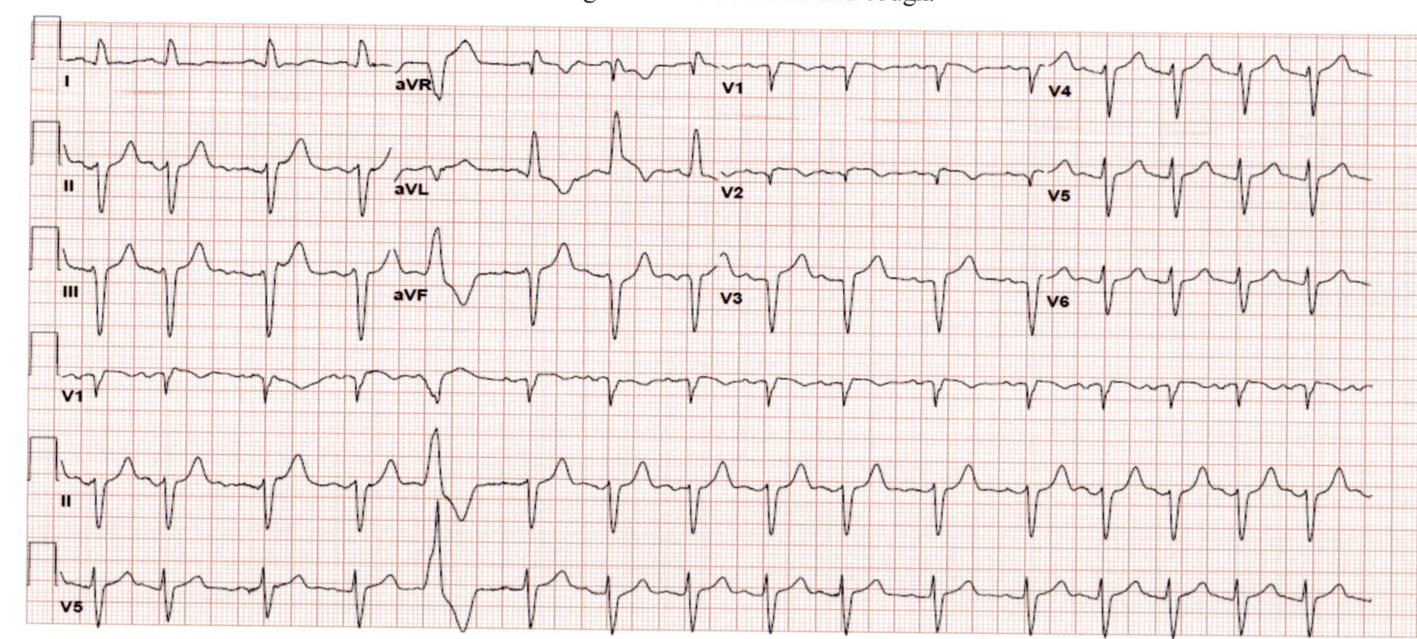

Additional Clinical History
The patient ran out of her medications three weeks ago and was unable to refill her prescriptions. She additionally reported a ten-pound weight gain associated with lower leg swelling and the inability to lie flat in bed.

Additional Information
On exam, the patient was tachypneic, with bilateral crackles, diminished breath sounds in the lung bases, jugular venous distention, and moderate pitting edema to the bilateral knees. Labs were notable for a mildly elevated troponin level and acute kidney injury.

ECG Interpretation

Rhythm: Sinus rhythm

Rate: 98 bpm.

Intervals: QRS = 90 ms QTc = 435 ms PR = 200 ms

Axis: Left axis deviation.

Abnormalities on the ECG

Premature atrial beats Left axis deviation.
   Left anterior hemiblock.
   Poor R wave progression.

ECG Test Answers
7, 13, 37, 59

ECG Synthesis

The ECG shows sinus rhythm with left anterior hemiblock and premature atrial complexes. It is difficult to decide whether this is indeed sinus rhythm or atrial tachycardia. The p waves are quite small but their axis is normal. In support of sinus rhythm is the presence of premature beats, seen as p waves that are premature and different in morphology than the usual p waves.

The ECG does not provide a clear explanation for this woman's symptoms and signs, and additional imaging is necessary.

A

B

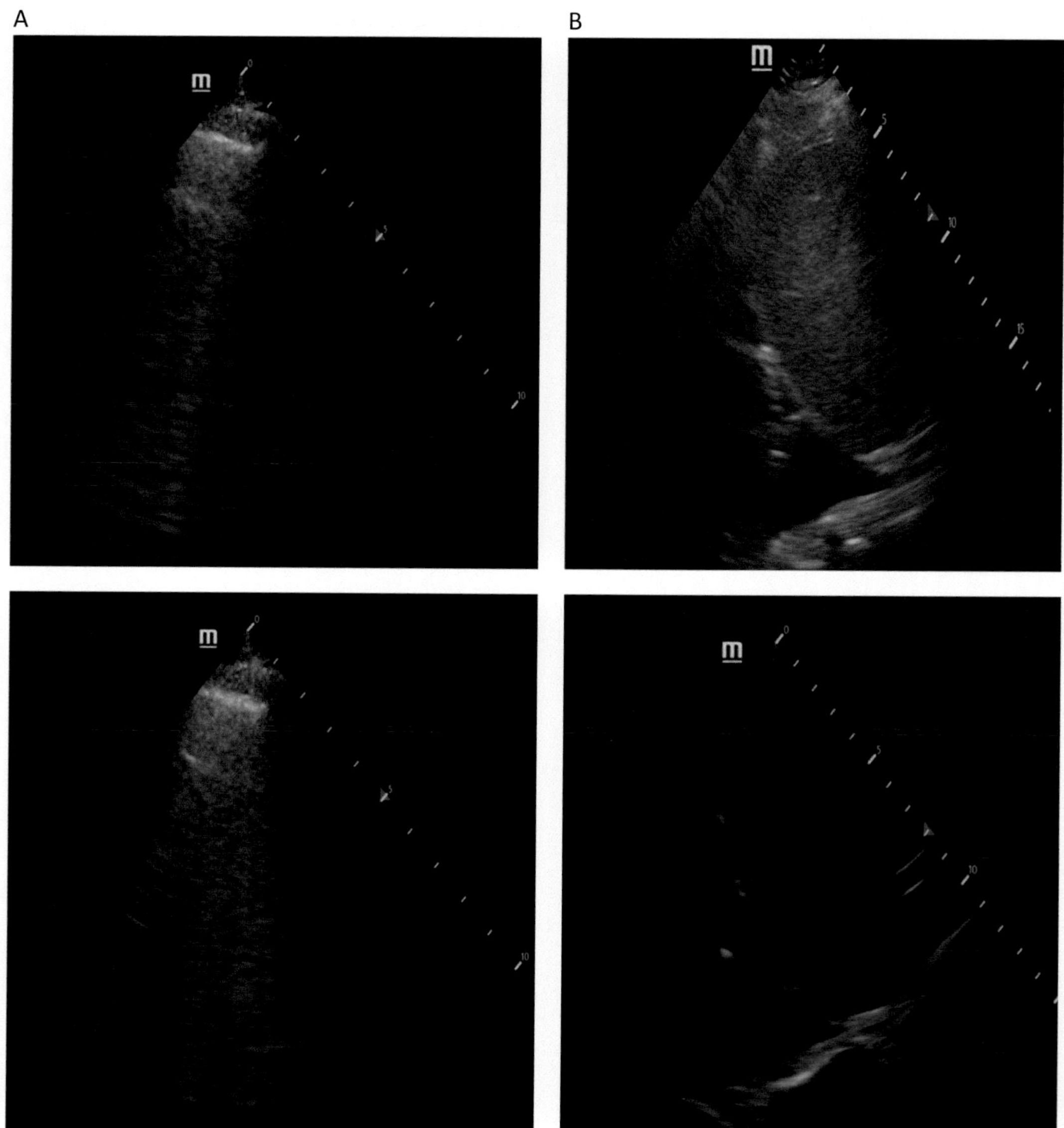

Panel A demonstrates B lines in the bilateral lung fields, with smooth-appearing pleura. Panel B shows small simple-appearing bilateral pleural effusions

Ultrasound Interpretation

The extensive B-line pattern, smooth pleura, and small bilateral effusions are most consistent with a fluid overload state. Given the patient's history and clinical presentation, the most likely explanation of the findings is decompensated heart failure.

Ultrasound Synthesis Given the patient's history and clinical presentation, the most likely explanation of the findings is decompensated heart failure.

Chest Electrosonography Synthesis

The ECG while abnormal, did not reveal any acute pathology. The chest ultrasound in conjunction with the patients history and physical findings confirmed a diagnosis of exacerbation of congestive heart failure. The patient was placed on non-invasive ventilation for respiratory support and started on intravenous furosemide, with gradual improvement in symptoms.

An 89-year-old woman with a past medical history of hypertension and receiving home supplemental oxygen for interstitial lung disease complicated by chronic bronchiectasis, presented with syncope and worsening hypoxia.

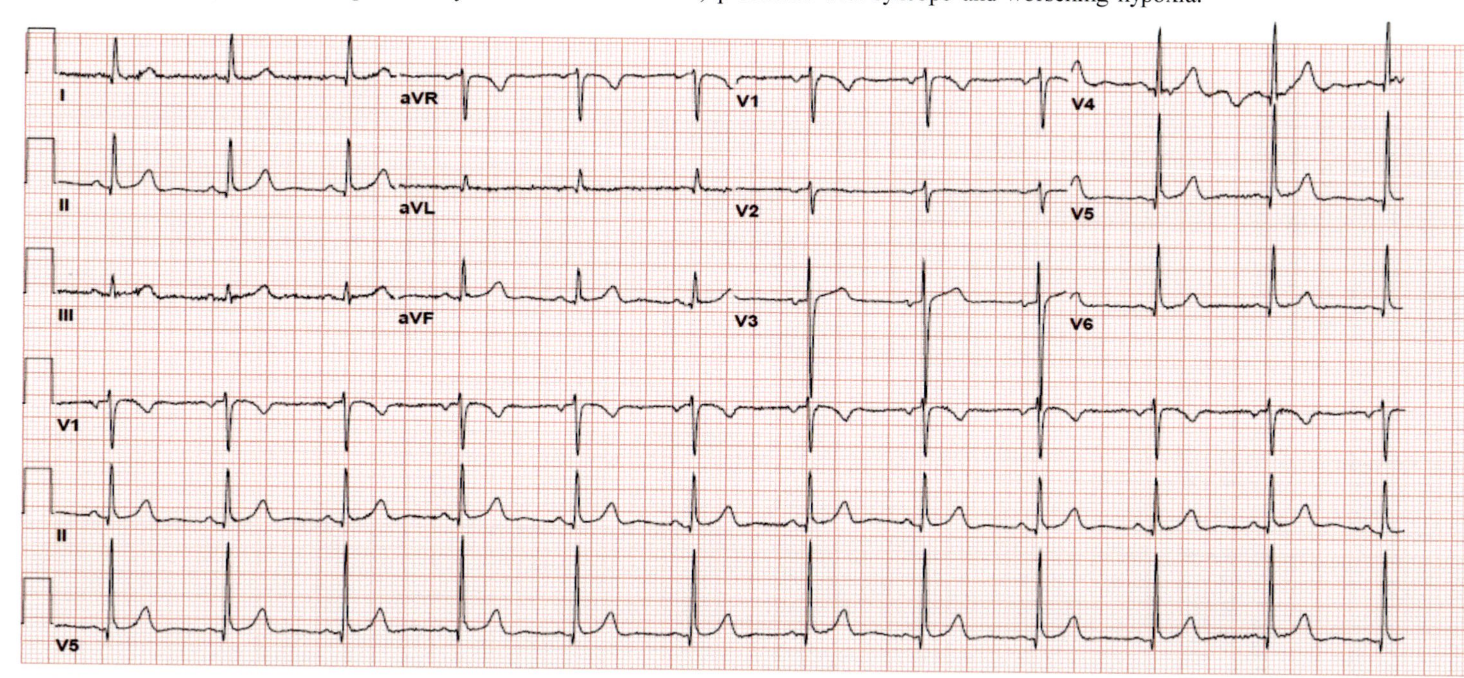

Additional Clinical History

On exam, she was cachectic, with bilateral crackles in the lung fields and warm extremities with no pedal edema.

Additional Information

Chest X-ray was notable for extensive fibrotic changes, with no obvious new focal consolidations. Chest CT angiogram was pertinent for a single subsegmental pulmonary embolism, with labs notable for chronic hypercapnia.

ECG Interpretation

Rhythm: Sinus rhythm.

Rate: 68 bpm.

Intervals: QRS = 80 ms   QTc = 407 ms   PR = 170 ms

Axis: Left axis deviation.

Abnormalities on the ECG
None.

ECG Test Answers
1

ECG Synthesis
This patient has a normal ECG.

Although the CT scan showed a subsegmental pulmonary embolus, there is no sinus tachycardia and no signs on ECG of right sided strain. It is therefore unlikely that the pulmonary embolus explains the clinical scenario in itself. The lack of any pathological findings on the ECG, suggested a pulmonary problem is more likely than a cardiac one, however additional imaging is required.

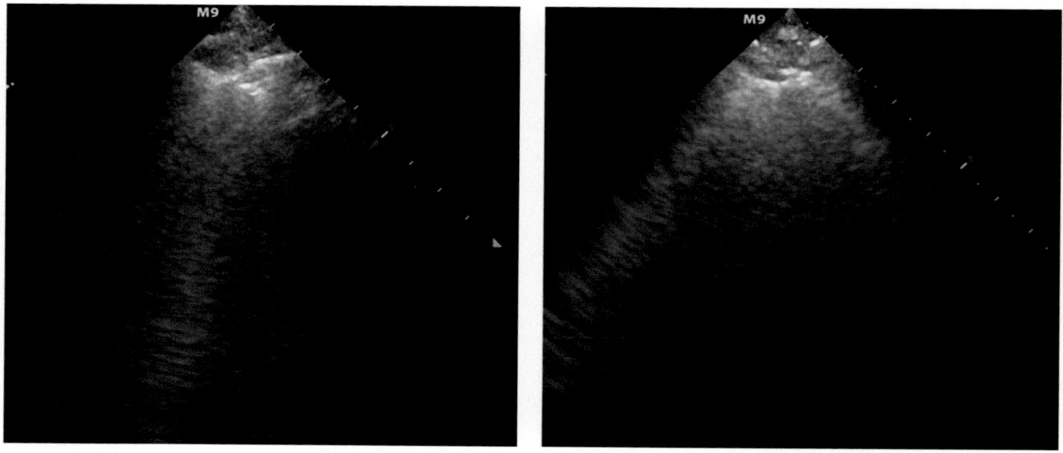

There are confluent B-lines seen in both the right and left lung fields, with no discernible A-lines present in either view. The pleura in both images appears irregular ("lumpy bumpy" appearance)

Ultrasound Interpretation

There are confluent B-lines seen in both the right and left lung fields, with no discernible A-lines present in either view. The pleura in both images appears irregular ("lumpy bumpy" appearance).

Ultrasound Synthesis

The extensive B-lines in both lung fields, as well as the irregular appearance of the pleura, is most suggestive of an extensive infectious or inflammatory process. Given the patient's history of underlying bronchiectasis, the findings are likely related to interstitial lung disease exacerbation.

Chest Electrosonography Synthesis

The lack of cardiac pathology on the ECG and the chest sonography findings suggested the patients symptoms were due to exacerbation of her underlying lung disease. The patient was started on steroids, standing nebulizer treatments, and antibiotics, with gradual improvement in symptoms.

6 Case 6

A 78-year-old woman with past medical history of chronic obstructive pulmonary disease, obstructive sleep apnea, and hypertension, presented with several days of dysuria, and was admitted for management of urosepsis. Upon arrival to the medical floor, the patient developed acute-onset shortness of breath, diaphoresis, and tachycardia.

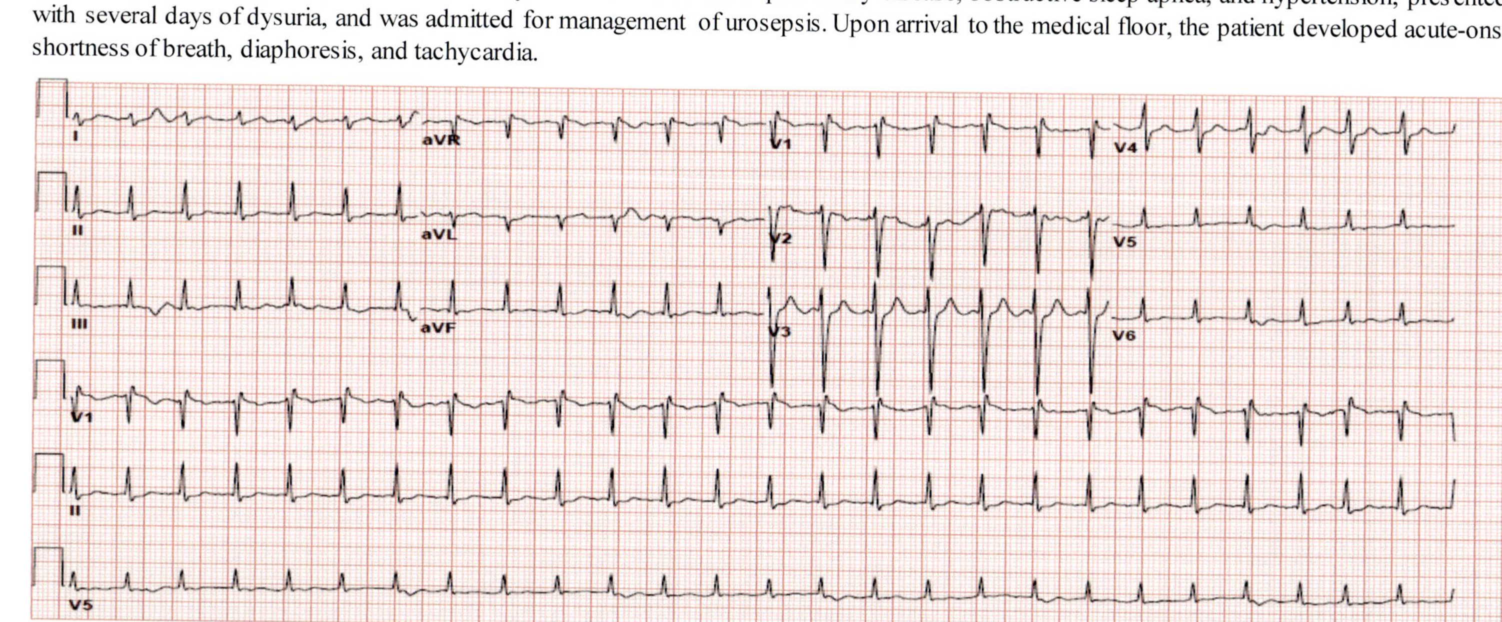

Additional Clinical History

On exam, the patient was uncomfortable-appearing and tachypneic, with diffuse bilateral crackles and mild suprapubic tenderness.

Additional History

Presenting labs were notable for mild leukocytosis and acute kidney injury. Chest X-ray was clear.

ECG Interpretation

Rhythm: Atypical atrial flutter.

Rate: 150 bpm.

Intervals: QRS = 90 ms QTc = 400 ms

Axis: Normal.

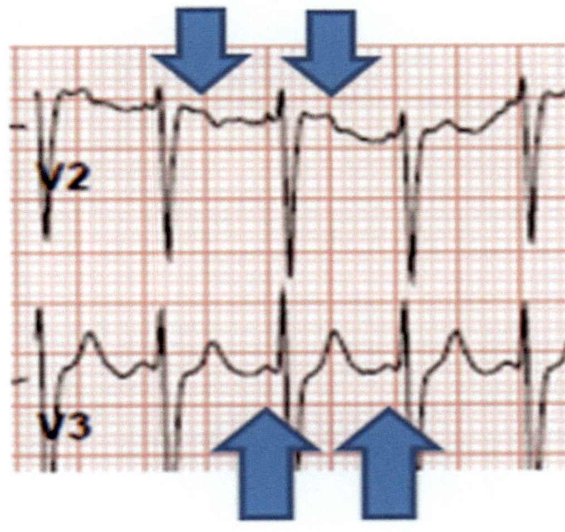

Abnormalities on the ECG

Atypical atrial flutter.

Incomplete right bundle branch block.

ECG Test Answers

17, 58

ECG Synthesis

The ECG shows a regular narrow complex tachycardia of 150 bpm. The p waves are difficult to define. However, in some leads a small atrial wave seems to appear at a constant position. An example is lead V3 where the atrial wave closely precedes the QRS complex. In lead V2, a small inscription is seen on top of the T waves. These atrial inscriptions may also be seen in leads III and aVF. Presuming these are truly signs of regular atrial activity, the tachycardia conducts to the ventricles at a 2:1 ratio. A rate of 300 bpm is typical of atrial flutter, therefore a rate of 150 bpm in a regular narrow complex tachycardia is typical of atrial flutter with 2:1 conduction.

Sudden onset atrial flutter with a rapid ventricular rate may explain the sudden onset of symptoms and deterioration in this patient. Other possibilities should be considered, such as a pulmonary embolus. This ECG does not show signs of right-sided cardiac strain typical of pulmonary embolism; nevertheless, additional imaging will provide essential information.

This patient was treated with a beta blocker which slowed her heart rate and improved her respiratory condition. It is important to note that beta blockers, especially long acting, should be used with extreme caution, if at all, in this setting due to their negative inotropic effects. Acute pulmonary edema due to tachyarrhythmia should usually be treated with emergency cardioversion.

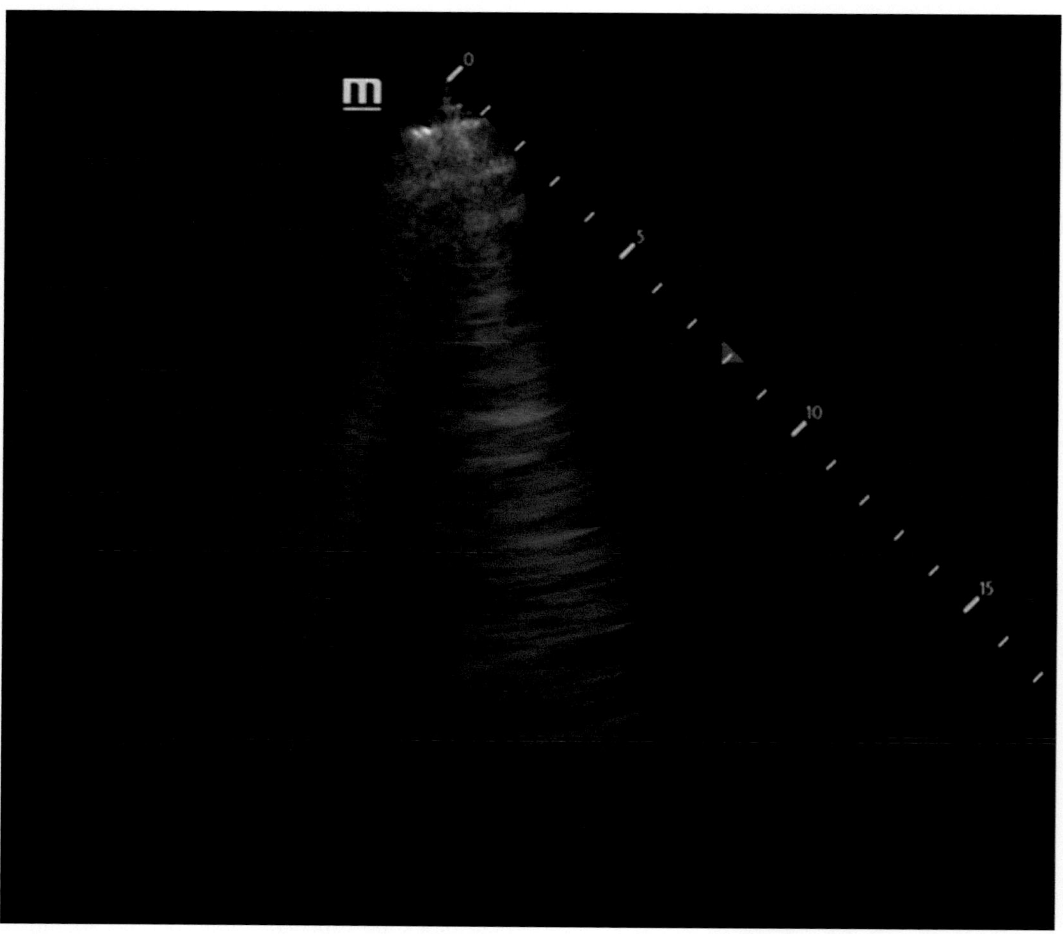

There are extensive B-lines in the bilateral lung fields, with a smooth-appearing pleura in both images

Ultrasound Interpretation

There are extensive B-lines in the bilateral lung fields, with a smooth-appearing pleura in both images.

Ultrasound Synthesis

The sudden onset of symptoms, as well as the B-line pattern on ultrasound, is most suggestive of flash pulmonary edema.

Chest Electrosonography Synthesis

The ECG revealed an atrial tachycardia which could certainly cause deterioration of her hemodynamic status, a finding confirmed by the emergent chest ultrasound. The patient was given a dose of intravenous metoprolol to slow her heart rate and intravenous furosemide, with rapid improvement in her respiratory symptoms.

A 66-year-old woman with a past medical history of dermatomyositis and interstitial lung disease (on immunosuppression), presented with shortness of breath and hemoptysis.

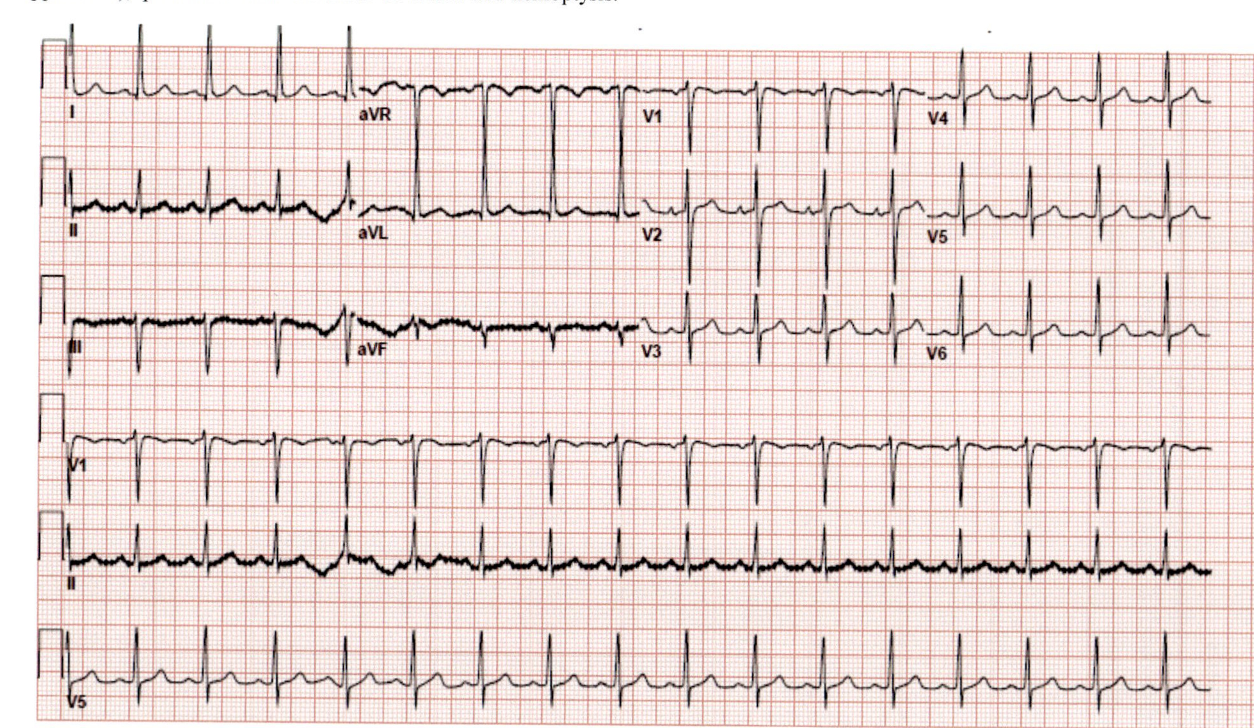

Additional Clinical History

The patient was intubated for management of worsening respiratory distress. Physical exam afterwards was notable for diffuse bilateral crackles.

Additional Information

Labs were notable for leukocytosis, worsened anemia, and mild hyperkalemia. Chest X-ray post-intubation showed extensive bilateral infiltrates, with no significant pleural effusions.

ECG Interpretation

Rhythm: Sinus tachycardia.

Rate: 101 bpm.

Intervals: QRS = 100 ms QTc = 413 ms PR = 110 ms.

Axis: Normal.

Abnormalities on the ECG
Sinus tachycardia.

Left ventricular hypertrophy.

ECG Test Answers
10, 40

ECG Synthesis
The ECG shows sinus tachycardia, a non-specific result of this patient's distress. There are several voltage criteria for left ventricular hypertrophy:

R wave in aVL + S wave in V3 is greater than 20 mV ('Cornell Criteria' for a woman), R wave in aVL greater than 12 mV, and R wave in lead I greater than 14 mV.

However, ST and/or t wave changes are not present and these findings are not specific. Therefore, these ECG abnormalities do not seem to account for the respiratory symptoms. Further imaging is necessary.

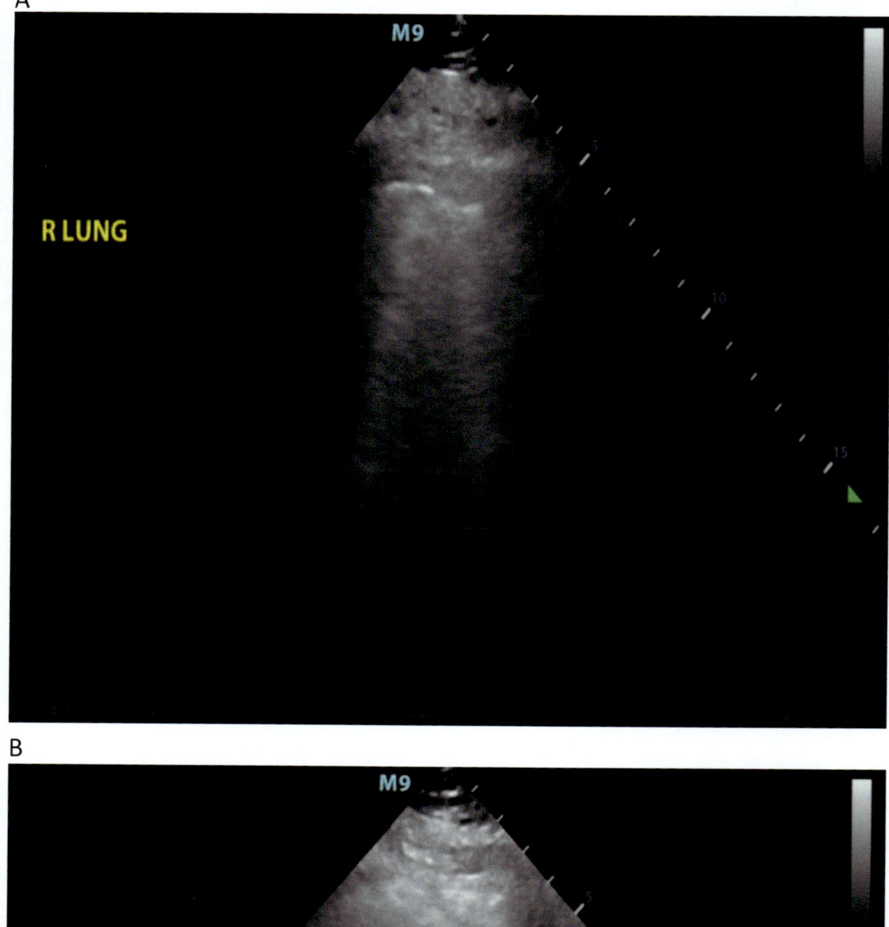

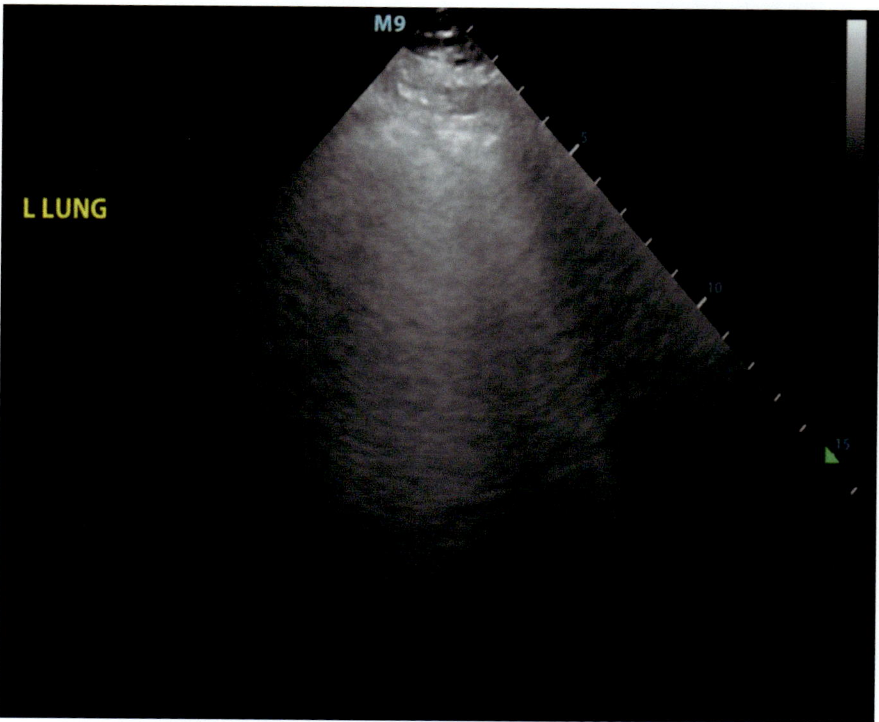

In the right anterior lung field (panel A), there are B-lines with irregular pleura. In the left anterior lung field (panel B), there are more confluent (extensive) B-lines, with a thickened pleura

Ultrasound Interpretation

In the right anterior lung field, there are B-lines with irregular pleura. In the left anterior lung field, there are more confluent (extensive) B-lines, with a thickened pleura.

Ultrasound Synthesis

The extensive B-lines, combined with an irregular appearance of the pleura, make an infectious or inflammatory etiology of the ultrasound findings most likely. Given the patient's history of dermatomyositis, her known underlying interstitial lung disease, and the history of hemoptysis, the clinical findings are most likely reflective of diffuse alveolar hemorrhage and an interstitial lung disease exacerbation.

Chest Electrosonography Synthesis

The ECG was not indicative of a cardiac cause of the patients symptoms. The clinical history and chest sonography established a diagnosis of diffuse alveolar hemorrhage. Subsequent bronchoscopy confirmed the diagnosis of diffuse alveolar hemorrhage. The patient was started on pulse-dose corticosteroids, with gradual improvement in her respiratory status.

8 Case 8

An 81-year-old man with past medical history of atrial fibrillation, diabetes, and recently treated Burkitt lymphoma, presented with altered mental status and worsening shortness of breath.

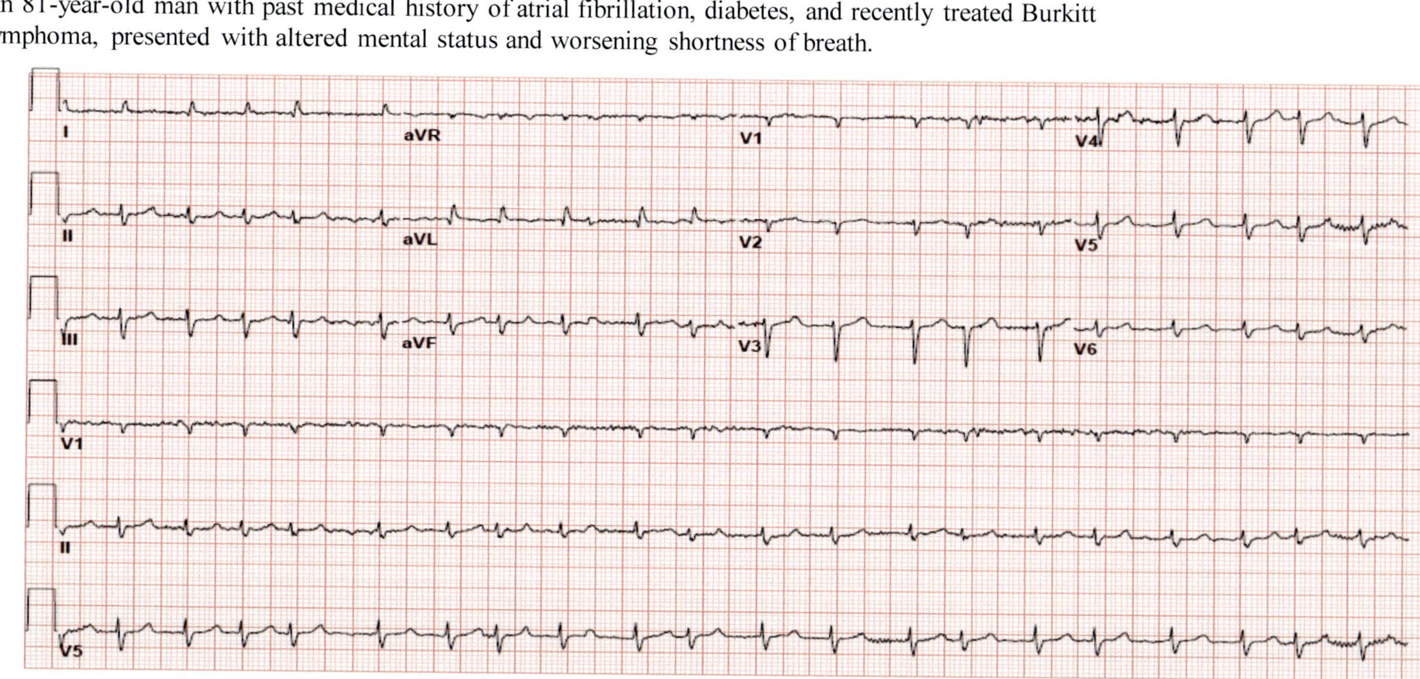

Additional Clinical History

Prior to symptom onset, the patient was seen having difficulty swallowing applesauce. He was intubated due to worsening hypoxia and respiratory distress. Post-intubation, the patient became hypotensive and febrile, with exam notable for left-sided rhonchi and a rapid irregular heart rate.

Additional Information

Labs were notable for anemia, thrombocytopenia, and mild hypernatremia. Post-intubation chest X-ray showed a left lower lung opacity with partial shift of the mediastinum to the left (the right hemithorax appeared clear).

ECG Interpretation

Rhythm: Atrial fibrillation.

Rate: 121 bpm.

Intervals: PR not measurable due to AF, QRS = 80 ms, QTc 380 ms.

Axis: Normal.

Abnormalities on the ECG

Atrial fibrillation.
Low voltage in limb leads.

ECG Test Answers
18, 35

ECG Synthesis
Atrial fibrillation is known and described in this patient's medical history. The rate is relatively high, presumably due to the hypoxia and respiratory distress.

Low voltage in limb leads should always raise the possibility of pericardial effusion, to be demonstrated or ruled out immediately by echocardiography.

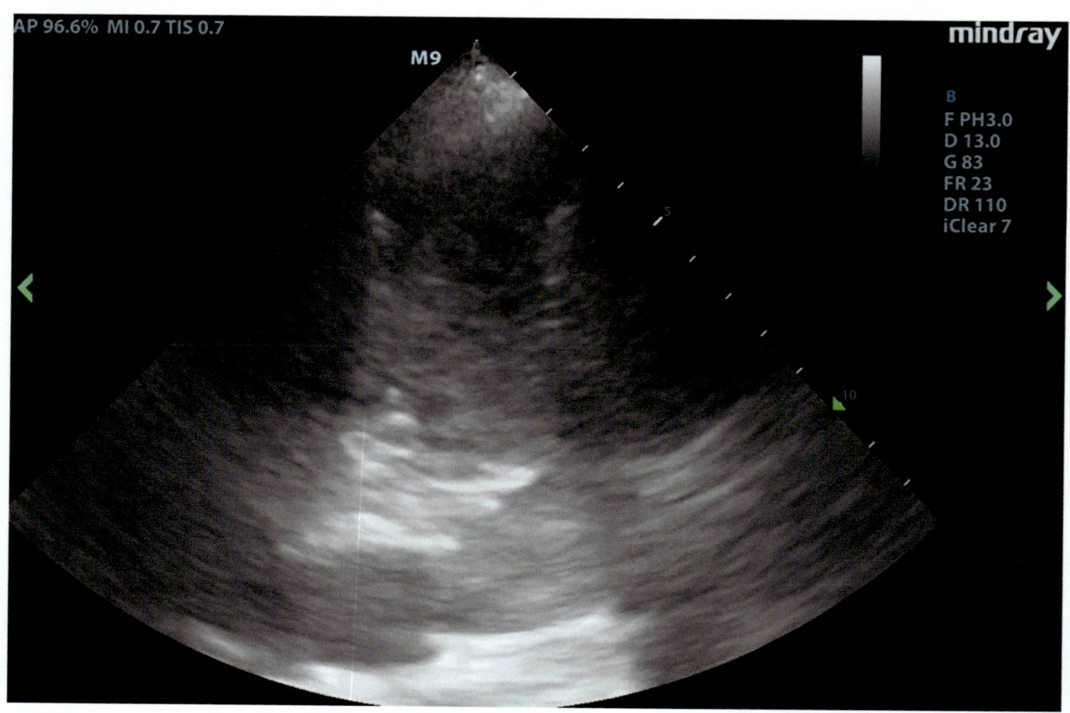

In this view of the left lung base, the curvilinear diaphragm can be visualized (in the center right). Cephalad to the diaphragm (in the left of the image), there is an extensive lung consolidation (hepatization), with no large pleural effusion seen

Ultrasound Interpretation

In this view of the left lung base, the curvilinear diaphragm can be visualized (in the center right). Cephalad to the diaphragm (in the left of the image), there is an extensive lung consolidation (hepatization), with no large pleural effusion seen. The hyperechoic air bronchograms move with respirations (dynamic air bronchograms) when visualized over time.

Ultrasound Synthesis

The large left lung consolidation, combined with the new respiratory distress, fever, and hypotension, are most concerning for new sepsis secondary to a left-sided pneumonia.

Chest Electrosonography Synthesis

The ECG showed rapid atrial fibrillation consistent with the clinical deterioration of the patient. Chest sonography revealed a new lung consolidation without evidence of effusion. The cause of the low voltage on ECG remained unclear. The patient was placed on broad-spectrum antibiotics, intravenous vasopressors, and mechanical ventilatory support.

A 75-year-old man with past medical history of hypertension, hyperlipidemia, diabetes, and advanced chronic obstructive pulmonary disease (COPD), presented with shortness of breath, productive cough, and chills.

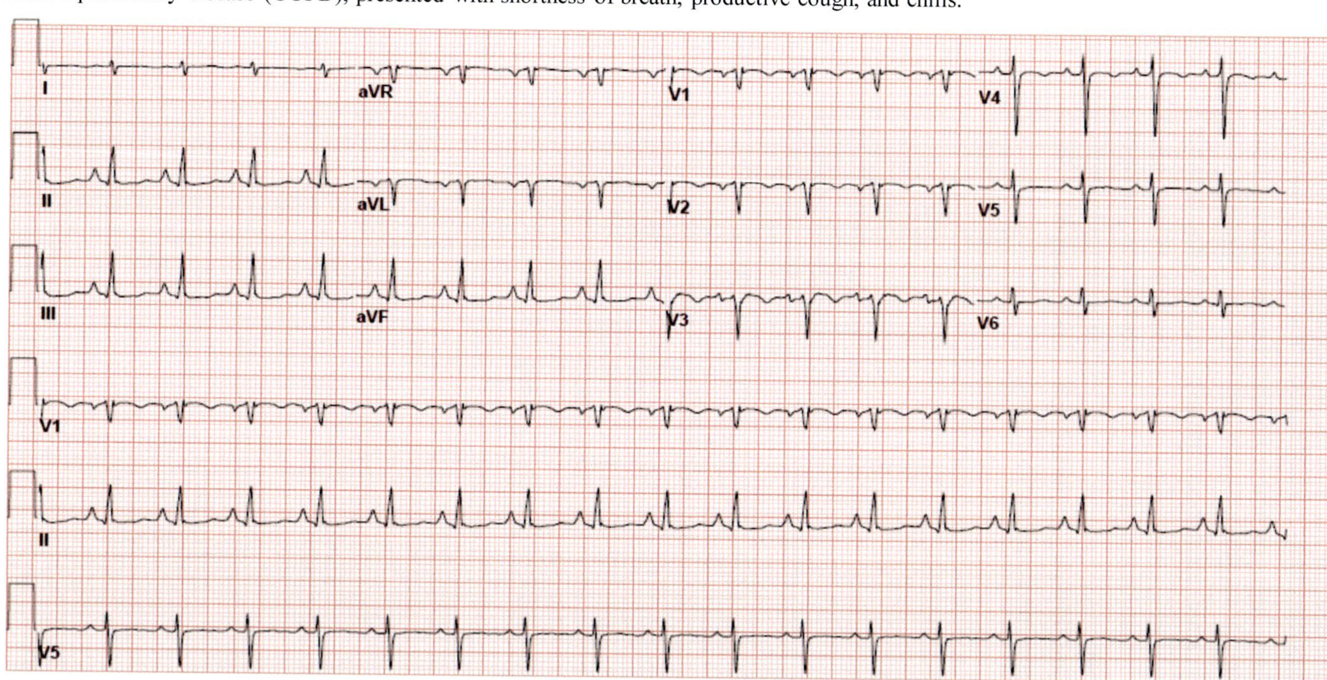

Additional Clinical History

The patient was hypoxic on room air and was placed on nasal cannula for oxygen support. On exam, the patient had bilateral expiratory wheezes and mild tachypnea, with increased accessory muscle use.

Additional Information

Chest X-ray showed no new infiltrates, with hyperinflated lungs. Labs were notable for mild leukocytosis, elevated hemoglobin, and venous blood gas with mild hypercapnea.

ECG Interpretation

Rhythm: Sinus tachycardia.

Rate: 107 bpm.

Intervals: QRS = 80 ms, PR = 100 ms, QTc = 467 ms.

Axis: Normal.

Abnormalities on the ECG

Sinus tachycardia.
Right atrial abnormality/enlargement (borderline).

Poor R wave progression ('clockwise rotation')—negative concordance of QRS in precordial leads.

ECG Test Answers
5, 10

ECG Synthesis
Sinus tachycardia is a non specific finding indicative of physiologic distress.

Right atrial abnormality (tall, peaked p waves in leads 2,3,F) is generally seen in chronic right heart strain. The differential diagnosis of poor R wave progression includes lead placement, antero septal myocardial infarction or advanced chronic pulmonary disease.

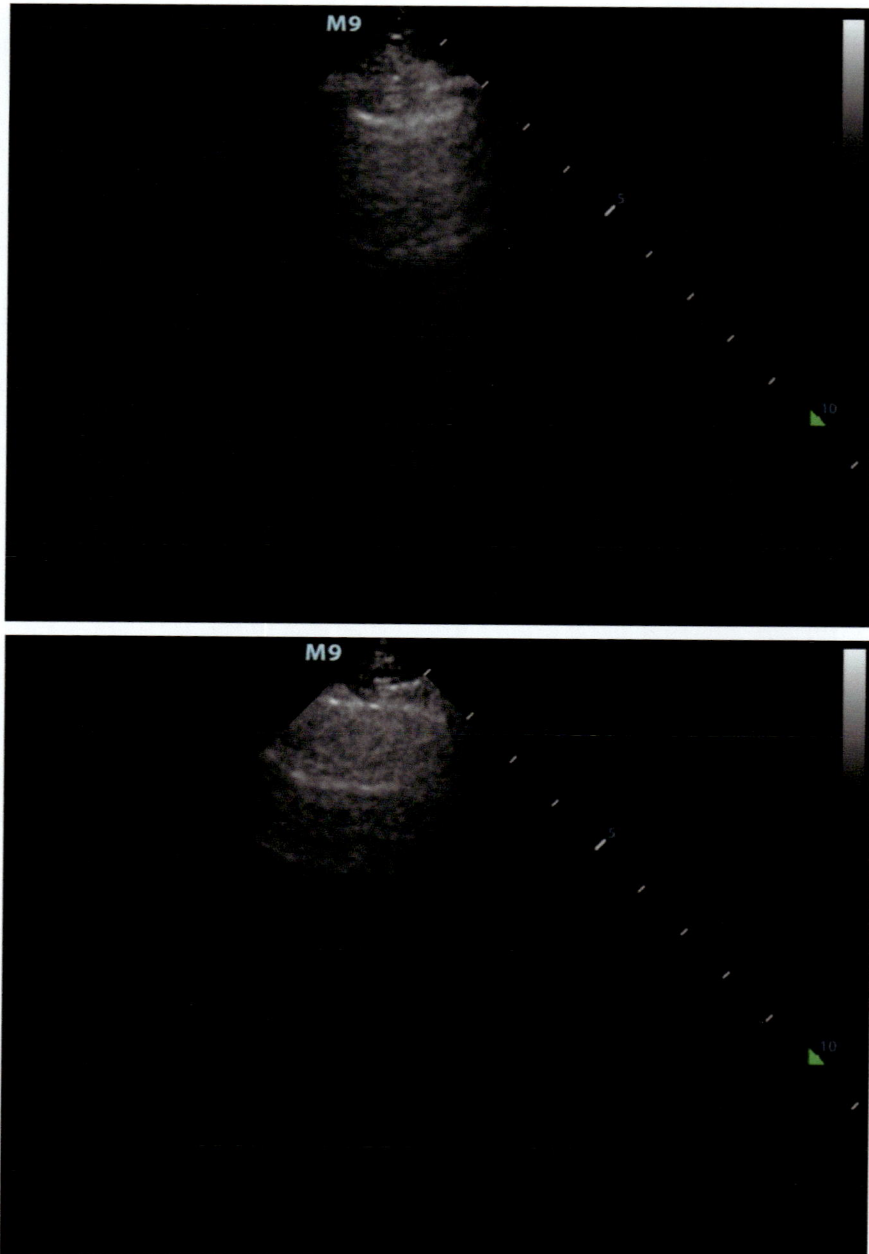

There is a normal A-line pattern in both lung fields

ECG Interpretation

Rhythm: Sinus tachycardia.

Rate: 111 bpm.

Intervals: QRS = 60 ms, PR = 170 ms, QTc = 408 ms.

Axis: Normal

Abnormalities on the ECG
Sinus tachycardia.

Low voltage in limb leads (<5 mV) and precordial leads (<10 mV).

ECG Test Answers
10, 35, 36

ECG Synthesis
Sinus tachycardia is non specific and is to be expected given the patient's respiratory and hemodynamic instability. The differential diagnosis of low voltage in limb and precordial leads includes pericardial effusion as well as pneumothorax. Emergent chest imaging is crucial to the assessment and management of this unstable patient.

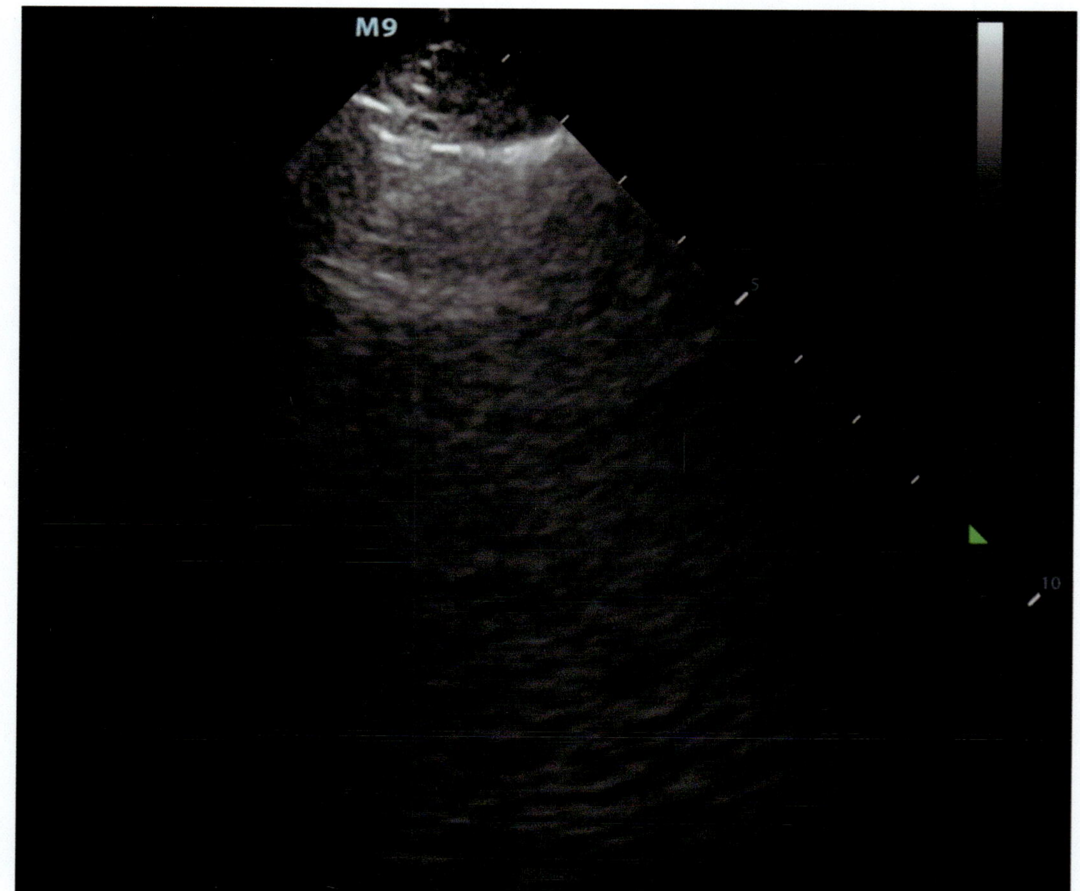

Ultrasound Interpretation

The pleura line left of center appears smooth, with repeated A-line pattern seen immediately deep to it. The pleura line right of center, however, appears coarse and thickened, with confluent B-lines emanating from it. These differences in pleural texture and the lung pattern below the pleura represent a lung point.

Ultrasound Synthesis

A lung point is pathognomonic of a pneumothorax, as it denotes its border, with the absence of lung sliding and A-line pattern immediately cephalad to it.

Chest Electrosonography Synthesis

The ECG findings of tachycardia and low voltage in the clinical context suggested the presence of a pneumothorax, a diagnosis confirmed by chest ultrasound. A small-bore chest tube was inserted into the left pleural space, with improvement in oxygenation, hemodynamics, and peak pressures on the ventilator.

References

Buda N, Masiak A, Smoleńska Ż, Gałecka K, Porzezińska M, Zdrojewski Z. Serial lung ultrasonography to monitor patient with diffuse alveolar hemorrhage. Ultrasound Quarterly 2017;33(1):86–89.

Cardenas-Garcia J, Mayo PH, Folch E. Ultrasonographic evaluation of the Pleura. Pleura. 2015;2.

Gargani L, Bruni C, Romei C, et al. Prognostic value of lung ultrasound B-lines in systemic sclerosis. Chest. 2020;158(4):1515–25.

Lichtenstein DA. Lung ultrasound in the critically ill. Ann Intensive Care. 2014;4:1. https://doi.org/10.1186/2110-5820-4-1.

Lichtenstein D, Mezière G, Seitz J. The dynamic air bronchogram. A lung ultrasound sign of alveolar consolidation ruling out atelectasis. Chest 2009;135 (6):1421–1425.

Mojoli F, Bouhemad B, Mongodi S, Lichtenstein D. Lung ultrasound for critically ill patients. Am J Respir Crit Care Med. 2019;199(6):701–14.

Patel KM, Ullah K, Patail H, Ahmad S. Ann Am Thorac Soc. 2021;18(5):749–56.

Picano E, Pellikka PA. Ultrasound of extravascular lung water: a new standard for pulmonary congestion. Eur Heart J. 2016;37(27):2097–104.

Qureshi NR, Rahman NM, Gleeson FV. Thoracic ultrasound in the diagnosis of malignant pleural effusion. Thorax. 2008;64:139–43.

Volpicelli G, Cardinale L, Garofalo G, Veltri A. Usefulness of lung ultrasound in the bedside distinction between pulmonary edema and exacerbation of COPD. Emerg Radiol. 2008;15(3):145–51.